The Johns Hopkins
High-Yield Review for
Orthopaedic Surgery

The Johns Hopkins High-Yield Review for Orthopaedic Surgery

EDITORS

Bashir A. Zikria, MD, MSc

Director of Sports Medicine
  Arthroscopy Education
Associate Professor of Orthopaedic
  Surgery
The Johns Hopkins School of Medicine
Team Physician
The Johns Hopkins School of Medicine
Johns Hopkins Department of Athletics
Baltimore, Maryland

Dawn M. LaPorte, MD

Vice Chairman of Education
Professor
Department of Orthopaedic Surgery
The Johns Hopkins School of Medicine
Baltimore, Maryland

A. Jay Khanna, MD, MBA

Professor
Division Chief
Department of Orthopaedic Surgery
The Johns Hopkins School of Medicine
Baltimore, Maryland

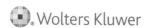 Wolters Kluwer

Philadelphia · Baltimore · New York · London
Buenos Aires · Hong Kong · Sydney · Tokyo

Executive Editor: Brian Brown
Development Editor: Stacey Sebring
Editorial Coordinator: Dave Murphy
Marketing Manager: Julie Sikora
Senior Production Project Manager: Alicia Jackson
Design Coordinator: Joseph Clark
Manufacturing Coordinator: Beth Welsh
Prepress Vendor: S4Carlisle Publishing Services

9 8 7 6 5 4 3 2 1

Printed in China

Library of Congress Cataloging-in-Publication Data

ISBN-13: 978-1-4963-8690-8

ISBN-10: 1-4963-8690-6

Library of Congress Control Number: 2019911831

CONTRIBUTORS

Rachab Abdie, BA
Villanova University
Villanova, Pennsylvania

Lara Atwater, MD
Resident
Department of Orthopaedic Surgery
The Johns Hopkins University School of
    Medicine
Baltimore, Maryland

Jaysson T. Brooks, MD
Assistant Professor
Department of Orthopaedic Surgery and
    Rehabilitation
Children's Hospital of Mississippi
University of Mississippi Medical Center
Jackson, Mississippi

E. Gene Deune, MD
Associate Professor
Division of Hand Surgery, Department of
    Orthopaedic Surgery
Hand Surgery, Microsurgery, and
    Reconstructive Surgery
The Johns Hopkins University School of
    Medicine
Baltimore, Maryland

Gregory K. Faucher, MD
Assistant Professor
University of South Carolina School of
    Medicine Greenville
Department of Hand Surgery
Prisma Health Upstate
Greenville, South Carolina

Matthew Hoyer, BS
Medical Student
The Johns Hopkins University School of
    Medicine
Johns Hopkins Hospital
Baltimore, Maryland

Nigel N. Hsu, MD
Assistant Professor
Department of Orthopaedic Surgery
The Johns Hopkins School of Medicine
Baltimore, Maryland

Casey Jo Humbyrd, MD
Chief, Foot and Ankle Division
Department of Orthopaedic Surgery
The Johns Hopkins School of Medicine
Baltimore, Maryland

Francis Hwang, MSN, CRNP
Orthopaedic Nurse Practitioner
Department of Orthopaedic Surgery
The Johns Hopkins School of Medicine
Baltimore, Maryland

A. Jay Khanna, MD, MBA
Professor
Division Chief
Department of Orthopaedic Surgery
The Johns Hopkins School of Medicine
Baltimore, Maryland

Kelly G. Kilcoyne, MD
Associate Professor, USUHS
Department of Orthopaedics
Walter Reed National Military
    Medical Center
Bethesda, Maryland

Thomas J. Kim, MD
Orthopaedic Resident
Orthopaedic Hand Surgeon
California Orthopaedics and Spine
Larkspur, California

David J. Kirby, MD
Department of Orthopaedic Surgery
New York University
New York, New York

Dawn M. LaPorte, MD
Vice Chairman of Education
Professor
Department of Orthopaedic Surgery
The Johns Hopkins School of Medicine
Baltimore, Maryland

Rushyuan Jay Lee, MD
Assistant Professor
Department of Orthopaedic Surgery
Johns Hopkins Bloomberg Children's Hospital
Baltimore, Maryland

Adam S. Levin, MD
Division of Orthopaedic Oncology
Department of Orthopaedic Surgery
The Johns Hopkins University School of
    Medicine
Baltimore, Maryland

Heather V. Lochner, MD, MSc
Director, Pediatric Hand Surgery
Department of Orthopaedic Surgery
Children's Hospital of Michigan
Detroit Medical Center
Assistant Professor, Clinician Educator
    Track
Department of Orthopaedic Surgery
Wayne State University School of
    Medicine
Detroit, Michigan

Michael McColl, BS
Medical Student
The Johns Hopkins University School of
    Medicine
Johns Hopkins Hospital
Baltimore, Maryland

Clifton G. Meals, MD
Assistant Professor
Department of Orthopaedics
Emory University School of Medicine
Atlanta, Georgia

Kenneth R. Means Jr, MD
Clinical Research Director
Department of Hand Surgery
Curtis National Hand Center at MedStar
    Union Memorial Hospital
Baltimore, Maryland

Louis C. Okafor, MD
Fellow
Department of Orthopaedic Surgery
Joint Preservation, Resurfacing, and
    Reconstruction
Washington University in St. Louis
St. Louis, Missouri

Greg Osgood, MD
Chief, Orthopaedic Trauma, Department
    of Orthopaedic Surgery
Associate Professor of Orthopaedic
    Surgery
Department of Orthopaedic Surgery
The Johns Hopkins School of Medicine
Baltimore, Maryland

Varun Puvanesarajah, MD
Department of Orthopaedic Surgery
Johns Hopkins Hospital
Baltimore, Maryland

Tina Raman, MD
Assistant Professor, Spine Surgery
NYU Langone Orthopaedic Hospital
New York, New York

Jay S. Reidler, MD, MPH
Department of Orthopaedic Surgery
The Johns Hopkins University School of
    Medicine
Baltimore, Maryland

Francis H. Shen, MD
Warren G. Stamp Endowed Professor
Division Head, Spine Division
Director, Spine Center
Department of Orthopaedic Surgery
University of Virginia Health Sciences
    Center
Charlottesville, Virginia

Yalda Siddiqui, BS
University of California Irvine
Department of Orthopaedic Surgery
Medstar Sports Medicine
Irvine, California

Uma Srikumaran, MD, MBA, MPH
Associate Professor
Department of Orthopaedic Surgery
The Johns Hopkins University School of
    Medicine
Baltimore, Maryland

Savyasachi C. Thakkar, MD
Department of Orthopaedic Surgery
MedStar Orthopaedic Institute at MedStar
    Georgetown University Hospital and
    MedStar Washington Hospital Center
Washington, District of Columbia

John E. Tis, MD
Associate Professor
Department of Orthopaedic Surgery
Johns Hopkins Bloomberg Children's
    Hospital
Baltimore, Maryland

Eric Wei, MD
Department of Orthopaedic Surgery
The Johns Hopkins University School of
    Medicine
Baltimore, Maryland

Bashir A. Zikria, MD, MSc
Director of Sports Medicine Arthroscopy
  Education
Associate Professor of Orthopaedic
  Surgery
The Johns Hopkins School of Medicine
Team Physician
The Johns Hopkins School of Medicine
Johns Hopkins Department of Athletics
Baltimore, Maryland

Ryan M. Zimmerman, MD
Greater Chesapeake Hand to Shoulder
  Clinic
Attending Surgeon
Curtis National Hand Center at MedStar
  Union Memorial Hospital
Baltimore, Maryland

FOREWORD

The Johns Hopkins High-Yield Review for Orthopaedic Surgery by Drs Bashir A. Zikria, A. Jay Khanna, and Dawn M. LaPorte delivers a concise and powerful, bullet-style review of orthopaedic surgery. This book is a "must-read" for any resident sitting for Part 1 of the American Board of Orthopaedic Surgery (ABOS) board examination. It may also be useful for seasoned clinicians studying for recertification examinations and for motivated students preparing for orthopaedic rotations.

Drs Zikria, LaPorte, and Khanna hold academic positions at The Johns Hopkins University School of Medicine and are recognized nationally and internationally as superb orthopaedic educators. Dr Zikria teaches worldwide as an authority in education and surgical skills. Dr LaPorte is a leader in American orthopaedic education through the Council of Orthopaedic Residency Directors and the Residency Review Committee. Dr Khanna has led a world-renowned orthopaedic review course for many years. As their chair, and an oral examiner and question writer for the ABOS, I am extremely pleased to introduce this informative text that represents the author's their collective commitment to education. This book is a testament to their dedication to resident education, and it brings together their experiences helping classes of residents prepare for and pass the written portion of the ABOS examination.

The book is organized by topic into short, approachable chapters. The senior author of each chapter is an expert in the corresponding field and has a strong interest in resident education. The bullet format used throughout the text is designed to be easy to follow. The use of boldface type highlights important, frequently tested topics. Within the text of each chapter are diagrams and anatomy and imaging illustrations that further elucidate high-yield concepts and tables that help tie together related groups of topics. The appendix at the end, Test-Taking Strategies, is particularly helpful in final preparations for the test. The appendix demonstrates strategies for taking multiple-choice tests, coping with test anxiety, and an examination preparation checklist.

This book is an excellent orthopaedic knowledge review for residents, students, and clinicians alike and is a fantastic addition to existing test preparation resources.

James R. Ficke, MD, FACS
Robert A. Robinson Professor
Director and Orthopaedic Surgeon-in-Chief
Department of Orthopaedic Surgery
Johns Hopkins University

Amit Jain, MD
Chief, Minimally Invasive Spine Surgery
Department of Orthopaedic Surgery
Johns Hopkins University

PREFACE

Orthopaedic surgery residents commit amazing resources such as time (5 or more intense years), money (in terms of opportunity costs, travel, tuition for courses, textbooks, and practice questions), and effort (with countless hours of studying, cramming, and stressing about examinations). Given this commitment, it is important to note that becoming an orthopaedic surgeon requires a two-pronged approach to learning. The first relates to a comprehensive, patient-centered, clinically oriented, and evidence-based training program, often over 5 or 6 years, that allows a recent medical graduate to acquire the requisite skills to become a practicing orthopaedic surgeon. The second is the acquisition of core knowledge that can be expected to be seen on board certification examinations (such as that administered by the American Board of Orthopaedic Surgery [ABOS]) and on the Orthopaedic In-Training Examination (OITE). The most frequent mistake that we have seen residents that perform poorly on these examinations make is to not recognize this distinction.

With this concept in mind and based on our experience in training numerous orthopaedic surgery residents in our program and through the various board review lectures and programs we give and run at our institution and others, we decided to help put together a book that would focus on the most "high-yield" and board-focused material and allow a resident, student, or practicing orthopaedic surgeon to only review information that will have the highest likelihood of being tested on a board or in-training examination. Of course, the contents of the ABOS examination are not available for anyone to review. However, it is well known that there are only a few ways of testing the key concepts in our field of orthopaedic surgery and, thus, there is a high degree of correlation between the questions seen on the OITE examinations, the American Academy of Orthopaedic Surgeons (AAOS) Self-Assessment Examinations (SAEs), other question banks, and the ABOS Part 1 examination.

Thus, we and our coauthors have all "worked backward" from these and other sources to sift, filter, cull, collate, and illustrate the material that we believe will best help a resident gain the greatest amount of knowledge per unit time in their quest to do well on one of the most important examinations of their career. The singular purpose of each chapter is to review the material that is most likely to be tested on an orthopaedic surgery board or in-training examination. Thus, none of the chapters focus on the authors' or editors' personal preferences or biases in terms of how the various conditions are treated. This book is not intended as a review of orthopaedics for your rotations but a high-yield review of the most commonly tested areas for the orthopaedic surgery board examination.

The book is organized into 10 chapters, with each chapter focused on a particular subspecialty of orthopaedic surgery such as hand surgery, sports medicine, and spine surgery. We have also included a targeted chapter on basic science that seeks to simplify this daunting body of material into a focused 20 pages with 15 illustrations so that an overwhelmed resident can review the material that is mostly likely to challenge her or him on a board or in-training examination. Only when this material is mastered should she or he consider reviewing more comprehensive (and, thus, less focused) reviews of musculoskeletal basic science. Finally, we have an appendix section that is focused on test-taking preparation.

In addition, *The Johns Hopkins High-Yield Review for Orthopaedic Surgery* contains more than 150 images and illustrations that have been carefully selected and created to help illustrate and teach the essential material that one must know when sitting for examinations. Thus, one study strategy may be to frequently review the images and illustrations along with the associated figure legends if the full text becomes too cumbersome and time-consuming in the days and weeks prior to an examination.

This book was envisioned to be a foundation for one of the most important examinations of your career. We realize that there are many other resources available to help with this process, including other review texts, comprehensive subspecialty textbooks, board review courses, webinars, websites, and question banks. The goal for each resident should be to try to find the optimal blend of these resources that works for them and allows them to be confident; the residents should start their board preparation by their third or fourth year of residency, so that they can avoid the eleventh-hour scramble and stress in the final months prior to the big examination. We wish you all the best with your studies and thank you for choosing *The Johns Hopkins High-Yield Review for Orthopaedic Surgery* and our team as your study partners.

Bashir A. Zikria, MD, MSc
Dawn M. LaPorte, MD
A. Jay Khanna, MD, MBA

CONTENTS

1 Basic Science

Adam S. Levin

MUSCULOSKELETAL GROWTH DEVELOPMENT

- Embryology
  - Initial **three layers** of embryologic development:
    - Endoderm
    - Mesoderm
    - Ectoderm
  - Musculoskeletal system and connective tissues **derive from the mesoderm.**
  - Limb bud development
    - 4 to 8 weeks' gestation
    - Central core becomes skeleton.
    - **Three cardinal axes (Figure 1.1):**
      - Proximal-distal
        - Largely governed by **apical ectodermal ridge** (overlying ectoderm)
        - Fibroblast growth factors, homeobox (HOX)
      - Anterior-posterior
        - Governed by **zone of polarizing activity**
          - Preaxial—radial, tibial
          - Postaxial—ulnar, fibular
        - Sonic hedgehog (SHH)
      - Dorsal-ventral
        - Bone morphogenetic proteins, **Wnt signaling**
  - Axial skeleton
    - Paired consolidations of mesoderm (**somites**) develop.
    - Somites consist of skeletal and dermatomal elements.

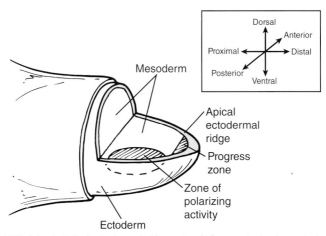

Figure 1.1 Limb bud. Apical ectodermal ridge extends from anterior to posterior along dorsal/ventral boundary of growing limb bud. Proximal to apical ectodermal ridge is the progress zone (an area of proliferating mesodermal cells). In posterior mesoderm is the zone of polarizing activity, an important signaling center. These centers are interconnected, so limb patterning and growth are partly dependent on coordinated function. From Donohue CM. Congenital digital deformities: ectrodactyly. In: Southerland JT, ed. *McGlamry's Comprehensive Textbook of Foot and Ankle Surgery*. Vol 2. 4th ed. Philadelphia, PA: Lippincott Williams & Wilkins; 2013:1109-1116. Redrawn after Jorde LB, Carey JC, Bamshad M, White RW. *Medical Genetics*. London, England: Mosby; 1999.

- Cartilage growth and development
  - Appendicular skeleton derives from **endochondral ossification.**
  - Cartilage differentiation at approximately 6 weeks' gestation
  - Vascular invasion into the cartilage by 8 weeks—primary ossification center
- Bone growth and development (Figure 1.2)
  - Bone is formed from remodeling of collagenous scaffold (**intramembranous ossification**), calcified cartilage (**endochondral ossification**), or other bone (**lamellar bone formation**).

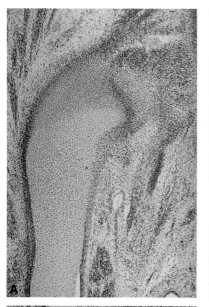
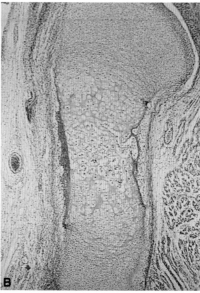
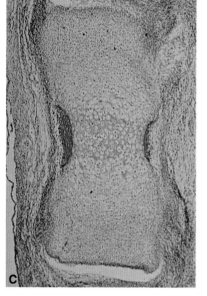

Figure 1.2 Photomicrographs demonstrating the development of a long bone. A, Essential dumbbell shape of the long bone organizes from the primitive mesenchymal tissue. B, Initially, the structure comprises cartilage. C, A calcified coliform in the mid-diaphysis, which is associated with vascular channels. D, Later, secondary ossification centers develop in the epiphysis. E, As skeletal maturation approaches, the physis attenuates and disappears. From Vigorita VJ. Basic science of bone. In: *Orthopaedic Pathology*. 3rd ed. Philadelphia, PA: Wolters Kluwer; 2016:1-54.

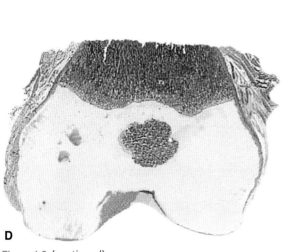
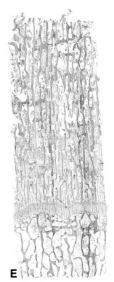

D

E

Figure 1.2 (*continued*)

- Endochondral development
  - **Periosteal sleeve** allows capillary invasion into the cartilage anlage.
  - Capillaries deliver osseous precursors to produce calcified cartilage.
    - **Primary ossification center**
    - As bone replaces cartilage, perichondrium is replaced by periosteum.
  - Development of physis (Figure 1.3)
    - **Secondary ossification center** at epiphysis
      - Secondary ossification center has largely **spherical growth pattern**, rather than longitudinal pattern.
- Intramembranous development
  - Osteoblasts form bone directly onto a collagen scaffold.
  - Typically flat bones (clavicle, pelvis)
- Physeal growth (see Figure 1.3)
  - Growth plate structure (Figure 1.4)
    - **Reserve zone**
      - Adjacent to epiphysis/secondary ossification center
        - Vascularity through epiphysis (epiphyseal artery branches)
        - Vessels pass through, but give little blood supply
        - **Low partial pressure of oxygen (PO_2)**, anaerobic metabolism
      - Minimal longitudinal growth
      - Relatively fewer cells in abundant matrix
        - **High type-II collagen**
    - **Proliferative zone**
      - **Columns of flat, ovoid cells**
      - Responsible for **longitudinal growth**
        - Based on rate of cell division
      - Nutrient supply from epiphysis, with diffusion through the matrix
      - **High PO_2, aerobic**
    - **Hypertrophic zone**
      - Plump, rounded cells
      - Responsible for **matrix production** and calcification

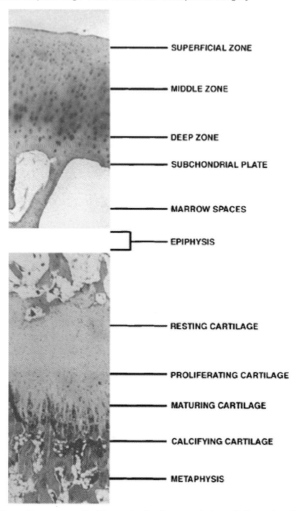

Figure 1.3 Sites of bone growth. The metaphysis grows in length from the physis (bottom) but the epiphysis itself grows radially in three dimensions from the deep zone of the articular cartilage (top). Both articular cartilage and physeal cartilage maintain a consistent architecture, which is critical for function. From Salter RB. Disorders of epiphyses and epiphyseal growth. In: *Textbook of Disorders and Injuries of the Musculoskeletal System*. 3rd ed. Baltimore, MD: Lippincott Williams & Wilkins; 1999:340.

- Essentially **lacks vascularity**
- Increasingly anaerobic toward metaphysis
- Three parts:
  - **Maturation zone**
  - **Degeneration zone**
  - **Zone of provisional calcification**
    - Attaches to the primary spongiosa of the metaphysis
- Vascularity from metaphyseal branches of the nutrient artery and metaphyseal arteries

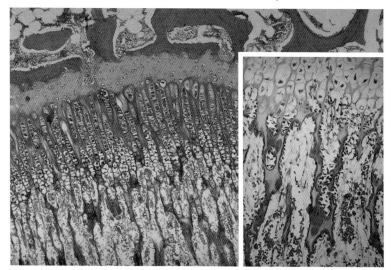

Figure 1.4 At the growth plate, resting cartilage at the subchondral plate begins to proliferate in columns. Following this incipient growth, cartilage cells begin to hypertroph, and following vascular penetration, undergo calcification forming a primary spongiosa or calcified cartilage zone (inset). This primary tissue remodels into bone or secondary spongiosa. From Vigorita VJ. Basic science of bone. In: *Orthopaedic Pathology*. 3rd ed. Philadelphia, PA: Wolters Kluwer; 2016:1-54.

- **Perichondrial ring of La Croix**
  - Ring of woven bone around the physis for **structural support**
- **Ossification groove of Ranvier**
  - Responsible for **appositional growth** of the physis/epiphysis
- Nerve growth and development
  - Nervous system originates from ectoderm.
    - **Neural crest**—sensory neurons
    - **Neural tube**—brain, spinal cord, motor neurons
  - Axonal growth guided by growth factors and matrix glycoproteins
- Abnormalities of musculoskeletal growth and development
  - Skeletal dysplasias
    - Many skeletal dysplasias and disorders of growth are related to the specific function within defined areas of the growth plate (Table 1.1).
  - Connective tissue disorders (Table 1.2)

BONE STRUCTURE AND FUNCTION

- Bone has multiple functions:
  - **Structural support**
  - Attachments for muscle activity
  - **Mineral homeostasis**
  - Hematopoiesis (bone marrow)
- Long bones
  - Epiphysis
    - Trabecular bone surrounded by thin cortical rim
    - Bordered by subchondral plate and physis/physeal scar
    - **Apophysis**—secondary ossification centers that are nonarticular (eg, greater trochanter, humeral epicondyles)

Table 1.1 Skeletal Dysplasias and Growth Disorders Related to Areas of the Growth Plate

Condition by Growth Plate Location	Genetic Mutation	Inheritance
Epiphysis		
Multiple epiphyseal dysplasia	COMP or type-IX collagen	AD
Reserve zone		
Pseudoachondroplasia	COMP	AD
Diastrophic dysplasia	Diastrophic dysplasia sulfate transporter	AR
Kniest dysplasia	COL2A1	AD
Proliferative zone		
Achondroplasia	FGFR3	AD
Hypochondroplasia	FGFR3	AD
Spondyloepiphyseal dysplasia	Type-II collagen	AD (congenital)
	Type-II collagen	AR (tarda)
	Unknown	XLD
Hypertrophic zone		
Mucopolysaccharidosis		
Hurler syndrome	Alpha-L-iduronidase	AR
Morquio syndrome	Beta-galactosidase	AR
Hunter syndrome	Iduronate sulfatase	XLR
Rickets (provisional calcification)	$1,25(OH)_2D_3$	
Primary spongiosa		
Metaphyseal chondrodysplasia		
Schmid type		AD
Jansen type	PTH receptor	AD
Secondary spongiosa		
Osteogenesis imperfecta		
Type I	COL1A1	AD
Type II	COL1A1	AR
Type III	COL1A1	AR
Type IV	COL1A1	AD
Osteopetrosis	M-CSF	AR

AD, autosomal dominant; AR, autosomal recessive; COL1A1, collagen type-I alpha-1 chain; COL2A1, collagen type-II alpha-1 chain; COMP, cartilage oligomeric matrix protein; FGFR3, fibroblast growth factor receptor-3; M-CSF, macrophage colony-stimulating factor; PTH, parathyroid hormone; XLD, X-linked dominant; XLR, X-linked recessive.

- Metaphysis
  - Trabecular bone surrounded by thin cortical rim
  - Typically a flare of the bone to connect the diaphysis to the epiphysis
  - Often a site of **ligamentous and tendinous attachments**, and site of **anastomosing vessels**
- Diaphysis
  - Frequently cylindrical tube of thick cortical bone, surrounding marrow and trabecular bone

Table 1.2 Connective Tissue Disorders and Associated Genetic Abnormalities

Condition	Genetic Mutation	Inheritance
Apert syndrome	FGFR2	AD
Ehlers-Danlos syndrome	Multiple subtypes—most commonly COL5A1	Varies
Marfan syndrome	Fibrillin-1	AD
Charcot-Marie-Tooth disease		
Type 1A	PMP22	AD
Type 1B	Myelin protein zero	AD
Type 2	Various defects in peripheral axon	Typically AD
Type 3 (Dejerine-Sottas)	PMP22 or myelin protein zero	AD
Type 4	Various defects	AR
X-linked	Connexin 32	XLR
Friedreich ataxia	Frataxin	AR
Spinal muscular atrophy	Survival motor neuron	AR
Duchenne muscular dystrophy	Dystrophin	XLR
Becker muscular dystrophy	Dystrophin	XLR

AD, autosomal dominant; AR, autosomal recessive; COL5A1, collagen type-V alpha-1 chain; FGFR2, fibroblast growth factor receptor-2; PMP22, peripheral myelin protein-22; XLR, X-linked recessive inheritance.

- - **Cortex bears most of mechanical load.**
  - Vascularity from branching **nutrient arteries** (medullary canal and inner 2/3 of cortex) and **periosteal vessels** (outer 1/3 of cortex)
- Bone architecture (Figure 1.5)
  - Cortical bone tissue
    - **Highly organized**, tightly packed bone
    - Organized into osteons
      - Central **Haversian canal**, containing neurovascular supply to the osteon
      - Ion channels allow currents for piezoelectric sensation of mechanical loads.
      - Circumferential organization of osteoid around the Haversian canals
      - **Volkmann canals** carry neurovascular supply between osteons.
      - **Canaliculi** are microscopic branching connections that route nutrients and electrochemical signals between osteons and between osteocytes within each osteon.
  - Trabecular bone
    - **Highly porous**, loosely organized network of osseous trabeculae
    - Marrow space is between trabeculae

BONE METABOLISM
- Bone cells (Figure 1.6)
  - **Marrow**—hematopoietic lineage cells
  - **Osteoblasts**—active in bone formation
    - Have **parathyroid hormone (PTH) receptors**
    - **Regulate osteoclastic activity**
  - **Osteocytes**—terminally differentiated osteoblastic cells within lacunae of the osteon
    - Responsible for mechanotransduction and **bone maintenance**

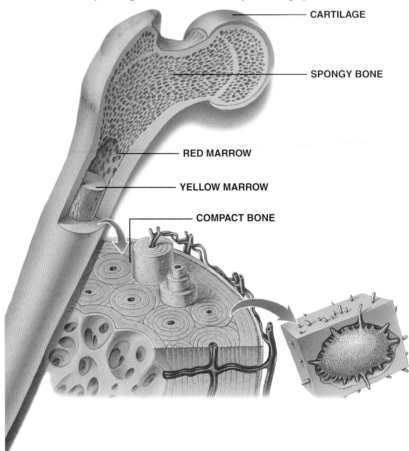

Figure 1.5 This graphical representation of the cortex of the femur bone demonstrates the organization of lamellar osteonic bone. Note the peripheral vascular supply and radially oriented canaliculi. Osteons are organized around a central Haversian canal. Osteocytes reside within lacunae of the osteon. Asset provided by Anatomical Chart Company.

- **Osteoclasts**—multinucleated cells derived from monocytes (hematopoietic lineage)
  - Responsible for **osseous resorption**
    - **Howship lacuna**—resorption pit of osteoclastic resorption
    - **Clear zone**—isolated acidic environment between osteoclast and mineralized matrix where demineralization occurs
    - **Ruffled border**—highly convoluted cell membrane to allow large surface area for excretion of acid and enzymes for matrix degradation
  - Stimulated by osteoblasts, through receptor activator of nuclear factor-kappa-B (**RANK**) receptor activator of nuclear factor-kappa-B ligand (**RANK-L**) signaling
  - Express tartrate-resistant acid phosphatase, cathepsin K
- Bone composition
  - Scaffold of organic matrix (approximately 25%) with mineral onlay (nearly 70%)
    - **Type-I collagen**—nearly **90% of the organic matrix**

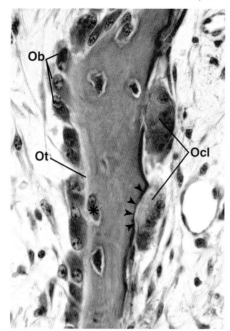

Figure 1.6 Intramembranous ossification. Osteoblasts (Ob) line the surface of the osteoid (Ot), the lighter pink-stained material that is interposed between calcified bone and the osteocytes. Additionally, note that the osteoblast marked with the asterisk is apparently nearly trapping itself in the matrix it is elaborating. Note the multinucleated osteoclasts (Ocl), which are responsible for bone resorption, resulting in Howship lacunae (arrowheads), which are shallow depressions on the bone surface. From Gartner LP, Hiatt JL. Cartilage and bone. In: *Color Atlas and Text of Histology*. 7th ed. Baltimore, MD: Lippincott Williams & Wilkins; 2018:88-119.

- Three alpha chains in a triple helix, connected by crosslinks
- Osseous degradation can be measured by **N-terminal or C-terminal telopeptides** of type-I collagen in serum or urine.
  - Secondary collagens (type III, type IV)
  - Adhesion proteins—fibronectin, vitronectin, osteonectin
  - Osteocalcin
  - Osteopontin
- Inorganic matrix
  - Mineral interdigitates into the type-I collagen helix to add axial compressive strength.
  - Hydroxyapatite: $Ca_{10}(PO_4)_6(OH)_2$
- Bone remodeling (Figure 1.7)
  - Bone constantly being remodeled
    - Rate of turnover
      - Up to 50% turnover per year in infants
      - Up to 5% turnover per year in adults
      - **Complete bone turnover every 2 to 20 years**
    - Turnover is for mineral homeostasis and mechanical stability.
    - **Wolff law**—remodeling to respond to mechanical forces
    - Trabecular remodeling
      - Higher rate than cortical remodeling
      - Osteoclastic resorption pits (Howship lacuna) filled in by osteoblasts

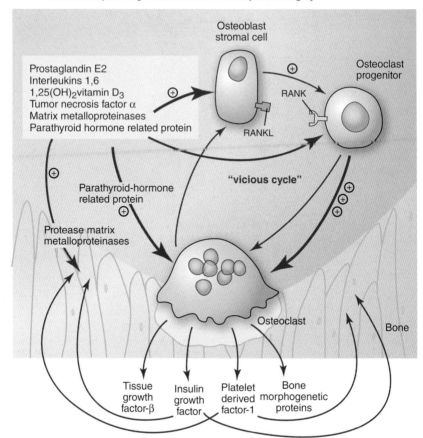

Figure 1.7 Key factors in the regulation of osteoblast/osteoclast bone remodeling. BMPs, bone morphogenetic factors; IGF, insulin growth factor; PDF-1, platelet derived factor 1; TGF-β, transforming growth factor-beta. From Vigorita VJ. Basic science of bone. In: *Orthopaedic Pathology*. 3rd ed. Philadelphia, PA: Wolters Kluwer; 2016:1-54.

- Cortical remodeling
  - Tunneled osteoclasts form cutting cones, followed by new vessels (Haversian canal), which bring osteoblasts behind (osteonic bone).
- Metabolic bone disease
  - In normal bone, tight coupling of osteoclastic resorption/osteoblastic formation, maintaining homeostasis
  - Calcium (Ca) homeostasis
    - **Tight control of Ca** between intracellular and extracellular compartments is important for action potentials.
    - Ca homeostasis involves:
      - Skeleton—**approximately 99% of total body Ca** stores as hydroxyapatite
      - Intestines—**only site of Ca intake** into the body
      - Kidneys—strict regulation of excretion and resorption

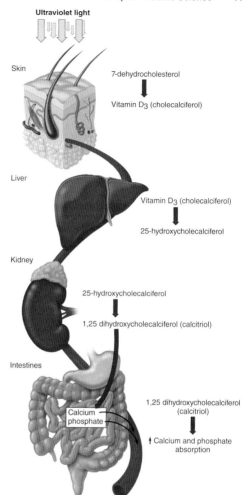

Figure 1.8 Synthesis of vitamin D and the role of various organs in its formation. From Premkumar K. Integumentary system. In: *The Massage Connection: Anatomy and Physiology.* 2nd ed. Baltimore, MD: Lippincott Williams & Wilkins; 2004:55-86.

- Vitamin D (Figure 1.8)
  - **Uptake through intestines** (vitamin D_3, cholecalciferol) or conversion in skin from cholesterol derivative
  - **Converted to $25(OH)D_3$ in the liver**
  - **Converted to active $1,25(OH)_2D_3$ in the proximal tubule of the kidney** in response to high PTH
  - Converted to inactive $1,24(OH)_2$-vitamin D_3 in response to low PTH
- Osteoporosis
  - Uncoupling of bone resorption and bone formation, with net decrease in bone formation
  - Typically associated with older age, postmenopausal state
  - Diagnosis via fracture risk assessment tool (**FRAX**) or **Z-score** on dual-energy X-ray absorptiometry (-2)

- Rickets/osteomalacia
  - Decreased or abnormal activity of 1,25(OH)$_2$-vitamin D$_3$
    - **Vitamin D–deficient rickets**—decreased vitamin D uptake, often related to malabsorption
    - **Vitamin D–dependent rickets**—defect in conversion to 25(OH)-vitamin D$_3$ (type I) or defect in receptor for 1,25(OH)$_2$-vitamin D$_3$ (type II)
    - **Vitamin D–resistant rickets**—phosphate wasting in kidneys
- Periprosthetic osteolysis
  - **RANK-L–mediated** osteoclastic resorption of bone
- Metastatic bone disease
  - Transforming growth factor-beta (**TGF-β**) stimulates cancer cell production of interleukin (**IL-11**) and parathyroid hormone–related peptide (**PTHrP**).
  - IL11 and PTHrP act upon osteoblasts to increase RANK-L and decrease osteoprotegerin.
  - RANK-L increases osteoclastic differentiation and activity, resulting in release of TGF-β—vicious cycle of feed-forward resorption of bone.
- Paget disease
  - **Uncoupled resorption and formation**
    - Osteolytic phase
    - Balanced phase
    - Osteosclerotic phase
  - One of the few indications for **lateral-view skull radiography** on orthopaedic examinations
- Osteopetrosis
  - Decreased bone resorption leads to an overall net production of bone.
- Renal osteodystrophy
  - A **group of conditions** leading to osseous resorption in patients with end-stage renal disease
  - **Secondary hyperparathyroidism**—because of increased phosphate (PO$_4$) and decreased Ca
  - Decreased conversion to 1,25(OH)$_2$-vitamin D$_3$ in diseased kidney
  - **Aluminum chelation** in dialysate may impair formation and resorption (adynamic bone disease).

FRACTURE HEALING

- Type of healing depends on rigidity of fracture
  - **Rigid**—direct healing through cutting cones
  - **Motion**—endochondral ossification (callus)
- Stages of fracture healing
  - **Hematoma/inflammation**—growth factors stimulate osteoprogenitor cells
  - **Early callus**—infiltration of osteoprogenitor cells
  - **Late callus**—collagen scaffold becomes a cartilaginous matrix (Figure 1.9)
  - **Endochondral ossification** of the cartilage anlage into bone
- **Too much motion** prevents ossification of the cartilage—becomes **hypertrophic nonunion** with pseudarthrosis
- **Impaired vascularity** leads to **atrophic nonunion**

CARTILAGE STRUCTURE AND FUNCTION

- Composition
  - **Chondrocytes**—mesenchymal cells embedded in cartilage matrix, responsible for extracellular matrix (ECM) production and maintenance
  - Matrix
    - Predominantly **water** (70%)—**decreases with age**
    - **Collagen type II**—60% of the organic ECM content

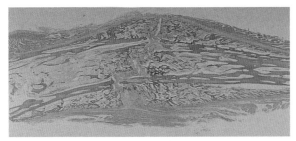

Figure 1.9 Callus (microanatomy). Low-power photomicrograph revealing periosteal new bone (external callus) as well as internal medullary callus. From Vigorita VJ. Skeletal and extraskeletal calcification and ossification syndromes. In: *Orthopaedic Pathology*. 3rd ed. Philadelphia, PA: Wolters Kluwer; 2016:55-113.

- Proteoglycans—approximately 20% to 30% of organic ECM content
  - **Fixed negative charge of proteoglycans** responsible for retention of water within the matrix
- Minor proteins—fibronectin, collagens (type VI, IX, X, XI)
- Articular cartilage orientation (Figure 1.10)
  - **Lamina splendens**—very thin acellular zone at the most superficial aspect of the cartilage
  - **Superficial-tangential zone**—superficial collagen-rich zone of fibers and flattened chondrocytes oriented tangential to the surface
    - Collagen fibers in tension under loading
  - **Intermediate zone**—random orientation of collagen fibers with rounded chondrocytes
  - **Deep zone**—deep zone of centrifugally oriented collagen fibers with columns of plump chondrocytes
    - Collagen fibrils in axial compression under load
    - Predominant production of ECM proteins and proteoglycans
    - Intermediate and deep zones show high proteoglycan concentration
- Function
  - Provide a low-friction bearing surface
    - High proteoglycan concentration allows high water content—responsible for axial load strength and some surface lubrication.
    - High surface tension improved with lubricin
  - **Anisotropic** mechanical properties—different mechanics depending on the direction of loading
- Degenerative joint disease (DJD)
  - Arthritis may have many underlying causes as follows:
    - Degenerative
    - Posttraumatic
    - Septic
    - Reactive—Reiter syndrome, after infection
    - Autoimmune—rheumatoid, psoriatic, idiopathic
    - Crystalline—gout, pseudogout
  - Radiographic findings of DJD
    - **Joint space narrowing**
    - Subchondral sclerosis
    - Periarticular osteophytes
    - Subchondral cyst formation
  - Ultrastructural changes in DJD
    - **Decreased proteoglycans**
      - Alterations in the mechanical stiffness of cartilage

Zones

Cells

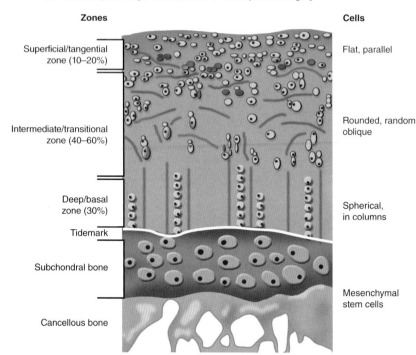

Superficial/tangential zone (10–20%)

Flat, parallel

Intermediate/transitional zone (40–60%)

Rounded, random oblique

Deep/basal zone (30%)

Spherical, in columns

Tidemark

Subchondral bone

Mesenchymal stem cells

Cancellous bone

Figure 1.10 The morphology of articular cartilage. The superficial zone comprises high-concentration collagen fibers oriented parallel to the articular surface, as well as flattened chondrocytes that are oriented parallel to the surface. The intermediate zone has collagen fibers that are less organized and are typically in an oblique orientation to the surface. Chondrocytes in this zone are more rounded than in the superficial zone. In the deep zone, chondrocytes and collagen fibers are oriented in vertical columns perpendicular to the surface. Collagen fibers traverse the tidemark, which represents a relative change from the deep zone to the zone of calcified cartilage. From Sandell LJ, Takebe K, Hashimoto S, Gill CS. Articular cartilage and labrum: composition, function, and disease. In: Clohisy JC, Beaulé PE, Della Valle CJ, et al, eds. *The Adult Hip: Hip Preservation Surgery.* Philadelphia, PA: Wolters Kluwer; 2015:31-41.

- **Collagen and fibronectin cleavage**
  - Matrix metalloproteinase (**MMPs**) and a disintegrin and metalloproteinase with thrombospondin motifs (ADAMTSs)
  - Mechanical
  - Loss of the superficial-tangential zone
    - Leads to fibrillation and further loss of proteoglycans
  - **Chondrocyte proliferation**
    - Clusters of cells in the proliferative zone
- Biochemical mediators of cartilage damage
  - MMPs—responsible for matrix degradation, mostly collagen
  - ADAMTS—responsible for matrix degradation, mostly proteoglycan
  - Tumor necrosis factor-alpha—proinflammatory, expressed in chondrocytes and synoviocytes in DJD
  - IL1—catabolic mediator in DJD
- Treatments
  - Physical therapy—maintains strength and range of motion, improves pain

- Nonsteroidal anti-inflammatory drugs—decrease inflammation and swelling
- Corticosteroids—typically via intraarticular injection, decrease inflammation and swelling
- Viscosupplementation—typically hyaluronic acid injections into the degenerative joint
  - Indications for use have been questioned in DJD
- **Arthroplasty**

MUSCLE STRUCTURE AND FUNCTION

- Muscle structure
  - Muscle fascicles, muscle fibers, myofibrils, sarcomeres, myofilaments
  - **Sarcomere (Figure 1.11)**—organizational structure of actin, troponin, tropomyosin, and myosin responsible for contraction

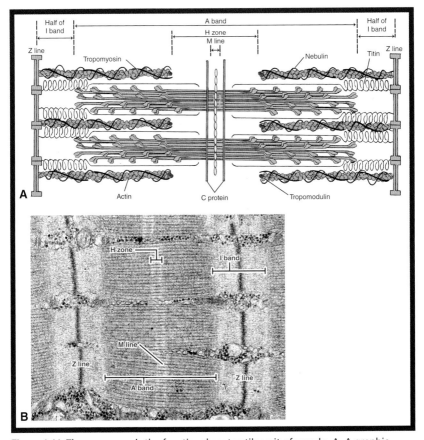

Figure 1.11 The sarcomere is the functional contractile unit of muscle. A, A graphic depiction of a sarcomere. B, An ATPase-stained micrograph. The myosin filaments (also called thick filaments) and the actin filaments (also called thin filaments) make up the sarcomere. One complete sarcomere runs from one Z line to the next Z line. When shortening occurs, the myosin and actin filaments slide over each other, causing the two Z lines of a sarcomere to come closer together. From Kraemer WJ, Fleck SJ, Deschenes MR. Skeletal muscle system. In: *Exercise Physiology: Integrating Theory and Application*. 2nd ed. Baltimore, MD: Wolters Kluwer; 2016:77-110.

- Muscle stimulation
  - **Acetylcholine (ACh)** from axon released to synaptic cleft
  - ACh causes depolarization at motor endplate.
  - Depolarization potential causes release of calcium from sarcoplasmic reticulum, promoting contraction.
- Fiber types
  - **Type I—slow twitch**, strong, endurance
    - High mitochondrial content
  - **Type II—fast twitch**, short bursts
    - More glycolytic than aerobic, fatigable
    - IIa: intermediate twitch
    - IIb: fast twitch
- Contraction types
  - **Isometric**—overall length of the muscle does not change (pushing a wall)
  - **Isotonic**—consistent force or resistance
  - **Concentric**—muscle shortens in the direction of contraction
  - **Eccentric**—muscle lengthens despite contraction
  - **Isokinetic**—constant speed (forces are changed to accommodate a constant velocity)
- Muscle injury—strains
  - Grade 1—tear of some muscle fibers
  - Grade 2—incomplete, with some functional loss
  - Grade 3—complete tear
- Tendons (Figure 1.12)
  - Dense fibrous connective tissue

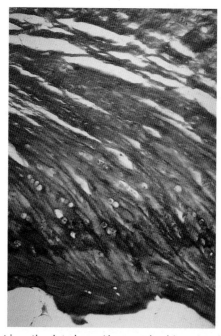

Figure 1.12 Ligament insertion into bone. Ligament (top) is eosinophilic and sparsely cellular, except at insertion into bone where chondroid cells appear. Note purple zone of calcification. From Vigorita VJ. Soft tissue pathology. In: *Orthopaedic Pathology*. 3rd ed. Philadelphia, PA: Wolters Kluwer; 2016:807-829.

- Low cellularity with relatively uniform organization of collagen fibers
- Blood supply
  - **Epitenon** and **endotenon** with **vascularity**
  - Increased vascularity at origin and insertion
  - **Some diffusion of nutrients from tenosynovium**
    - Areas of decreased blood supply
- Tendon repair
  - **Inflammation**—up to 5 days; cytokine release and early granulation
  - **Proliferation**—5 days to 6 weeks
    - Fibroblastic migration and immature collagen scaffold
    - Low tension; repetitive loading improves tensile strength of repair
  - **Remodeling**—after 6 weeks; reorganization to improve mechanical strength

NERVE STRUCTURE AND FUNCTION

- Structure (Figure 1.13)
  - **Epineurium**—**outermost** layer
    - Collagen and elastin **framework** to protect the nerve fascicles
  - **Perineurium**—surrounds each fascicle
    - **Tensile strength** to protect from stretch
  - **Endoneurium**—surrounds nerve fibers
  - **Neurons**—individual cells of the nerve
    - **Dendrites**—receptive cell processes for signaling to the cell body
    - **Cell body in dorsal root ganglion** (sensory) or **anterior horn cells** (motor)
    - **Axons**—long process to distribute action potentials along a distance
    - **Terminal end**—terminal processes for release of neurotransmitters

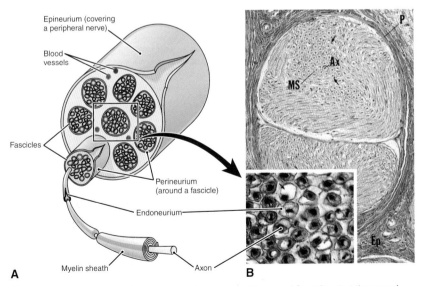

Figure 1.13 A, Structure of a nerve showing neuron fibers and fascicles. B, Micrograph of a nerve (×132). Two fascicles are shown. Perineurium (P) surrounds each fascicle. Epineurium (Ep) is around the entire nerve. Individual axons (Ax) are covered with a myelin sheath (MS). Inset shows myelinated axons surrounded by endoneurium. From Cohen BJ, Hull KL. The nervous system: the spinal cord and spinal nerves. In: *Memmler's The Human Body in Health and Disease*. 14th ed. Philadelphia, PA: Wolters Kluwer; 2019:200-225.

- **Schwann cells—myelination** along an axon to increase propagation of action potential
- **Node of Ranvier—unmyelinated junctions** between Schwann cells; allows **saltatory conduction** along myelinated axons

● Nerve injury
  - **Neurapraxia**
    - **Preserved axons**, but altered conduction across a segment (stretch or pressure)
  - **Axonotmesis**
    - **Axonal disruption**, but endoneurium is intact
    - Nerves undergo **Wallerian degeneration**—distal axons degenerate and new axonal growth required within the neuronal architecture
  - **Neurotmesis**
    - **Complete disruption** of the nerve (laceration)
    - Nerves undergo **Wallerian degeneration** but can recover only if surgically repaired.

● Nerve repair/regeneration
  - Axons regenerate at approximately **1 mm/d**.
  - Repair is by sprouting at the proximal aspect of the injury.
    - If scaffold intact, then sprouting is along the intact connective tissue
    - If scaffold disrupted, then can form a **neuroma**
  - **Grouped fascicle repair** aligns proximal fascicle with distal fascicle so that innervation and distal function/sensation are aligned.
  - **Epineurial repair** recreates the epineurial structure to allow nerve regeneration along the nerve course.
  - Decreased functional return if nerve repair performed under tension
    - **Nerve grafts**—allow repair across a gap, without tension of direct repair for segmental injuries
    - **Nerve tubes or vein grafts**—protect the epineurial repair and allow for directional sprouting

BIOMECHANICS

● Biomechanics: the study of the **effects of energy and forces** on biologic systems
  - Orthopaedics focuses on the effects (motions and deformations) of forces and moments acting on musculoskeletal tissues.
● **Kinematics:** the study of **motions** within the musculoskeletal system
● Diarthrodial joints (eg, hip, knee, shoulder)
● Locomotion
● Gait
● **Biotribology:** the study of **friction, lubrication, and wear** resulting from the interaction of apposed articular surfaces in relative motion
● **Newton laws**
  - **First law** (inertia): Every object in a state of uniform motion tends to remain in that state of motion unless an external force is applied to it.
  - **Second law:** force, mass × acceleration (F, ma)
  - **Third law:** For every action there is an equal and opposite reaction.
● Vectors—have both magnitude and direction (velocity, force)
  - Each vector can be broken down into directional parts, resulting in a summative, resultant vector.
● **Moment**—action of a force applied to an object, which tends to **rotate** the object about an axis
  - Magnitude of moment (torque), force × distance from the center of rotation
● Free body (Figure 1.14)
  - At equilibrium, all net forces and net moments are 0.
  - The forces acting on any limb or body part may be identified by isolating that body part as a free body.

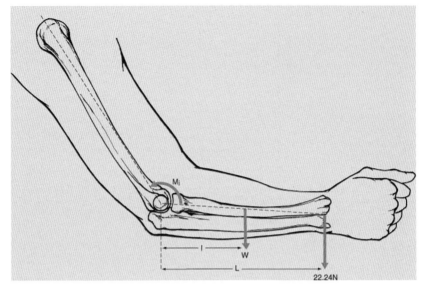

Figure 1.14 Free-body diagram of the elbow for the task of lifting a 5-lb load, indicating the external loads and the internal moments. The free-body diagram reduces the muscle forces and their moment arms to a single internal moment (M_i). From Oatis CA. Analysis of the forces at the elbow during activity. In: *Kinesiology: The Mechanics and Pathomechanics of Human Movement*. 2nd ed. Baltimore, MD: Lippincott Williams & Wilkins; 2009:243-252.

- Forces and moments each in three dimensions, six potential degrees of freedom
- On examination, free-body diagrams for forces and moments can be made under the assumption of equilibrium for nearly all biomechanics questions.
- When a rigid body is both rotating and translating (eg, femur during gait):
  - Motion at any instant of time can be described as rotation around a moving center of rotation (instant center of rotation).
- Biomaterials
- Stress—**stress, force/area**
- Strain—proportional **change in length** (change in length over original length)
  - Strain has no units
- Stress-strain curve
  - Describes the material properties
  - **Young modulus of elasticity**—the slope of the linear part of the stress-strain curve (Figure 1.15)
    - Cancellous bone
    - Polymethyl methacrylate
    - Cortical bone
    - Titanium
    - Stainless steel
    - Cobalt chrome alloy
    - Ceramic
  - **Yield point**—the point at which plastic deformation occurs
    - Stress-strain curve is no longer linear, and **deformation** results.
    - **Brittle materials** may **break** at this point, rather than deform.
  - **Failure point**—the maximal stress that can be applied before failure of a material
  - Toughness—the area under the stress-strain curve

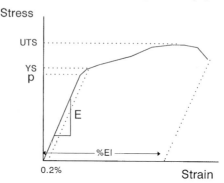

Figure 1.15 Schematic stress-strain curve for a typical metal. Note the elastic region with Young modulus (E), proportional limit (P), yield strength (YS), ultimate tensile strength (UTS), and percent elongation (%El). From Gilbert JL. Basic science of metals. In: Callaghan JJ, Rosenberg AG, Rubash HE, et al, eds. *The Adult Hip: Hip Arthroplastic Surgery.* Vol 1. 3rd ed. Philadelphia, PA: Wolters Kluwer; 2016:224-239.

- **Fatigue failure**—material failure after cyclic loading
- **Isotropy**—equal material properties in all directions
  - **Anisotropy**—different mechanical properties, **depending upon the direction of testing**
- **Viscoelasticity**—stress-strain curve is **dependent upon time/rate of testing**
  - **Creep**—change in strain over time
- **Corrosion**
  - **Galvanic**—**different metals** in a conductive medium
  - **Fretting**—**micromotion** at metallic junctions
  - **Crevice**—**imperfections** on the surface of materials

2 Adult Reconstruction

Savyasachi C. Thakkar
and Louis C. Okafor

BIOMATERIALS

- Wear mechanisms
  - **Radiostereometric analysis** is the most sensitive method to measure wear in total hip arthroplasty (THA).
  - Polyethylene (PE) wear
    - **6-mm minimum thickness for ultrahigh-molecular-weight PE** in total knee arthroplasty (TKA) and THA
    - Types of wear
      - Adhesive wear—primary wear mechanism for the hip; osteolytic process of wear
      - Abrasive wear—a hard third body gets between two surfaces, leading to scratches, gouges, and scoring marks on the worn surface
      - Third-body wear
    - Wear rate is measured by either volumetric (volume) or linear wear (depth of wear into the PE).
      - **Non–cross-linked PE has linear wear of 0.1 to 0.2 mm/y, and highly cross-linked has lower linear wear rate, smaller particles, and reduced toughness**.
      - Younger and more active patients have more wear.
      - **At risk for osteolysis if linear wear rate is more than 0.1 mm/y**
  - Ceramic wear
    - **Ceramic-on-ceramic has the lowest wear rate.**
    - Stripe wear is unique to ceramic heads, in which femoral head liftoff separation from cup during ambulation leads to wear in form of markings on the head.
  - Metal-on-metal wear
    - In fluid-film lubrication, metal-on-metal has less wear than metal-on-PE.
    - Ability to achieve fluid-film lubrication is inhibited by component position.
      - **Acetabulum with abduction greater than 55° leads to edge loading.**
    - **Titanium is too soft to use for bearing surface and leads to higher failure rates.**
- Osteolysis
  - Wear particles act via **receptor activator of nuclear factor kappa-B ligand pathway to stimulate bone resorption**.
  - Effective joint space
    - Circumferentially coated femoral implants can seal the rest of the femur from wear particles and osteolysis.
    - Acetabular components with screws are all part of the effective joint space.
- Cross-linking/sterilization
  - **Irradiation should be done in an inert environment to create cross-links and minimize free radicals.**
    - Free radicals can be quenched with annealing or remelting.
    - Remelting leads to a decrease in the amount of free radicals compared to annealing but increases the risk for crack propagation.
  - **Irradiation in air leads to greatest amount of oxidation and worse outcomes.**
    - Increased shelf-life of these products is associated with more rapid failure.
    - Oxidation causes increased elastic modulus and decreased strength.
  - Increased irradiation leads to more cross-links and less volumetric wear but lower tensile and fatigue strength.

- Metals
  - **Nickel allergy cannot use cobalt chrome, which is made from chromium, molybdenum, and cobalt.**
  - Zirconium femoral head failure is due to its material properties, which often leads to component fracture.
- Polymethylmethacrylate (PMMA) components
  - Methacrylate—liquid monomer
  - PMMA—polymer powder
  - N,N-dimethyl-p-toluidine—activator
  - Benzoyl peroxide—initiator of the reaction

HIP RECONSTRUCTION

- Anatomy
  - **Deep branch of medial femoral circumflex artery is critical to maintain femoral head vascularity.**
  - Dysplastic hips have excessive femoral neck anteversion and a posterior greater trochanter.
  - Marfan syndrome has increased prevalence of acetabular protrusio.
  - **Sciatic nerve crosses anterior to the piriformis between ischial tuberosity and** greater trochanter (Figure 2.1).
  - **Acetabulum is the safe zone for screws (Figure 2.2).**

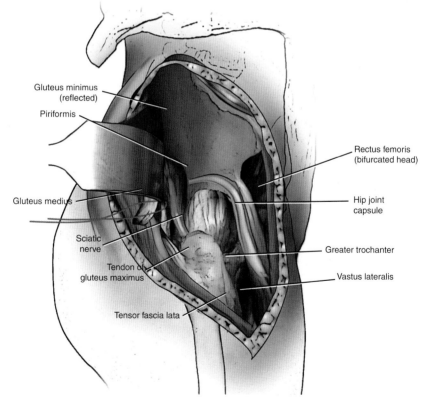

Figure 2.1 Sciatic nerve anatomy at hip. From Helfet DL, Sen MK, Bartlett CS, et al. Acetabular fractures: extended iliofemoral approach. In: Wiss DA, ed. *Master Techniques in Orthopaedic Surgery: Fractures.* 3rd ed. Philadelphia, PA: Lippincott Williams & Wilkins; 2013:885-910.

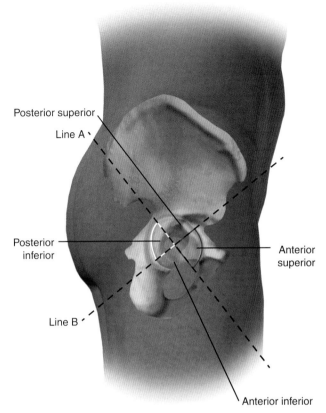

Figure 2.2 The acetabular quadrant system can be used to identify the "safe zone" for screw fixation. Placing hardware in the superior-posterior quadrant minimizes risk. From Klein GR, Levine HB. Neurovascular injury following total hip arthroplasty. In: Callaghan JJ, Rosenberg AG, Rubash HE, et al., eds. *The Adult Hip: Hip Arthroplasty Surgery*. 3rd ed. Philadelphia, PA: Wolters Kluwer; 2016:1062-1076.

- Diseases
  - Ankylosing spondylitis
    - Pelvic positioned in fixed hyperextension that leads to exaggerated anteversion in standing and can put at risk for anterior dislocations.
  - Osteonecrosis
    - **Associated with steroids, alcohol, and HIV—Most common reason in the United States is alcohol abuse.**
    - Treatment with bisphosphonates in early stages decreases risk of collapse of the femoral head.
    - **Core decompression for precollapse**
  - Sickle cell disease
    - Tight medullary canals and may need to be reamed for femoral component placement
  - Rheumatoid arthritis

- Discontinue biologics that affect tumor necrosis factor-alpha pathway (ie, etanercept) 1 to 2 weeks preoperatively
- Can continue methotrexate
- Protrusio acetabuli common in rheumatoid hip
- Femoral neck fractures
  - Healthy, active, elderly—THA
  - Sick, inactive, elderly—hemiarthroplasty

Surgical Treatment

- Arthrodesis
  - **Preferred fusion position is 20° hip flexion, 0° abduction, and 5° external rotation (ER).**
  - **In conversion to a THA, abductor function is predictive of better postoperative walking ability.**
- Approaches
  - Anterior (Smith-Petersen approach)—lateral femoral cutaneous nerve at risk
    - Superficial internervous plane: sartorius (femoral nerve) and tensor fascia lata (superior gluteal nerve)
    - Deep internervous plane: indirect head of rectus femoris (femoral nerve) and gluteus medius (superior gluteal nerve)
  - Lateral
    - Partial removal of gluteus medius insertion from greater trochanter
    - Lower rate of posterior hip dislocation since short external rotators are not detached
  - Posterior
    - **Psoas protects the anterior retractor from causing damage to the iliac vessels.**
    - **Highest risk of dislocation**
- THA implants
  - Bearings
    - Metal-on-metal
    - Metal-on-poly
    - Ceramic-on-poly
    - **Ceramic-on-ceramic (ceramic has fracture risk)**
  - Fixation
    - Acetabulum: cemented versus cementless (standard)
    - Femur
      - Cemented (risk of embolism during cement pressurization)
        - At least 2-mm mantle is necessary and cement restrictor 2 cm distal to stem.
        - Third-generation cementing uses cement mixing in vacuum, cement pressurization, and cleaning of femoral canal with pulse lavage.
      - Cementless—Prior radiation for cancer increases aseptic loosening risk.
        - **Bony ingrowth requires surface with pores 50 to 150 μm, 40% to 50% porosity, and <50 μm gaps—Fibrous ingrowth may occur if these conditions are not achieved.**
        - Fixation location metaphyseal or diaphyseal—Diaphyseal has increased stress shielding of greater trochanter and proximal femur and may lead to greater trochanter fracture. For example, anatomic medullary locking stem with significant stress shielding of proximal femur.
  - Implant positioning considerations
    - Offset
      - High offset also correlates with decreased joint reaction force.
      - If the offset is too low, abductor weakness and hip instability can result.
    - Leg length
      - Increased neck length increases leg length and offset.
      - **Large amount of leg lengthening can lead to sciatic palsy.**

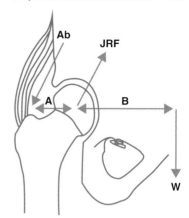

Figure 2.3 Hip implant positioning. Inadequate offset leads to worse lever arm for abductors and positive Trendelenburg sign. A, abductor moment arm; Ab, abductor force; B, moment arm of body weight; JRF, joint reaction force; W, body weight. Adapted from Mirza SB, Dunlop DG, Panesar SS, et al. Basic science considerations in primary total hip replacement arthroplasty. *Open Orthop J*. 2010;4:169-180.

- Stability
    - Increase soft-tissue (abductor) tension by **increasing offset (Figure 2.3).**
        - Inadequate offset leads to worse lever arm for abductors and positive Trendelenburg sign.
    - **Increased head-to-neck ratio**
    - Female sex is an independent risk factor for dislocation
    - Posterior dislocation—flexion, adduction, and internal rotation (IR)
    - Anterior dislocation—extension and ER
- Vancouver classification of periprosthetic fractures (Figure 2.4)

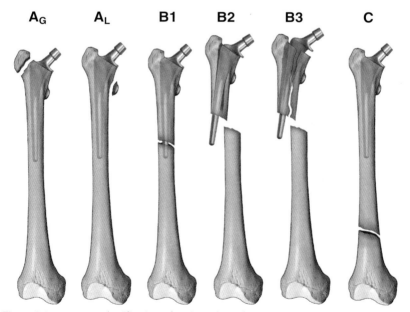

Figure 2.4 Vancouver classification of periprosthetic fractures. From Nauth A, Stevenson I, Smith MD, Schemitsch EH. Fixation of periprosthetic fractures about/below total hip arthroplasty. In: Parvizi J, Rothman RH, eds. *Operative Techniques in Joint Reconstruction Surgery*. 2nd ed. Philadelphia, PA: Wolters Kluwer; 2016:258-269.

- Type A—fracture around trochanter; treatment is conservative or surgical if associated with a loose stem
  - Type A_G—around greater trochanter
  - Type A_L—around lesser trochanter
- Type B—fracture around or just distal to stem
  - Type B1—stable stem; treated with open reduction and internal fixation (ORIF) with cerclage, struts, and plate
  - Type B2—loose stem; treated with long-stem revision with or without ORIF
  - Type B3—loose implant with substantial bone loss; treated with revision and structural allograft
- Type C—fracture well below the implant; treated with ORIF with plate systems
- THA complications
  - **Chronic dislocation**
    - **Recurrent dislocation with malpositioned components requires revision THA.**
    - **Late dislocation primarily caused by poly wear**
  - Deep venous thrombosis
  - Limb length discrepancy
    - **Most common reason for lawsuits after THA**
    - Patient may feel it is greater than the actual difference due to weak hip abductors.
      - Abduction contracture lowers affected side, leading to feeling of longer leg.
      - Adduction contracture raises affected side, leading to feeling of shorter leg.
  - Osteolysis
    - Paprosky classification of acetabular bone loss (Figure 2.5)
      - Type I—minimal bone loss; no migration, minimal lysis; supportive rim
      - Type II—columns intact and supportive
        - Type IIA—superior migration <2 cm; teardrop intact and no ischial lysis; superior dome deficient, but superior rim intact
        - Type IIB—superolateral migration <2 cm; teardrop intact and no ischial lysis; superior rim compromised
        - Type IIC—medial migration; teardrop obliterated; medial wall absent
      - Type III—columns nonsupportive
        - Type IIIA—superolateral migration >2 cm ("up and out"); teardrop obliterated; rim deficiency at 10 to 2 o'clock
        - Type IIIB—superomedial migration >2 cm ("up and in"); teardrop obliterated; rim deficiency at 9 to 5 o'clock
    - Femoral defect classification (Figure 2.6)
      - Type I—minimal defects; similar to primary THA
      - Type II—metaphyseal damage; minimal diaphyseal damage
      - Type IIIA—metadiaphyseal bone loss; 4-cm scratch fit can be obtained at isthmus
      - Type IIIB—metadiaphyseal bone loss; 4-cm scratch fit cannot be obtained
      - Type IIIC—extensive metadiaphyseal damage; thin cortices and widened canals
    - Acetabular osteolysis with well-fixed and well-positioned modular components can have lesion bone grafted with liner exchange.
  - Sciatic nerve palsy
    - **Excessive retraction in posterior approach on piriformis and short external rotators by retractors**
    - Leg lengthening
    - Risk in dysplastic hips
    - **Peroneal branch is most likely to be affected.**
    - **Manage with immediate hip extension and knee flexion.**
  - Squeaking prosthesis—Extreme anteversion increases contact between the metal of the trunnion and the ceramic/cup
  - Iliopsoas impingement

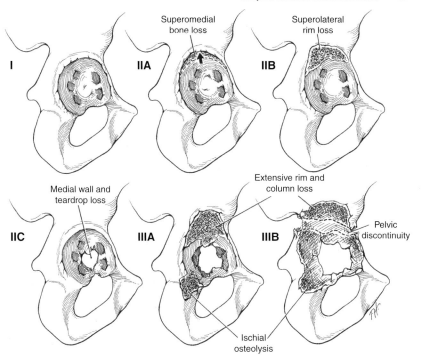

Figure 2.5 Paprosky classification of acetabular bone loss. Reprinted with permission from Craig EV. *Clinical Orthopedics.* Philadelphia, PA: Lippincott Williams & Wilkins; 1999.

- Presents as persistent groin pain after THA, possibly due to acetabular component impingement
- Diagnosed by injection steroid into iliopsoas
- Treated by revising acetabular component if it is causing impingement, or consider iliopsoas tenotomy if component is well positioned
- Intraoperative fracture
  - **Femur calcar fracture with femoral stem placement—Remove implant and cerclage cable above lesser trochanter and require partial weight bearing for 6 weeks.**
- Heterotopic ossification—prophylaxis with indomethacin or radiation (equivalent)
- Pseudotumor formation
  - Often due to metal-on-metal wear products from either trunnion or other modular junction as well as head/cup articulation
  - Granulomatous lesion or destructive cystic lesion affecting soft tissue and bone
- Revision THA
  - Indications
    - Chronic dislocations
    - Periprosthetic fractures
    - Infections
    - PE wear

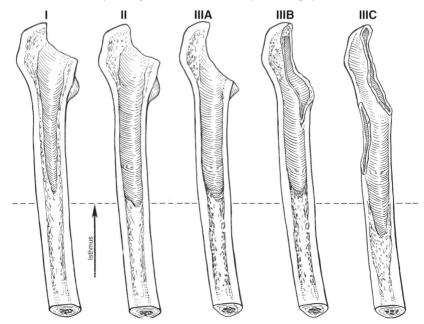

Figure 2.6 Femoral defect classification. Reprinted with permission from Craig EV. *Clinical Orthopedics*. Philadelphia, PA: Lippincott Williams & Wilkins; 1999.

- Symptoms—start-up pain
  - Thigh pain—related to femoral component
  - Groin pain—related to acetabular component
- Surgical approach
  - Trochanteric osteotomy—for revision or difficult exposures. Rarely used in primary total hip replacement
  - Trochanteric slide osteotomy
  - Extended trochanteric osteotomy—vastus lateralis remains attached—revision settings for removing femoral stem
  - Pelvic discontinuity and instability—treat with a triflange cup/acetabular component.
- Hip resurfacing
  - Relative contraindication—coxa vara
  - Complication—femoral neck fracture

KNEE RECONSTRUCTION

- Anatomy
  - **Epicondylar axis is perpendicular to Whiteside line (anteroposterior axis) and 3° ER from the posterior condylar line (Figure 2.7).**
    - Aligning the femoral component rotation with the transepicondylar axis places it in 3° of ER.
  - **Valgus knees require extra care because of posterior lateral condylar hypoplasia.**
    - Joint line
      - Goal is to restore ligament tension.
      - 8 mm is maximum elevation/depression.

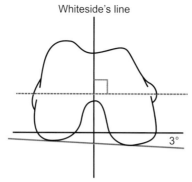

Whiteside's line

3°

Figure 2.7 Anatomic relationships in the knee. The transepicondylar axis (blue) connects the medial and lateral epicondyles and is perpendicular to Whiteside line (AP axis) and in 3° of external rotation from the posterior condylar line (red). AP, anteroposterior.

- **Joint line elevation can cause:**
  - **Mid-flexion instability**
  - **Patellar tracking problems**
  - **Patella baja**
- **Joint line depression can cause:**
  - **Lack of full extension**
  - **Flexion instability**
- Saphenous nerve is on posterior border of sartorius at medial aspect of the knee.
- Lateral release can compromise patellar blood supply.
- Screw home mechanism
  - Popliteus contracts to unlock the knee from full extension by IR of the tibia.
  - Tibia goes into IR in beginning of flexion from full extension to accommodate the different radii of curvature for the femoral condyles.
  - In deep flexion, the tibia goes into more IR.
- Diseases
  - Spontaneous osteonecrosis of the knee
    - Typically occurs in female patients older than 55 years and involves one condyle—medial femoral condyle most common
    - Sudden onset of pain without a history of injury—idiopathic
    - Imaging
      - Radiographs are initially normal, but as the disease progresses, flattening or a radiolucency bordered by a sclerotic halo may be identified in the weight-bearing portion of the affected condyle.
      - Bright on T2 magnetic resonance imaging (MRI) and increased isolated bone scan uptake on the affected side of joint
      - In the late stage of disease, subchondral collapse with secondary osteoarthritic changes may be seen.
  - Osteoarthritis—nonoperative interventions
    - **Weight loss, activity modifications, exercise regimen**
    - **Quadriceps strengthening**
    - **Arthroscopy always the wrong answer for arthritic knee**

Surgical Treatment

- Osteotomies
  - Valgus osteotomies for proximal tibia (lateral closing or medial opening) lead to patella baja

- Varus osteotomies for distal femur—high tibial osteotomy (Figure 2.8)
  - Indications
    - **Young, active patient (<50 years)**
    - Neurovascularly intact
    - **Only one knee compartment is affected.**
    - Preoperative arc of motion is at least 90°.
    - Not more than 10° to 15° varus
  - Contraindications
    - **Inflammatory arthritis**
    - Obese patient body mass index > 35
    - Flexion contracture > 15°
    - Knee flexion < 90°
    - Patellofemoral arthritis
    - Ligament instability
    - Varus thrust
- Unicompartmental knee arthroplasty (UKA)
  - Indications
    - Older (>60) patient
    - Lower demand patient
    - Thin (<82 kg) patient
  - Contraindications
    - Inflammatory arthritis
    - Anterior cruciate ligament deficiency
    - Fixed varus deformity > 10°
    - Fixed valgus deformity > 5°
    - Arc of motion < 90°
    - Flexion contracture > 5° to 10°
    - Prior meniscectomy in other compartment
    - Tricompartmental arthritis
    - Young high-activity patients and heavy laborers
    - Obese patients
    - Grade IV patellofemoral arthritis

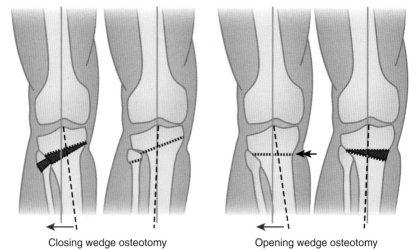

Closing wedge osteotomy   Opening wedge osteotomy

Figure 2.8 High tibial osteotomy for varus malalignment.

- TKA
  - Implant designs (least to most constrained)
    - Cruciate retaining (CR)—unpredictable femoral rollback during flexion
    - Cruciate substituting (CS)—deep dish PE, which adds constraint to the articulation
    - **Posterior stabilized (PS)—use for patients who have undergone patellectomy**
    - Constrained condylar knee—for varus/valgus constraint
    - Hinge
      - Most often used when collateral ligaments are not functional
      - Increases the component constraints by applying a hinge
      - Reduces the instability of the components
      - Increased forces to be transmitted to fixation and implant interfaces, which can result in premature aseptic loosening
  - **Balancing flexion and extension gaps (Table 2.1)**
    - **Increasing slope increases flexion gap.**
    - **Distal femur cut only affects extension gap.**
    - **Proximal tibia cut affects both flexion and extension gaps.**
    - **Component size only affects flexion gap.**
  - Balancing varus/valgus
    - Varus
      - **Remove osteophytes, meniscal and capsular attachments**
      - Deep medial collateral ligament (MCL) and capsule
      - Posteromedial corner (semimembranosus)
      - Superficial MCL
      - Posterior collateral ligament (PCL)
    - Valgus
      - Remove osteophytes
      - Lateral capsule
      - IT band (if tight in extension)
      - Popliteus (if tight in flexion)
      - **Lateral collateral ligament—is important to know that the last structure to be released**
  - Patellar resurfacing
    - Decreased anterior knee pain
    - Decreased need for secondary reoperation
    - **Increased patient satisfaction**
    - **Rheumatoid arthritis is an absolute indication.**

Table 2.1 Balancing Flexion and Extension Gaps in Knee Arthroplasty

	Extension Loose	Extension Normal	Extension Tight
Flexion Loose	Use thicker polyethylene insert	Shift femoral component posterior Posterior augmentation	Resect distal femur Use larger femoral component
Flexion Normal	Distal femoral augmentation	Nothing needed	Resect distal femur Release posterior capsule
Flexion Tight	Use smaller femoral component and augment distally Shift femoral component anterior and augment distally	Use thinner polyethylene insert Resect proximal tibia	Use smaller polyethylene insert Resect proximal tibia

- Postoperative care—Continuous passive motion may improve early range of motion (ROM), but **does not improve final ROM**.
- Biomechanics—Increased PE conformity leads to decreased femoral rollback during flexion.
- Outcomes—Mobile-bearing versus fixed-bearing TKA show no difference in survivorship.
- Theoretical advantage of conformity that should decrease wear
  - Complications
    - UKA—tibial plateau stress fractures
    - TKA
      - Complex regional pain syndrome
      - Inadequate metaphyseal fixation—aseptic loosening
      - **Peroneal nerve palsy**
        - **Associated with valgus knees**
        - **Treat with knee flexion and removal of compressive dressings**
      - Patellar clunk syndrome
        - **PS knees in which scar tissue develops under patella and gets stuck in box**
        - Initially treated nonoperative and, if no improvement, then treated with arthroscopic debridement
      - Patellar maltracking
        - Intraoperatively, release the tourniquet and reevaluate tracking.
        - **IR of femoral component, IR of tibial component, and lateralization of patella more medial component position predispose to maltracking. (When the patella is lateralized, Q angle is increased).**
        - Evaluate component rotation with computed tomography or MRI
      - **Patellar tendon rupture (recurrent)—reconstruction using an Achilles tendon bone/tendon allograft**
      - Popliteal snapping—snapping posterolateral joint line
      - Stiffness
        - Aggressive PT
        - Early and late manipulation under anesthesia (MUA) improves pain and flexion.
        - **Early MUA improves extension.**
      - Infection
      - Vascular injury—requires emergent vascular surgery consult and arteriogram and is a consideration for fasciotomy
      - PCL insufficiency in a CR knee
      - Joint line discrepancy—8 mm is the maximum acceptable joint line elevation.
- Revision TKA
  - Exposure techniques
    - **Quadriceps snip—no restrictions on postoperative rehabilitation**
    - Patellar turndown (VY turndown)—difficulty with quadriceps strength. Slows down postoperative rehab due to quad repair.
    - **Tibial tubercle osteotomy—Strongest indication is patella baja.**
  - Wound coverage after revision—no available soft-tissue coverage
    - Medial gastrocnemius rotational flap with skin graft
    - Most common flap for total knee replacement
    - Blood supply is medial sural artery and vein.
- Anderson Orthopaedic Research Institute classification of bone defects
  - Important points about the classification and treatment
  - **Type 1—key point is that component is stable**
  - Type 2—metaphyseal bone that compromises stability and needs augmentation for stability

- Type 3—metaphyseal bone defect—major component that occasionally includes collateral or patella ligament insufficiency
- Rules for management
  - Less than 5 mm contained—cement (PMMA) fill
  - 5 to 10 mm—cement with reinforcement
  - >10 mm—need to bone graft the contained lesion
  - 10 to 15 mm uncontained—modular stem or augments
  - >15 mm uncontained—need structural allograft

PERIPROSTHETIC JOINT INFECTION

- Common mechanisms
  - **_Staphylococcus aureus_ and coagulase-negative _Staphylococcus_ cause most infections.**
  - Biofilm formation
    - Adhere to implants and elude antimicrobial therapy
    - **Produce exopolysaccharide glycocalyx**
- Diagnosis—2011 AAOS Guidelines recommend aspiration if erythrocyte sedimentation rate (ESR) and/or C-reactive protein (CRP) elevated for knees and more selective approach for hips (Tables 2.2 and 2.3).
  - Acute infection
    - Any active infection <4 weeks
    - Presentation of effusion, pain on ROM both passive and active, fevers, or chills
    - Labs if CRP and/or ESR elevated, then aspiration recommended
    - WBC > 1100
  - Chronic infection
    - >4 weeks
    - More likely to be an indolent bacteria, specifically _Staphylococcus epidermidis_
- Treatment
  - **Acute infection within 4 weeks—incision and drainage and poly exchange**
  - Single stage
    - Not recommended for chronic infections
    - **Never answer single stage for any infection over 4 weeks**
  - **Two stage**
    - **Removal of implant and antibiotic spacer**
    - **Elution of antibiotics from a cement spacer is increased by porosity of the PMMA.**

Table 2.2 Definition of Periprosthetic Joint Infection

Major criteria—One of the following must be present:

- Two positive periprosthetic cultures with phenotypically identical organisms

- A sinus tract communicating with the joint

Alternatively

Minor criteria—Three of the following must be present (for thresholds, see Table 2.3):

- Elevated serum C-reactive protein and erythrocyte sedimentation rate

- Elevated synovial fluid white blood cell count or ++ change on leukocyte esterase (LE) test strip

- Elevated synovial fluid polymorphonuclear neutrophil percentage

- Positive histologic analysis of periprosthetic tissue

- A single positive culture

Adapted from Parvizi J, Gehrke T. Definition of periprosthetic joint infection. _J Arthroplasty._ 2014;29:1331.

Table 2.3 Threshold for Minor Diagnostic Criteria for Periprosthetic Joint Infection (PJI)

Major Criteria (At Least One of the Following)	Decision
Two positive cultures of the same organism	Infected
Sinus tract with evidence of communication to the joint or visualization of the prosthesis	

		Minor Criteria	Score	Decision
Preoperative Diagnosis	Serum	Elevated CRP or D-Dimer	2	≥6 infected
		Elevated ESR	1	
	Synovial	Elevated synovial WBC count or LE	3	2–5 possibly infected[a]
		Positive alpha-defensin	3	
		Elevated synovial PMN (%)	2	0–1 not infected
		Elevated synovial CRP	1	

	Inconclusive Pre-op Score or Dry Tap[b]	Score	Decision
Intraoperative Diagnosis	Preoperative score	-	≥6 infected
	Positive histology	3	4–5 inconclusive
	Positive purulence	3	
	Single positive culture	2	≤3 not infected

[a]For patients with inconclusive minor criteria, operative criteria can also be used to fulfill definition for PJI.
[b]Consider further molecular diagnostics such as next-generation sequencing.
HPF, high-power field (×400).
Adapted from Parvizi J, Gehrke T. Definition of periprosthetic joint infection. *J Arthroplasty*. 2018;29:1309–1314.

3 Pediatrics

John E. Tis, Jaysson T. Brooks, and Rushyuan Jay Lee

PEDIATRIC MULTITRAUMA

General Principles

- More elastic bone
- Thicker periosteum—easier to hold reduction
- Remodeling
  - Correction of deformity with growth
  - Highest in younger children, plane of motion, and when fracture is near physis
- Injury to growth plate
  - Most relevant in lower extremity—leg length discrepancy (LLD)
  - More likely to occur with displaced fracture through physis
  - Treatment
    - **Bar excision**
      - **>2 years growth remaining**
      - **<50% physeal involvement**
    - **Epiphysiodesis: >2 cm growth remaining** in contralateral physis (lower extremity)
- Salter-Harris classification (Figure 3.1)
  - Risk of growth arrest related to amount of displacement
  - Type V—rare crush injury—high risk of growth arrest
- Nonaccidental trauma (NAT) (child abuse)
  - Most common fracture is isolated long-bone fracture.
  - **Suspect NAT** in:
    - Any **fracture before walking age**
    - **Femur fracture before age 3**
    - Multiple, unwitnessed injuries
  - Get skeletal survey
  - Full examination for burns/bruising, sexual abuse, and retinal hemorrhages
  - Failure to report—10% mortality

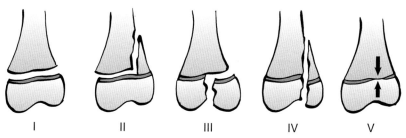

Figure 3.1 Salter-Harris classification of physeal fractures. Type I: fracture line is entirely within the physis. Type II: fracture line extends from the physis into the metaphysis. Type III: fracture enters the epiphysis from the physis and almost always exits the articular surface. Type IV: fracture extends across the physis from the articular surface and epiphysis, to exit in the margin of the metaphysis. Type V: crush injury to the physis with initially normal radiographs with late identification of premature physeal closure. From Rathjen KE, Kim HKW. Physeal injuries and growth disturbances. In: Flynn JM, Skaggs DL, Water PM, eds. *Rockwood and Wilkins' Fractures in Children*. 8th ed. Philadelphia, PA: Wolters Kluwer Health; 2015:133-163.

Multitrauma

- Epidemiology
  - **Most common cause of death in children >1 year**
  - Mortality up to 20%
  - Falls
  - Motor vehicles
    - **Children <8 years—high risk of C-spine injury**
      - Large/heavy head
      - Inability to restrain head
- Positioning for transport—cutout in board or padding under back
- Assessment
  - Primary/secondary
  - Glasgow Coma Scale (3-15)
    - <8 indicates higher mortality.
  - Look for **abdominal bruising (lap belt)**
- Resuscitation
  - Large physiologic reserve hides fluid loss (vitals may be normal).
  - If venous access unsuccessful, use intraosseous.

UPPER EXTREMITY FRACTURES

Clavicle Fractures

- Classification
  - Medial
    - Last physis to close (age 23-25)
    - May be mistaken for sternoclavicular dislocation
  - Shaft
  - Lateral
- Treatment—sling for 4 to 6 weeks
- **Operative indications**
  - Open fractures
  - **Medial fracture** with **posterior displacement and mediastinal impingement**—percutaneous with towel clip or open
  - Severely displaced lateral fractures (controversial)

Proximal Humerus Fractures

- Assessment: careful neurovascular assessment
- Classification: Neer and Horowitz
  - Grade 1: displacement ≤ 5 mm
  - Grade 2: displacement ≤ one-third of humeral diameter
  - Grade 3: displacement ≤ two-thirds of humeral diameter
  - Grade 4: displacement > two-thirds of humeral diameter
- Treatment
  - Sling/immobilizer/coaptation splint or hanging arm cast for all grades 1 and 2
  - Reduce grades 3 and 4 fractures, especially in adolescents (90° abduction and external rotation [ER])
- Operative indications (closed or open reduction and pinning)
  - Open
  - Irreducible grades 3 and 4 fractures in adolescents

Humeral Shaft Fractures

- Current treatment—sling, hanging arm cast, coaptation splint, fracture brace
- Operative indications
  - Open
  - >30° angulation in adolescent
  - Flexible nails or plate

Distal Humerus Fractures

- **Supracondylar**
  - Epidemiology
    - **Half of pediatric elbow fractures**
    - 95% extension type
    - Vascular injuries (1%)
    - Neurologic
      - **Acute interstitial nephritis—most common**
      - Ulnar—rare; iatrogenic from medial pin
  - Assessment
    - Careful neurologic and vascular examination
    - **If well perfused (good color and capillary refill), no vascular intervention indicated even if pulses are absent.**
  - Classification (modified Gartland)
    - Type I—nondisplaced; long arm cast 3 to 6 weeks
    - Type II—intact posterior hinge
    - Type III—completely displaced, no hinge
    - Type IV—completely displaced, unstable flexion and extension
  - Treatment
    - **Vascular injury—reduce**
      - **If poor perfusion after reduction, then emergent vascular intervention is indicated.**
    - Type I: long arm cast
    - Type II: long arm cast if:
      - Anterior humeral line intersects capitellum
      - No coronal plane malalignment
      - Closed reduction and percutaneous pins (CRPP) if above criteria not met
    - Type III: CRPP
    - Type IV: CRPP
    - **Lateral pins confer equivalent clinical stability to crossed pins** but without 3% to 8% ulnar nerve injury
    - Divergent configuration—most stable
    - Open reduction if inadequate closed reduction or perfusion does not return after closed reduction
  - Complications
    - **Volkmann ischemic contracture—avoid casting in >90° flexion**
    - Malunion
      - Varus (Gunstock)—lower in type 2 fractures if reduced and pinned
        - If severe, increases incidence of lateral condyle fractures
        - Requires corrective osteotomy if severe
      - Recurvatum
- Lateral condyle
  - Assessment—need oblique view
  - Classification—fracture displacement

- Type I: <2 mm displacement
- Type II: 2 to 4 mm displacement
- Type III: displaced > 4 mm
- Treatment
  - Type I: Long arm cast for 6 weeks
    - Need frequent follow-up with oblique views to check for displacement
  - Type II: Closed or open reduction and pinning
    - Need arthrogram to check articular congruity if treated closed
  - Type III: Open reduction and pin or screw fixation
  - Lateral approach preferred: Avoid posterior dissection
    - Visualize joint surface
- Complications:
  - **Osteonecrosis—from posterior dissection**
  - Nonunion—from posterior dissection or inadequate stability
    - May lead to valgus and tardy (late) ulnar nerve palsy
    - Treat with screw fixation and bone graft
- Medial epicondyle
  - Epidemiology
    - 50% associated with elbow dislocations
  - Assessment
    - Look for **entrapped fragment in the ulnohumeral joint**
    - Ulnar palsy—usually transient from stretch
  - Treatment
    - Remove entrapped fragment using supination, valgus, and finger extension
    - Early motion (3-5 days)
    - Surgery
      - Absolute—entrapped fragment
      - Relative (controversial)—weight-bearing athlete (gymnast) or dominant elbow in throwing athlete
      - Open reduction with screw ± suture anchor for comminuted fragments
    - Complications
      - Stiffness—common with closed or open treatment
      - Instability
- **Transphyseal fracture**
  - Epidemiology
    - Most common in age < 3 years
    - Often **associated with NAT in children < 3 years of age**
  - Assessment
    - Differential includes elbow dislocation
      - In transphyseal fracture, capitellum is in line with radius.
      - Arthrogram definitive
  - Treatment—similar to supracondylar fractures
    - Closed reduction, percutaneous pinning
  - Complications
    - Malunion—from late diagnosis
    - Closed reduction not indicated >7 days postinjury

Other Elbow Injuries

- Radial neck fractures
  - Classification
    - Nondisplaced, minimally displaced
    - Displaced >4 mm or angulated >30°
  - Treatment
    - Nondisplaced: 3 to 7 days splinting followed by mobilization
    - Displaced

- Closed reduction (multiple techniques)
- Percutaneous reduction with K-wire
- Retrograde flexible nail (Metaizeau)
- Open reduction—rare
- Usually are stable following reduction using any technique
- Avoid implant across radiocapitellar joint
- Olecranon fracture
  - Assessment—look for radial displacement from capitellum (Monteggia) on lateral
  - Classification and treatment
    - Nondisplaced—casting in 45° of flexion
    - Displaced (>2 mm)—open reduction and internal fixation (ORIF) with tension band or plate (comminuted)
- **Monteggia fracture—dislocation**
  - Radial head dislocation matches direction of ulnar apex angulation
    - Recognition is paramount.
    - May occur with plastic deformation of ulna
    - **Differential: congenital dislocation of radius** (do not reduce)
      - Often bilateral
      - Convexity of radial head and deformity of capitellum
  - Treatment
    - Closed reduction and casting
      - Radial head reduces and is stable once ulna is reduced.
      - **Cast in supination if dislocation is anterior or lateral**
      - Cast in neutral or pronation if dislocation is posterior (uncommon)
    - ORIF
      - Only needed in open/unstable fractures
      - Intramedullary (IM) flexible nail
      - Plate for comminuted fractures
    - Complications
      - Delayed treatment leads to arthritis and lack of motion.
      - Reduce all dislocations <12 months old
      - May need osteotomy and reconstruction for chronic, unrecognized dislocations

Forearm Fractures

- **Diaphyseal or distal (metaphyseal)**
  - **Almost all can be treated nonoperatively.**
  - Treatment
    - Diaphyseal
      - Look for compartment syndrome
      - Reduction and long arm cast for 6 weeks
      - Surgery
        - Open fracture, grades 2 and 3
        - Angulation after reduction >15° in any child
        - Angulation after reduction >10°/bayonet apposition in children >10 years of age
        - IM nail or plate
      - High refracture rate
    - Distal
      - Reduction and short arm cast 4 to 6 weeks
      - Most remodel
      - Surgery
        - Open fractures (avoid plate near physis—smooth pins usually sufficient)
        - Significant displacement or angulation after reduction in child with <2 years growth remaining

- Complications
  - Compartment syndrome
  - Loss of rotation (especially with loss of normal radial bow)
  - Physeal arrest (displaced Salter-Harris fractures)

Hand Fractures

- Similar principles as in adults—almost all are treated nonoperatively
- Less stiffness than in adults
- Fractures in the distal part of the phalanges cannot remodel and so require near anatomic closed or open reduction.

PELVIC AND LOWER EXTREMITY FRACTURES

General Concepts

- Fractures adjacent to physis can **remodel**, and fracture through physis can cause **growth disturbance.**
  - Both dependent on contribution of growth from particular physis.
- Surgical fixation
  - Avoid physis if possible
  - If crossing physis, use smooth pins or plan on removing fixation
  - **If nearing skeletal maturity, may use adult options for fixation**, that is, rigid nailing
- External fixators—an option for damage control

Pelvic Fractures

- Stable fractures treated with protected weight bearing
- Unstable fractures—external fixation or ORIF
- Premature triradiate closure results in LLD.

Pelvic Avulsion Fractures

- From sprinting other explosive maneuvers
- Treatment
  - Activity modification and gradual return to activities
  - Surgery uncommon

Hip Dislocation (Figure 3.2)

- Usually posterior
- Require timely closed reduction, to reduce osteonecrosis risk
- **Open reduction for nonconcentric reduction**, entrapped fragments

Hip Fractures

- Delbet classification (Figure 3.3)
- **Types I to III require urgent closed reduction** and internal fixation
  - *Osteonecrosis risk higher with more proximal fractures*
  - Consider **needle decompression or capsulotomy for hematoma evacuation** to decrease osteonecrosis risk
- Possible coxa vara and nonunion with nonsurgically treated fractures

Femoral Shaft Fractures

- *Consider Child Protective Service evaluation for young and nonambulatory patients*

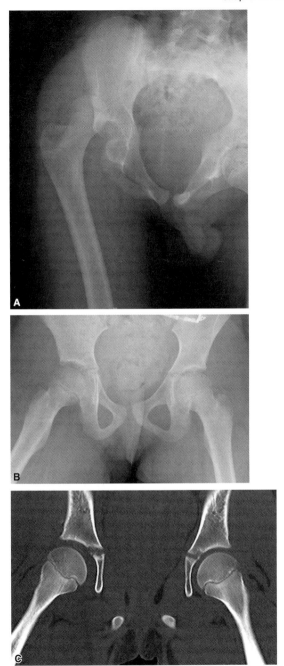

Figure 3.2 Nonconcentric reduction of left hip. A, Injury. B, Postreduction radiograph. C, Postreduction computed tomography (CT) demonstrating entrapped bony fragments. Copyright R. Jay Lee.

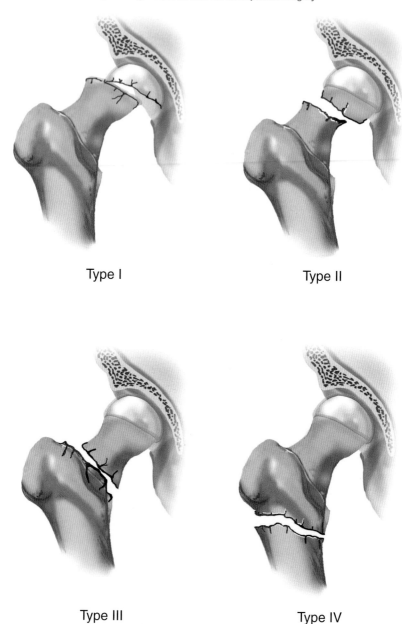

Type I

Type II

Type III

Type IV

Figure 3.3 Delbet classification of pediatric hip fractures. Type I: transepiphyseal fracture. Type II: transcervical fracture. Type III: cervicotrochanteric fracture. Type IV: intertrochanteric fracture. From Epps HR. Pediatric lower extremity injuries. In: Brinker MR, ed. *Review of Orthopaedic Trauma*. 2nd ed. Philadelphia, PA: Lippincott Williams & Wilkins; 2013:467-486.

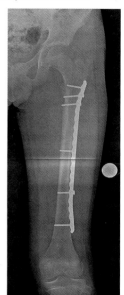

Figure 3.4 Submuscular bridge plating for displaced diaph-yseal femur fracture. From Sink EL, Ricciardi BF. Submuscular plating of femoral shaft fractures. In: Flynn JM, Sankar WN, eds. *Operative Techniques in Pediatric Orthopaedic Surgery.* 2nd ed. Philadelphia, PA: Wolters Kluwer; 2016:202-206.

- Treatment
  - <6 months—Pavlik harness
  - 6 months to 5 years—spica cast
  - 5 to 11 years—flexible nails, submuscular plating for comminuted (Figure 3.4)
  - 10 to 11+ years—rigid nailing, **avoid piriformis** starting point
  - External fixator for open fractures, polytrauma, and damage control
- Expect overgrowth up to 1 to 2 cm
- Rotation does not correct, varus/valgus less well tolerated than procurvatum/recurvatum

Distal Femur Fractures

- Distal femur metaphyseal fractures
  - Long leg cast
  - Surgical treatment if unstable or irreducible
- Physeal fractures
  - **Vascular examination important**
  - Long leg cast for extra-articular fractures
  - Surgical treatment for displaced intra-articular fractures
  - Avoid physes if possible; if crossing physes, use smooth pins
  - *High rate of growth arrest 50%*

Patella Fractures

- Bipartite patella (Figure 3.5)
  - **Anatomic variant—leave alone if asymptomatic**
  - Usually superior lateral pole, with round edges
  - Can be symptomatic and require excision

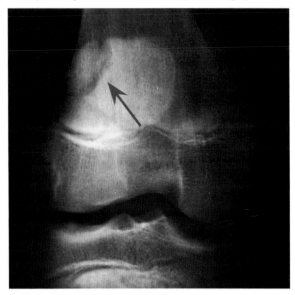

Figure 3.5 Bipartite patella, superolateral location (arrow). From Staheli LT. Knee and tibia. In: *Fundamentals of Pediatric Orthopedics*. 5th ed. Philadelphia, PA: Wolters Kluwer; 2016:185-200.

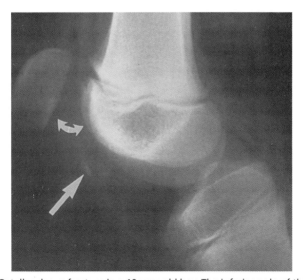

Figure 3.6 Patellar sleeve fracture in a 10-year-old boy. The inferior pole of the patella is displaced anteriorly (curved arrow). The bone fragment seen (straight arrow) was avulsed by, and remains attached to, the patellar tendon. From Thompson RW, Kim Y-J, Lee LK. Musculoskeletal trauma. In: Bachur RD, Shaw KN, eds. *Fleisher and Ludwig's Textbook of Pediatric Emergency Medicine*. 7th ed. Philadelphia, PA: Wolters Kluwer; 2016:1195-1237.

- Patellar sleeve fractures (Figure 3.6)
  - Can be missed
  - Chondral sleeve avulsion without bony component
  - **Radiographs show only patella alta** after trauma.
  - ORIF, reduce chondral surfaces if significant
- General
  - Casting if extensor mechanism intact, less than 2-mm step off at articular surface
  - Otherwise ORIF as in adults

Tibial Tubercle Fractures

- Classification (Figure 3.7)
  - Type I: distal avulsion
  - Type II: exiting before tibial articular surface
  - Type III: exiting in tibial articular surface
  - Type IV: though proximal tibial physis
  - Type V: multiple variants
- Treatment
  - Cast if nondisplaced
  - **Surgical fixation for any displacement and/or extensor lag, with screw fixation**
  - *Compartment syndrome risk with injury to recurrent branch of anterior tibial artery*

Tibial Spine Fractures

- Traditionally the pediatric anterior cruciate ligament (ACL) injury
  - Classification: Meyers and McKeever (Figure 3.8)
    - Type I: minimally displaced
    - Type II: posterior hinge
    - Type III: completely displaced without hinge
    - Type IV: completely displaced and comminuted

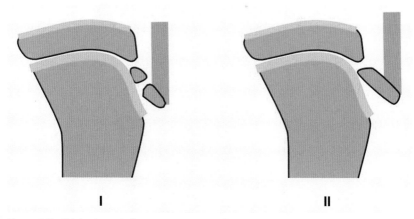

I   **II**

Figure 3.7 Tibial tubercule fractures. Type I is a fracture within the tubercle. It may be minimally displaced, designated A, which is difficult to differentiate from chronic Osgood-Schlatter condition, or displaced, designated B. Types II and III may be subdivided into A without or B with fragmentation of the displaced fragment. In type IV, force lifts tibial tubercle, then continues along the proximal physis of tibia. From Diab M, Staheli LT. Trauma. In: *Practice of Paediatric Orthopaedics*. 3rd ed. Philadelphia, PA: Wolters Kluwer; 2016:147.

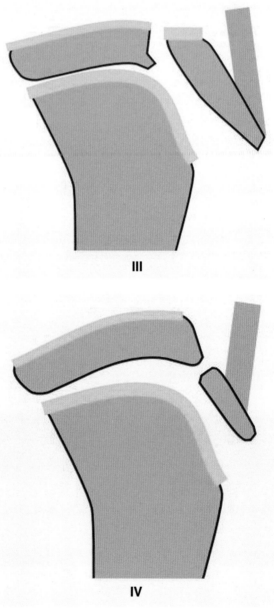

Figure 3.7 (*continued*)

Type I

Type II

Type III

Type IV

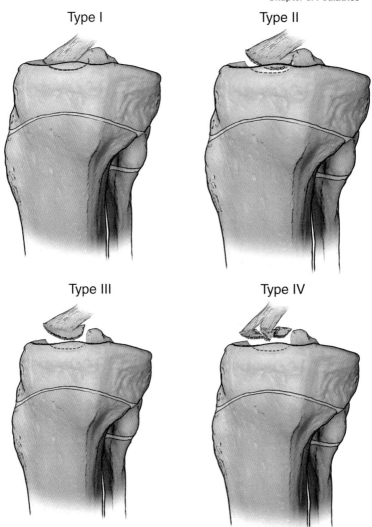

Figure 3.8 Meyers and McKeever classification with Zaricznyj modification. Type I has minimally displaced fragments. Type II has displacement through the anterior portion of the fracture with an intact posterior hinge. Type III has complete displacement of the fracture fragments. Type IV has complete displacement and comminution of the fracture fragments. From Gans I, Ganley TJ. Arthroscopy-assisted management or open reduction and internal fixation of tibial spine fractures. In: Flynn JM, Sankar WN, eds. *Operative Techniques in Pediatric Orthopaedic Surgery*. 2nd ed. Philadelphia, PA: Wolters Kluwer; 2016:396-404.

- Treatment
  - Casting for type I, closed reduction and casting for type II
  - Surgical fixation for unreducible type II and most types III and IV, avoid physis
  - ***Block to reduction, most commonly medial meniscus***
- Arthrofibrosis risk, ACL laxity not always clinically significant, impingement with malunion

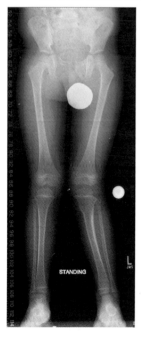

Figure 3.9 Patient with a proximal tibial Cozen fracture. From Lamont LE, Garner MR, Widmann RF. Salter-Harris distal femur and proximal tibia fractures. In: Cordasco FA, Green DW, eds. *Pediatric and Adolescent Knee Surgery*. Philadelphia, PA: Wolters Kluwer; 2015:274-283.

Proximal Tibial Fractures

- Physeal
  - **Vascular examination** for popliteal artery injury
  - Casting for reducible fractures, ORIF irreducible fractures
- Metaphyseal
  - *Cozen fracture*, or late genu valgum (Figure 3.9)—**should remodel**, so observe
  - Casting for most

Tibial and Fibular Shaft Fractures

- Toddler fractures
  - Low-energy minimally displaced fractures
  - Brief immobilization 3 to 4 weeks
- General tibial and fibular fractures
  - Most amenable to casting
  - Surgical fixation for unstable fractures, unacceptable angulation >5° to 10°, shortening

Distal Tibial and Fibular Physeal Fractures

- Suspected distal fibular physeal injuries are more commonly lateral ankle sprains.
- Distal tibial physis closes centrally, medially, and, finally, lateral, giving to distinct transition injuries.
- **Computed tomography (CT) can better demonstrate articular displacement if radiographs unclear.**

- Tillaux fractures (Figure 3.10)
  - **Salter-Harris type III**—anterolateral tibial epiphysis
  - 12 to 14 years, slightly younger
  - Amenable to casting if minimally displaced <2 mm
  - Reduction and epiphyseal screw fixation if displaced
- Triplane fractures (Figure 3.11)
  - **Salter-Harris type IV**—anterolateral tibial epiphysis with metaphyseal fragment
  - 13 to 15 years, slightly older
  - Can be comminuted
  - Amenable to casting if minimal displaced <2 mm

Foot Fractures

- **Accessory ossification centers are common** in the foot and may be mistaken for a fracture.
  - If symptomatic, treat with period of immobilization
- Most minimally displaced pediatric foot and toe fractures may be treated with casting.
- **Suspected occult fractures in a limping child**, brief immobilization, repeat examination, or radiograph
- Exclude infection, neoplastic process

SPINE CONDITIONS
Congenital Torticollis

- Diagnosis
  - Examination—tight sternocleidomastoid muscle
  - **Head tilted to same side and rotated to the opposite side**
  - May have associated mass in muscle

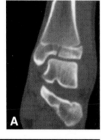
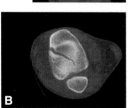
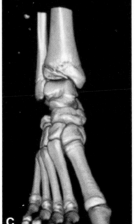
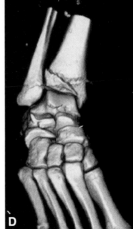

Figure 3.10 Three-dimensional computed tomography (CT) reconstruction of juvenile Tillaux fracture. A, Coronal CT image of minimally displaced juvenile Tillaux fracture. B, Sagittal CT image of minimally displaced juvenile Tillaux fracture. C and D, Three-dimensional reconstruction of juvenile Tillaux fracture. From Shea KG, Frick SL. Ankle fractures. In: Waters PM, Skaggs DL, Flynn JM, eds. *Rockwood and Wilkins' Fractures in Children*. 9th ed. Philadelphia, PA: Wolters Kluwer; 2020:1120-1172.

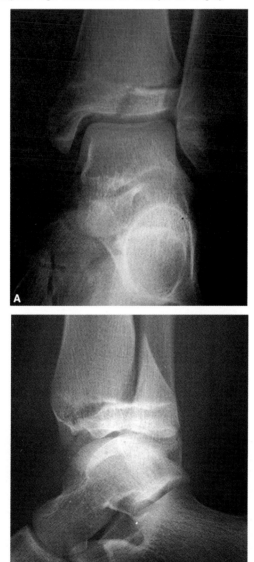

Figure 3.11 Triplane fracture of the distal tibia in a 12-year-old girl with computed to-mography (CT) evaluation. A, The anteroposterior radiograph shows a Salter-Harris type III fracture. B, The lateral radiograph shows an apparent Salter-Harris type II fracture. This indicates a triplane injury. C, Three-dimensional reconstruction demonstrates the fracture from the anterolateral and the posteromedial views. D, Closed reduction was unsuccessful. Arthroscopically assisted open reduction was performed. The fracture was stabilized with a single anterolateral cannulated screw inserted percutaneously. From Sink EL, Flynn JM. Thoracolumbar spine and lower extremity fractures. In: Weinstein SL, Flynn JM, eds. *Lovell and Winter's Pediatric Orthopaedics*. Vol 2. 7th ed. Philadelphia, PA: 2014:1773-1829.

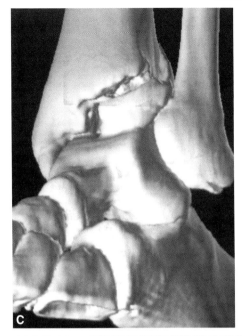

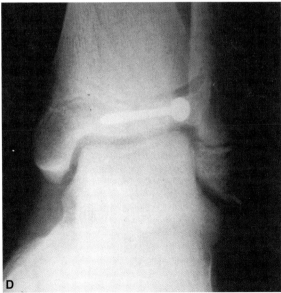

Figure 3.11 (*continued*)

- Differential diagnosis
  - Congenital scoliosis or other vertebral anomaly
  - Ophthalmologic abnormality
  - Tumor
  - Vestibular abnormality
- Associated conditions
  - **Hip dysplasia** (5%-20%)
  - Metatarsus adductus
- Etiology
  - Sternocleidomastoid compartment syndrome
  - Must rule out other causes with careful examination and ophthalmologic consult
- Treatment
  - **Stretching** 90% successful if initiated within the first year of life
  - Surgical treatment
    - Indicated if nonoperative treatment fails after 12 to 24 months
    - Unipolar or bipolar release of sternocleidomastoid muscle from distal attachments
- Complications
  - Plagiocephaly/facial asymmetry—if torticollis is left untreated or deformity persists

Atlantoaxial Rotatory Subluxation

- Etiology
  - Upper respiratory infection (Grisel syndrome)
  - Trauma (may be minor)
- Classification
  - Fielding I to IV: based on facet subluxation (Figure 3.12)
- Diagnosis
  - Examination: may demonstrate spasm or fibrosis of sternocleidomastoid muscle on the same side as the chin, in contrast to torticollis that has spasm on opposite side as chin
  - Differential diagnosis (nonidiopathic associated with atlantoaxial instability)
    - Down syndrome—occiput-C2 fusion for neurologic symptoms and atlanto-dens interval (ADI) >5 mm
    - Klippel-Feil syndrome
    - Skeletal dysplasias
    - Mucopolysaccharidoses
- Imaging—dynamic rotatory CT
  - **In atlantoaxial rotatory subluxation, the relationship of C1 on C2 is unchanged when the head is rotated in opposite directions**

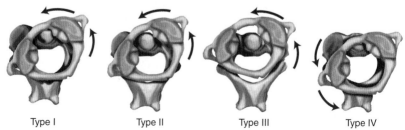

Type I   Type II   Type III   Type IV

Figure 3.12 Fielding classification of atlantoaxial rotatory subluxation. Greenleaf R, Richman RD, Altman DT. General principles of vertebral bony, ligamentous, and penetrating injuries. In: Brinker MR, ed. *Review of Orthopaedic Trauma*. 2nd ed. Philadelphia, PA: Lippincott Williams & Wilkins; 2013:406-417.

- Treatment
  - Subluxation <1 week
    - Soft collar
  - Subluxation 1 week to 1 month (or failure of soft collar for 2 weeks)
    - Halter traction
  - Subluxation > 1 month
    - Halter traction followed by halter vest
  - Subluxation > 3 months, neurologic deficits, or failed halo traction
    - C1 to C2 fusion

Scoliosis

- Treatment based largely on etiology: congenital versus neuromuscular versus idiopathic
- Terminology
  - Congenital—vertebral structural abnormality at birth
  - Idiopathic
  - Other: neuromuscular and syndromic
- Congenital
  - Types
    - Failure of formation (hemivertebra)
    - Failure of segmentation (bar)
    - Combined (worst prognosis)
  - Congenital kyphosis—often associated with scoliosis
    - Similar surgical indications—include progression of kyphosis
  - **Associated conditions (61%)**
    - Cardiac (26%)
    - Urogenital (21%)
    - Limb abnormalities
      - Sprengel
      - Hip dysplasia
      - Limb hypoplasia
    - Anal atresia
    - Hearing deficits
    - Facial asymmetry
    - Neural axis abnormality (40%)
  - Imaging
    - **Magnetic resonance imaging (MRI) of the spine and kidneys (Figure 3.13)**
    - **Echocardiogram**
  - Treatment
    - Nonoperative (observation) indications
      - No neurologic symptoms
      - No progression >10°
      - No kyphosis >40°
    - Surgical
      - Indications (general)
        - Bracing not effective
        - Significant progression
        - Decreasing pulmonary function
        - Neurologic deficit
      - Hemivertebra excision
        - Truncal imbalance
        - Age <6 (relative)
        - Higher risk in curves >50° and for excision above the level of the conus
      - Early in situ arthrodesis
        - Minimal deformity
        - Usually reserved for failures of segmentation

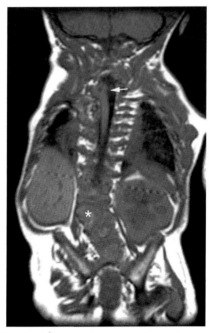

Figure 3.13 Coronal T1-weighted image showing scoliosis, absence of the right kidney, and vertebral anomalies at the apex of the spinal curvature (asterisk marks a hemivertebra). The sacrum is absent. From Schwartz ES, Barkovich AJ. Congenital anomalies of the spine. In: Barkovich AJ, Raybaud C, eds. *Pediatric Neuroimaging*. 5th ed. Philadelphia, PA: Lippincott Williams & Wilkins; 2012:857-922.

- Hemiepiphysiodesis
  - Age < 5
  - Curve <70°
  - <5 segments involved
- Thoracostomy—may benefit patients with multiple fused ribs and thoracic insufficiency syndrome
- Growing rod—may be combined with hemivertebra excision and thoracostomy to release fused ribs
- Idiopathic
  - Infantile
    - **>90% of curves >30° progress; many curves <30° spontaneously resolve**
    - Imaging
      - Plain x-ray—**rib vertebral angle difference (RVAD)** >20° predictive of progression (Figure 3.14)
      - Excessive rotation phase 2 (overlap) rib-vertebra relationship
      - **MRI**—need in all patients with curves > 20° due to high incidence of intraspinal anomalies (20%)
    - Nonoperative treatment:
      - Observation—indicated for curves < 30°
      - Indicated for patients with curves 20° to 50° that have progressed or at high risk for progression based on excessive rotation seen on plain x-rays
      - Cast treatment—indicated for patients with curves 30° to 50° that have progressed or at high risk for progression based on excessive rotation seen on plain x-rays

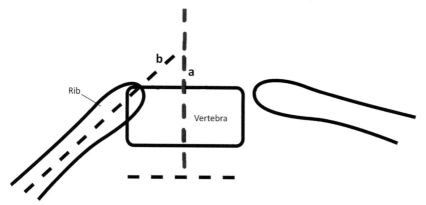

Figure 3.14 The rib vertebral angle difference (RVAD) helps in predicting curve progression. A line (a) is drawn perpendicular to the endplate of the apical vertebra. A second line (b) is drawn from the midpoint of the neck of the rib at the apical vertebra through the midpoint of the head of the same rib and extending to the perpendicular on the convex side. The angle between those two lines is calculated, as is the angle on the concave side. The RVAD is obtained by subtracting the angle on the convex side from the angle on the concave side of the curve. A difference of more than 20° suggests a high likelihood of a progressive form of idiopathic infantile scoliosis (IIS), according to Mehta.

- Mehta derotational technique—serves to straighten spine in younger/flexible patients
  - May be used as a temporizing measure before surgery in more rigid patients
- Bracing
  - To reduce progression in incompletely corrected curves after casting
  - Older patients who will not tolerate a cast
- Surgical treatment—avoid early fusion (before age 10)
  - Growing rods—dual construct that allows for thoracic growth through regular lengthening
  - Vertical expandable prosthetic titanium rib (VEPTR)—a growing construct attached to the ribs—may be combined with growing rods in patients with thoracic insufficiency or fused ribs
  - Shilla technique—short apical fusion with proximal and distal anchors—does not require periodic lengthening
- Juvenile
  - **MRI—indicated for all patients aged < 10**
  - Brace treatment—for patients with > 20° curve and > 5° documented progression
  - Surgical treatment—indicated for all curves > 50°
    - Growing rods are used for patients with significant thoracic growth remaining.
    - Fusion may be considered for large/rigid curves in patients aged > 8.
      - Age <10 leads to some pulmonary compromise.
      - Anterior and posterior fusion both equally effective
      - Some investigators advocate adding anterior fusion to posterior fusion for rigid curves >70° and in patients with open triradiate cartilage to avoid crankshaft.
      - Crankshaft may be avoided using multiple pedicle screws (fixation of anterior column).

- Adolescent: >age 10
  - **Indications for MRI**—atypical curve
    - Abnormal neurologic examination
    - Left thoracic or right lumbar curve
    - Sharp angular curves
    - Hyperkyphosis
  - **Bracing**
    - Indications
      - **Progression > 5°**
      - **Curve > 25°**
      - **Risser 0, 1, 2**
    - Wear > 16 hours/d until spinal growth complete or curve > 45°
  - **Surgery curves > 50°**
    - Anterior or posterior fusion of all structural curves (any curve that does not correct to < 25° on bending films or has abnormal sagittal contour)
- Associated diagnoses—**Marfan** and neurofibromatosis
  - Must have MRI to evaluate for **dural ectasia**
  - Indications for bracing and fusion are the same as idiopathic.

Spondylolysis and Spondylolisthesis

- General
  - 25% of patients with spondylolysis have associated spondylolisthesis.
  - Level
    - **Most common—L5** (90%) > L4 > L3
  - Wiltse classification
    - **Isthmic** most common—males > females, but females more likely to develop high-grade slip
    - Dysplastic—higher risk of neurologic compromise
- Imaging—spot lateral radiograph
  - Oblique radiographs aid diagnosis of spondylolysis.
  - Single-photon emission CT **scan most sensitive** modality used to detect occult spondylolysis.
- Spondylolisthesis classification
  - Low grade (≤50% slip)
  - High grade (>50% slip)
- Nonoperative treatment
  - Observation
    - Asymptomatic spondylolysis
    - Low-grade spondylolisthesis
  - Bracing (lumbosacral orthosis) and therapy
    - Symptomatic spondylolysis
    - Symptomatic or progressive low-grade spondylolisthesis
  - **Surgical indications**
    - Neurologic symptoms
    - High-grade spondylolisthesis
    - Progressive, symptomatic low-grade spondylolisthesis
    - Persistent pain > 6 months nonoperative treatment
  - Surgical treatment
    - Spondylolysis
      - Pars repair (numerous techniques)
      - L5 to S1 fusion (with or without instrumentation)
    - Spondylolisthesis
      - L4 to S1 for high-grade slips
      - Consider translumbar interbody fusion for high-grade slips

- Consider decompression in the presence of neurologic symptoms
- Reduction is controversial and carries risk of L5 nerve root damage.

Scheuermann Kyphosis

- **Criteria**
  - **>45° thoracic** kyphosis or **>30° thoracolumbar** kyphosis
  - **>5° wedging in at least three vertebrae**
  - **Endplate irregularities**
- Diagnosis
  - Standing full-length lateral and posteroanterior (PA) radiograph
  - 25% associated scoliosis
  - May be associated with increased body mass index (BMI)
  - Rigid—does not correct with hyperextension over bolster
- Nonoperative treatment
  - Observation—nonprogressive curves < 55°
  - Bracing
    - Curves 55° to 70°
    - Brace above the shoulders for apex T8 or above
    - >1-year growth remaining—works best in skeletally immature patients
  - Surgery—instrumented posterior fusion
    - Curves >75°
    - Neurologic deficit
    - Progression despite bracing
    - Pain despite bracing and therapy
    - Need preoperative MRI to evaluate for herniated disk
    - Most can be managed posteriorly with osteotomies
    - Add anterior release for rigid curves or herniated disks

Spinal Trauma

- General
  - C3—occiput most common in children <8
  - **Noncontiguous** trauma common
  - Up to 20% fractures due to blunt trauma have normal initial examination.
  - Bony fractures usually immobilized nonoperatively.
- Treatment principles
  - **Immobilize with head slightly posterior** (special board or towels underneath chest)
  - **Halo** immobilization requires **8 to 12 pins with low torque** (4 ft lb) in young children
  - **Up to 34%** spinal cord injuries have no radiographic abnormality **(SCIWORA)**
  - Need MRI—most sensitive at 48 hours
  - SCIWORA—spinal cord injury without radiographic damage
    - The immature boney column can stretch 5 cm.
    - Need MRI to evaluate
    - Spinal cord can only stretch 6 mm.
    - 12 weeks immobilization
- Cervical trauma
  - Occipitoatlantal injuries
    - Powers ratio >1—anterior displacement of occiput
    - <0.55—posterior displacement
    - Treatment:
      - Initial = halo
      - Definitive = fusion of occiput to C1 or C2
  - Atlas fracture: axial load
    - Treatment—halo or cast

- Dens fracture: may spontaneously reduce
  - Treatment: halo or rigid collar
- Subaxial fractures
  - Initial treatment—traction
  - Definitive—usually collar or halo unless unstable
  - Exception—endplate dissociation from body is unstable and may need fusion.

NEUROMUSCULAR DISORDERS
Cerebral Palsy
- Definition
  - **Nonprogressive, permanent brain injury**
  - Musculoskeletal manifestations can be progressive.
  - Seizures with cerebral palsy can contribute to loss of function.
  - Progressive stiffness and weakness in a family, should think familial spastic paraparesis
  - Can be spastic (most commonly benefit from orthopaedic procedures), dyskinetic, or ataxic
  - Quadriplegia, diplegic, hemiplegic
  - Gross Motor Function Classification System
    - Level I—most functional; walks with no limitations
    - Level II—walks with some limitations
    - Level III—requires cane-type mobility device
    - Level IV—is self-mobile with limitations
    - Level V—most limitations; requires wheelchair
- Developmental evaluation
  - Sit by 9 months
  - Cruise by 14 months
  - Walk by 18 months
- Examination
  - Evaluation of contractures
    - Duncan-Ely test for rectus femoris
    - Thomas test for hip flexion
    - Silfverskiold for ankle equinus
  - Gait analysis
- Medical treatment
  - Mobility, with therapy, assistive aids, brace
    - Supramalleolar orthosis (SMO) for coronal plane foot pronation supination
    - Ankle-foot orthosis (AFO) for ankle dorsiflexion/plantarflexion
    - Knee-ankle-foot orthosis for knee stabilization
  - Prevention of contractures with bracing and stretching
  - Occupational therapy for activities of daily living
  - Speech and swallowing therapy
  - Antispasticity medications
    - Baclofen, oral or intrathecal for spasticity
    - Diazepam
    - Botox for dynamic contractures
- Surgical treatment
  - Multilevel surgery
  - Tendon lengthening for contractures, osteotomy for torsional or angular deformities, tendon transfers for over active or weak muscles units.
  - Spine brace for sitting posture, not effective for preventing scoliosis progression.
  - Posterior spinal fusion **(PSF) to pelvis**, high risk of infection
- Upper extremity
  - Contractures, splinting, and Botox
  - Osteotomies, tendon lengthening, and tendon transfers

- Hip
  - Problems more common in quadriplegic than ambulatory patients.
  - Dislocation posterior-superior and can be painful.
  - Goal of treatment is to prevent dislocation and assist with care.
  - Reimer migration index
  - **Adductor tenotomy** for young children with minimal subluxation
  - Add varus **derotational osteotomies (VDROs), pelvic osteotomy** for young children with more severe subluxation, or older children
    - Open triradiates—Dega osteotomy
    - Closed triradiates—Ganz or triple osteotomy
    - Salvage—Chiari or shelf reconstruction
    - Failed—femoral head resection
- Knee
  - Crouch gait from contracture hamstrings or weak ankle plantar flexors
  - Lengthen hamstring and advance quadriceps for mild case
  - Distal femoral extension osteotomy and advance quadriceps for severe cases
- Foot and ankle
  - Equinus deformity—bracing, stretching, and release of gastrocnemius with/without soleus based on Silfverskiold. Achilles can also be lengthened, but overlengthening can lead to crouch gait.
  - Equinovarus, from overactive tibialis anterior, tibialis posterior, and contracted gastroc-soleus—split tibialis anterior or posterior transfers to correct flexible, osteotomies for rigid
  - Equinovalgus, contracted gastroc-soleus and peroneals, weak tibialis posterior—SMO or AFO, or osteotomies and tendon lengthening
  - Pes planus—SMO or AFO, osteotomies
  - Hallux valgus—splinting or metatarsophalangeal (MTP) fusion
- Fractures
  - High risk for fractures due to poor bone mineral density
  - Consider bisphosphonate

Myelomeningocele and Spina Bifida (Figure 3.15)

- **Failure of neural crest closure**
- Spina bifida, failure of posterior vertebral elements to close, no neurologic involvement

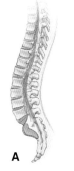 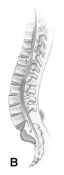 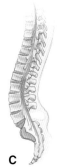 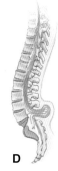

Figure 3.15 A, Normal spine. B, Spina bifida occulta. C, Meningocele. D, Myelomeningocele. From Ricci S, Kyle T, Carman S. Nursing care of the child with an alteration in mobility/neuromuscular or musculoskeletal disorder. In: *Maternity and Pediatric Nursing*. 3rd ed. Philadelphia, PA: Wolters Kluwer; 2017:1672-1740.

- Meningocele, dura through bony defect, spinal cord contained within unfused posterior vertebral elements
- Myelomeningocele, spinal cord uncontained
- Diagnosis with alpha fetal protein, ultrasound (US), amniocentesis
- **Supplement with folic acid, risk with certain drug exposures, maternal diabetes**
- Classification by level of cord involvement—L4 needed to walk
- Nonorthopaedic treatment
  - Mobility, skin checks for pressure sores, gastrointestinal and urinary regimens
  - Closure of myelomeningocele, VP shunt, untethering of cord
- Spine—fusion for scoliosis and correction of kyphosis
- *Hip—dysplasia and instability left unreduced*, unless unilateral dislocation in ambulator
- Lower extremity—contractures released or corrected with guided growth. Angulation and torsional deformities also surgically addressed
- Foot and ankle—rigid clubfoot and other deformities depending on spinal cord level, treated surgically
- *Fractures—erythema, swelling, warmth, and may be misdiagnosed as infection*

Muscular Dystrophy (Duchenne)

- **Dystrophin, absent, stabilizes cell membrane—abnormal but present in Becker dystrophy**
- X-linked recessive
- **Calf pseudohypertrophy**, difficulty in running or climbing stairs, Gower sign, loss of ambulation by age 10
- **Gower sign (Figure 3.16)**
- Steroids delay progression of symptoms
- **Scoliosis >20° treated early, prior to pulmonary and cardiac dysfunction**
- Malignant hyperthermia risk

Spinal Muscular Atrophy

- *Progressive proximal to distal weakness*
- Autosomal recessive
- **Survival motor neuron, loss of alpha motor neurons in anterior horn**
- Spinal muscular atrophy type 1 (SMA 1) (Werdnig-Hoffman)
  - Onset at birth
  - Respiratory failure and death at 2 years
- SMA 2
  - Onset 6 to 18 months
  - Life expectancy >15 years
  - Hip contractures, scoliosis, joint contractures
- SMA 3
  - Onset >18 months
  - Normal life expectancy
  - Like SMA 2, but can stand
- Scoliosis, bracing for sitting posture, VEPTR for thoracic insufficiency, or *PSF for curve >40 or decreasing pulmonary function*, forced vital capacity <40% normal
- Hip dysplasia, treat if painful to maintain hip reduction, tenotomy, osteotomies
- Contractures

Hereditary Sensory Neuropathies

- Chronic, progressive sensory neuropathies
- Distal hand and foot weakness, decreased sensation, areflexia
- Type 1 or Charcot-Marie-Tooth type 1 (CMT 1)

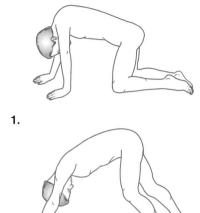

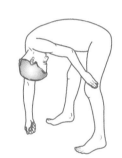

1.

2.

Figure 3.16 Gower sign. The individual walks up the front of the legs and thighs when asked to stand from a seated position. From Forgach JL, Washington AL. Muscular dystrophy. In: Atchison BJ, Dirette DP, eds. *Conditions in Occupational Therapy: Effect on Occupational Performance.* 5th ed. Philadelphia, PA: Wolters Kluwer; 2017:69-81.

3.

- • PMP22
- • Autosomal dominant (AD), with some exceptions
- • Slow motor nerve conduction
- ● Type 2 or CMT 2
  - • Decreased motor and sensory nerve condition
  - • AD, with some exceptions
  - • Normal to slightly prolonged muscle action potential
- ● Type 3 or Dejerine-Sottas
  - • Severely decreased motor nerve conduction
  - • Autosomal recessive
  - • Presents in infancy
  - • Enlarged peripheral nerves, ataxia, nystagmus
- ● Hip dysplasia
- ● Cavus foot (Figure 3.17)
  - • Tight intrinsics, contracture of plantar fascia, weak tibialis anterior and peroneals
  - • Posterior tibialis transfer for weak tibialis anterior
  - • Plantar fascial release and osteotomies

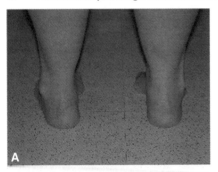

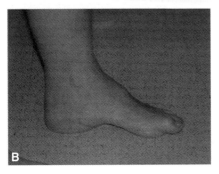

Figure 3.17 Clinical photographs of foot deformity in Charcot-Marie-Tooth disease. A, Posterior view shows hindfoot varus. B, Medial view shows high arch and hallux clawing. From Pateder DB. Charcot-Marie-Tooth disease. In: Frassica FJ, Sponseller PD, Wilckens JH, eds. *The 5-Minute Clinical Consult*. 2nd ed. Philadelphia, PA: Lippincott Williams & Wilkins; 2007:69.

- Achilles lengthening for hindfoot equinus
- Calcaneal osteotomy for hindfoot varus
- Claw toes, interphalangeal fusion, and Jones transfers
- Scoliosis, try brace, but PSF
- Intrinsic weakness, tendon transfers, contracture release, and arthrodesis

Friedrich Ataxia

- Spinocerebellar disorder
- Frataxin (FXN) and cellular iron homeostasis
- Younger age of onset with more base sequence repeats in FXN
- Ataxia, areflexia, Babinski sign
- Pes cavus, lengthening and transfers, or arthrodesis
- Scoliosis, PSF without pelvis extension

Rett Syndrome

- X-linked dominant, from de novo mutation
- Methyl-CpG–binding protein 2 methylates DNA
- Typically female, as lethal in males

LOWER EXTREMITY AND FOOT DEFORMITIES
Normal Alignment and Rotation

- The terms "version" and "torsion" are often erroneously used interchangeably in the literature:
  - Version: describes the axial measurement of the proximal femur or tibia
  - Torsion: describes the overall "twist" of the femoral or tibial shafts

- *The mechanical axis, defined as a line drawn from the center of the femoral head to the center of the ankle*, passes just medial to the center of the knee in most individuals. The anatomic axis of a bone is defined as a mid-diaphyseal line traversing the entire bone segment.
- When the mechanical axis line crosses a joint line, specific joint angles are created where "m" stands for mechanical: lateral proximal femoral angle, lateral distal femoral angle, medial proximal tibial angle, and the lateral distal tibial angle (Figure 3.18).

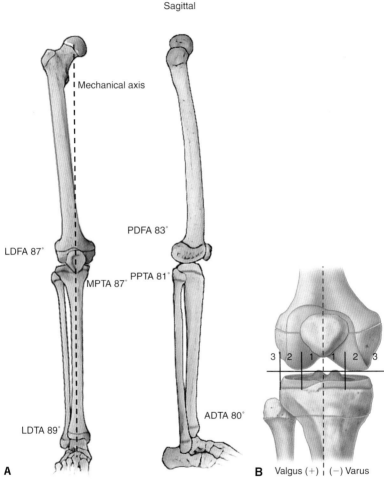

Sagittal

Mechanical axis

PDFA 83°

LDFA 87°

PPTA 81°

MPTA 87°

ADTA 80°

LDTA 89°

A

B Valgus (+) ¦ (−) Varus

3 | 2 | 1 | 1 | 2 | 3

Figure 3.18 A, The mechanical axis is a straight line drawn from the center of the femoral head to the center of the ankle joint. The normal angles for LDFA, MPTA, and LDTA will assist in identifying the location of deformity in the coronal plane, and PDFA, PPTA, and ADTA likewise will locate deformity in the sagittal plane. B, Dividing the knee into zones, the mechanical axis should pass through the central one-third of the joint. Deviation into zone 2 or 3 indicates deformity that may require surgical intervention. ADTA, anterior distal tibial angle; LDFA, lateral distal femoral angle; LDTA, lateral distal tibial angle; MPTA, medial proximal tibial angle; PDFA, posterior distal femoral angle; PPTA, posterior proximal tibial angle. From Muchow RD, Noonan KJ. Guided growth to correct limb deformity. In: Flynn JM, Sankar WN, eds. *Operative Techniques in Pediatric Orthopaedic Surgery*. 2nd ed. Philadelphia, PA: Wolters Kluwer; 2016:550-557.

Limb Length Discrepancy

- Normal growth
  - **Boys are expected to stop growing at age 16 and girls at age 14.**
  - Most lower limb growth occurs at the knee, with the **femur contributing 10 mm/y of growth and the tibia 6 mm/y of growth.**
- Etiologies
  - Various diagnoses that are associated with shortened limbs, including fibular hemimelia, tibial hemimelia, previous septic arthritis, and Blount disease.
  - LLD can be also secondary to limb overgrowth, which is often caused by increased blood flow to the leg (ie, posttraumatic/postinfectious, arteriovenous malformations). Klippel-Trenaunay and Beckwith-Wiedemann syndrome (**must screen for Wilms tumor**) are also **associated with hemihypertrophy.**
- Evaluation
  - Accurate measurement of the LLD is paramount. Clinically, a tape measure from the anterior superior iliac spine to the medial or lateral malleolus is used.
  - **CT scanograms** are the gold standard when determining limb length in the presence of **joint contractures**.
  - Teleroentgenography consists of a single shot standing x-ray of both limbs.
  - Orthoroentgenography consists of separate x-rays of the bilateral hips, knees, and ankles, which are put together later on one film.
- Predicting discrepancy at maturity
  - In congenital LLD, the length ratio of the short limb to the long limb is constant throughout growth.
  - Skeletal, not chronological, age is used as the starting age.
  - Although various methods are used to predict the LLD, in general, the predicted LLD is the sum of the current LLD and the expected growth in the bone.
- Treatment
  - Treatment is based on the current and/or expected LLD:
    - **0 to 2 cm:** observation
    - **2 to 6 cm:** nonoperative management with shoe lift or operative management involving epiphysiodesis or limb shortening
    - **6 to 20 cm:** limb lengthening
  - Epiphysiodesis can be accomplished via percutaneous drilling, stapling (less effective), physeal bar formation by placement of a rectangular bone block, or transphyseal screws as described by Metaizeau.

Angular Deformities

- Physiologic bowing versus Blount disease
  - The metaphyseal–diaphyseal (MD) angle differentiates between these two diagnoses.
  - The MD angle is measured by drawing a line along the anatomic axis of the tibia, then drawing a line perpendicular to this anatomic axis line. The final line is drawn along the slope of the metaphysis. The MD angle is created by the intersection of the perpendicular line and the line traversing the slope of the metaphysis (Figure 3.19).
    - Normal is 11°.
    - *Patients with MD angles > 16 have a 95% probability of having Blount disease.*
    - An MD angle can similarly be drawn on the femur. The ratio of femoral MD angle to tibial MD angle is > 1 in physiologic bowing and < 1 in Blount disease.
- Infantile Blount disease
  - Common in overweight children who ambulate before 10 months old
  - Results in osteochondrosis of the proximal medial tibial physis; the distal femoral physis is usually not involved.
  - Correction of the varus deformity can reverse changes at the proximal medial physis.

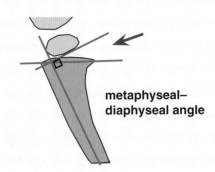

**metaphyseal–
diaphyseal angle**

Figure 3.19 The measurement of the metaphyseal–diaphyseal angle is important in the management of children with Blount disease. From Staheli LT. Lower limb. In: *Fundamentals of Pediatric Orthopedics*. 5th ed. Philadelphia, PA: Wolters Kluwer; 2016:135-156.

- *Treatment is guided by the patient's age and radiographic changes at the medial physis as classified by Langenskiöld (*Figure 3.20*).*
  - Age < 3 years old (stages I and II): Brace treatment
  - Age < 3 years old (worsening stage II or stage III): Growth modulation via lateral tibial physeal plate or staple
  - Age > 3 years old (worsening stage II or stage III): Valgus producing proximal tibial osteotomy
  - Age > 3 years old (stages IV-VI): Resection of physeal bar, elevation of medial joint line, valgus producing proximal tibial osteotomy
- Juvenile Blount disease
  - In contrast to infantile Blount disease, usually both the proximal medial tibial physis and the distal femoral physis are involved.
  - Treatment is often surgical, involving corrective distal femoral and/or proximal tibial osteotomies.

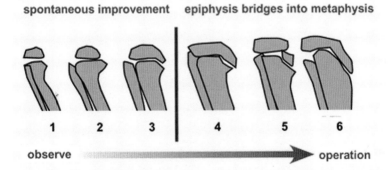

spontaneous improvement   epiphysis bridges into metaphysis

1   2   3   4   5   6

observe   operation

Figure 3.20 The Langenskiöld classification describes the severity of pathology seen at the proximal medial tibial physis in Blount disease and helps to guide treatment. An osteotomy is usually required in stages IV to VI. From Staheli LT. Lower limb. In: *Fundamentals of Pediatric Orthopedics*. 5th ed. Philadelphia, PA: Wolters Kluwer; 2016:135-156.

- Genu valgum
  - Physiologic genu valgum should peak by age 4 and normalize to 5° to 7° of valgus by age 8.
  - Evaluate for history of proximal medial tibial fracture *(Cozen fracture), which results in a valgus limb alignment that eventually resolves.*
  - If genu valgum is severe enough, corrective osteotomies can be performed.

Rotational Deformities

- Tibial torsion
  - Internal tibial torsion resulting in intoeing is common in toddlers and associated with physiologic tibial bowing, both which resolve usually around 6 to 7 years of age.
  - Nonsurgical interventions, such as bracing, do not change the natural history of intoeing for most children.
  - There is no correlation in the literature between variations in rotation and the risk of lower extremity arthritis as an adult.

Tibial Bowing

- Anterior
  - Associated with fibular hemimelia
- Anterolateral (Figure 3.21)
  - **Associated with congenital pseudoarthrosis of the tibia (CPT)**
  - **50% of patients with anterolateral bowing also have neurofibromatosis.**
  - First line of treatment for anterolateral bowing is full-time bracing. Surgical treatment is not advised until a CPT presents itself and usually once patient has reached skeletal maturity.

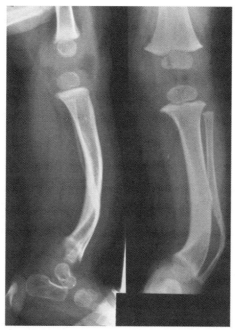

Figure 3.21 Anterolateral bowing. From Alman BA, Goldberg MJ. Syndromes of Orthopaedic importance. In: Weinstein SL, Flynn JM, eds. *Lovell and Winter's Pediatric Orthopaedics.* Vol 1. 7th ed. Philadelphia, PA: Lippincott Williams & Wilkins; 2014:218-277.

- Posteromedial
  - Best prognosis with *resolution of bowing over time*
  - Associated with a calcaneovalgus foot deformity (Figure 3.22)
  - Although treatment is nonoperative, *parents should be counseled that a residual LLD is usually present after skeletal maturity is reached.*

Limb Deficiencies

- Proximal focal femoral deficiency (PFFD)
  - Historically, prenatal use of thalidomide was a common cause of PFFD.
  - Up to 80% associated with ipsilateral fibular deficiency
  - Clinically, the proximal femur is flexed, abducted, and externally rotated (Figure 3.23).
  - Nonoperative treatment is usually preferred in patients with bilateral PFFD.
  - Surgical options include knee arthrodesis with amputation of the foot, a Van Nes rotationplasty, and limb lengthening.
  - All surgical procedures are postponed until 2.5 to 3 years of age.
- Fibular deficiency
  - Clinically patients have:
    - Rigid equinovalgus foot
    - *Absent foot rays (usually fourth and fifth)*
    - Genu valgum
    - Anterior bowing of the tibia
  - Most patients are treated surgically with the options of amputation or limb lengthening.

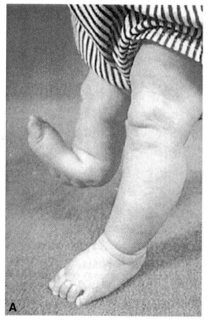
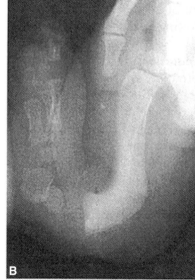

Figure 3.22 Posteromedial bowing. From Schoenecker PL, Rich MM, Gordon JE. The lower extremity. In: Weinstein SL, Flynn JM, eds. *Lovell and Winter's Pediatric Orthopaedics*. Vol 1. 7th ed. Philadelphia, PA: Lippincott Williams & Wilkins; 2014:1261-1340.

- Most frequent amputations are Syme and Boyd amputations.
  - Syme: amputation through the tibiotalar joint
  - Boyd: similar to Syme, but the calcaneus is preserved and fused to the tibia, sparing the underlying heel pad.
- Tibial deficiency
  - Unlike fibular deficiency, tibial deficiency is genetically inherited, with the most common mode of inheritance being AD.
  - Rigid equinovarus is the most common foot deformity.
  - Decision-making is guided by the presence of an intact extensor mechanism and thus a proximal tibia that is present.
  - Without an intact extensor mechanism, a knee disarticulation is preferred.

Congenital Dislocation of the Knee

- The spectrum of congenital dislocation of the knee includes simple subluxation to full dislocations.
- Associated with a breech presentation at birth
- The quadriceps tendon is often severely contracted and is central to treatment.
- **Initial treatment includes gentle stretching/manipulation with serial casting**—Goal is knee flexion beyond 90°.
- Surgical treatment for severe dislocations or those recalcitrant to serial casting involves release of the quadriceps and the surrounding retinaculum.

Clubfoot (Congenital Talipes Equinovarus)

- Congenital foot deformity
- Those associated with syndromes are more severe.
- Normally, the axis of the talus and calcaneus are divergent on an anteroposterior (AP) foot radiograph; however in clubfoot, they are parallel. Some parallelism is also seen in the clubfoot lateral foot x-ray.
- Deformity can be remembered by CAVE:
  - **C**avus
  - Forefoot **A**dductus
  - Hindfoot **V**arus
  - **E**quinus
- Serial casting, Ponseti method
  - Correct in CAVE order
  - **Most will need Achilles tenotomy to correct equinus.**
  - The final cast is held in 20° of dorsiflexion and 75° of ER.
  - **Boot and bar afterward for maintenance**
  - Okay to repeat serial casting for recurrence of clubfoot deformity
  - An anterior tibialis transfer to the dorsum of the foot can be performed for residual supination foot during "swing phase" of gait.
- Although plaster of Paris is still used, semirigid fiberglass (aka "soft casts") is now known to be superior when performing serial manipulations and casting.
- Casts should be applied every 5 to 7 days until further improvement ceases.
- Surgical correction—for late presentation, resistance to serial casting.

Congenital Vertical Talus

- The deformity is defined by a *dorsolateral dislocation at the talonavicular joint* with plantar-flexion of the talus in relation to the midfoot.
- The deformity is completely resistant to manipulation, unlike congenital oblique talus (COT).

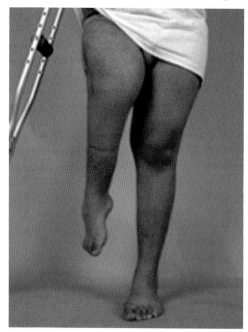

Figure 3.23 Proximal focal femoral deficiency. From Bowen RE, Otsuka NY. The child with a limb deficiency. In: Weinstein SL, Flynn JM, eds. *Lovell and Winter's Pediatric Orthopaedics*. Vol 1. 7th ed. Philadelphia, PA: Lippincott Williams & Wilkins; 2014:1596-1660.

- *Radiographically, differentiate from COT using a plantarflexion lateral radiograph* (Figure 3.24).
  - In congenital vertical talus (CVT), there is persistent dorsal dislocation of the fore-foot on the hindfoot.
  - Do not confuse with the lateral foot radiographs in clubfoot, which show parallel-ism of the talus and calcaneus.
- Serial casting is the initial treatment choice in most cases.

Congenital Oblique Talus

- Talus plantarflexed in relation to midfoot similar to CVT.
- Differentiate from CVT on plantarflexion lateral radiograph, where normal midfoot relationship restored
- Main treatment is serial casting.

Positional Calcaneovalgus Foot

- Clinically, the dorsum of the foot is resting against the anterior surface of the leg.
- Can be confused with CVT or with the foot deformity seen in posteromedial bowing of the tibia, however:
  - **The hallmark of positional calcaneovalgus is the flexibility of the deformity, which differentiates it from CVT.**
  - Also, there is no tibial deformity that differentiates it from posteromedial bowing of the tibia.
- Treatment is always nonsurgical.

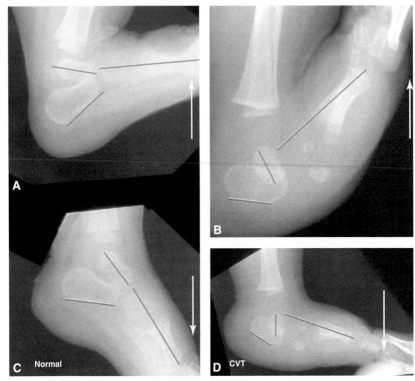

Figure 3.24 A-C, Normal foot in maximum dorsiflexion and then maximum plantarflexion. B and D, show the same views in a patient with congenital vertical talus (CVT). Notice how the head of the talus does not align with the first metatarsal during maximum plantarflexion. This finding is pathognomonic for CVT. From Mosca VS. Foot and ankle deformities. In: *Principles and Management of Pediatric Foot and Ankle Deformities and Malformations*. Philadelphia, PA: Wolters Kluwer Health; 2014:61-118.

Cavus Foot Deformity

- Unlike pes planovalgus, the presence of cavus is related to an underlying neuromuscular disorder unless proven otherwise.
- CMT is most commonly associated with the development of a cavus foot deformity.
- *The Coleman block test is helpful in diagnosis (Figure 3.25).*
  - *If the hindfoot varus corrects, then the cavus is driven by plantarflexion of the first ray only.*
  - *If the hindfoot varus does not correct, then it is also involved in the cavus deformity, indicating the need for a corrective calcaneal osteotomy.*
- Orthotic treatment for flexible deformities involves posting of the lateral forefoot and hindfoot.

Pes Planovalgus (Flexible Flatfoot)

- Characterized by a valgus hindfoot, retained mobility at the subtalar joint, and an absent longitudinal arch that is capable of returning when tested

Metatarsus Adductus

- Characterized primarily by forefoot adductus and a neutral hindfoot (in reality, a small amount of hindfoot valgus may be present)

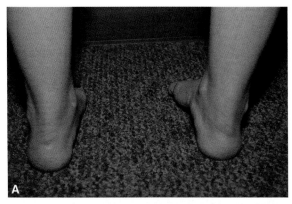

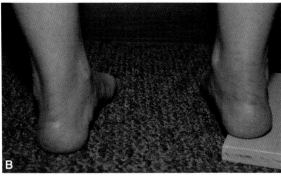

Figure 3.25 In the Coleman block test, the patient bears weight with the lateral border of the foot on a 2-cm block while the first metatarsal is allowed to drop down off the edge of the block. Note the hindfoot position without the block (A) and with the block (B), the hindfoot varus corrects to neutral position, suggesting the hindfoot is flexible and the medial forefoot is the source of hindfoot varus. From Schwend RM, Olney B. Surgical treatment of cavus foot. In: Flynn JM, Sankar WN, eds. *Operative Techniques in Pediatric Orthopaedic Surgery*. 2nd ed. Philadelphia, PA: Wolters Kluwer; 2016:1044-1055.

- The severity can be determined by which toe is intersected by the heel bisector line.
  - **Prognosis has no relation to the severity as determined by the heel bisector line.**
- **Spontaneous correction occurs in most children.** Data are inconclusive on whether stretching or bracing is useful.

Skewfoot

- Characterized primarily by forefoot adductus and a *valgus hindfoot deformity*
- The hindfoot is never neutral like in metatarsus adductus.

Idiopathic Toe Walking

- Often habitual with resolution before the age of 3 years
- Persistence of toe walking after the age of 3 years is abnormal, and treatment begins with patient and parental education and development of a heel-cord stretching regimen.
- Serial casting is started if stretching exercises fail.
- Persistence of toe walking past the age of 7 years will likely not resolve nor respond to further nonoperative methods. Heel-cord lengthening is then the definitive treatment.

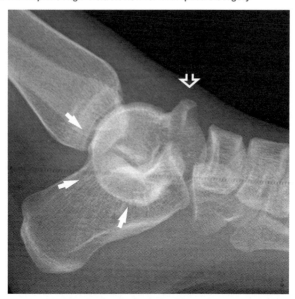

Figure 3.26 The C-sign (arrows) is formed superiorly by the medial talar dome and inferiorly by the sustentaculum tali. From Greenspan A, Beltran J. Anomalies of the upper and lower limbs. In: *Orthopedic Imaging: A Practical Approach*. 6th ed. Philadelphia, PA: Wolters Kluwer Health; 2015:1057-1099.

Tarsal Coalition

- Calcaneonavicular and middle facet talocalcaneal coalitions are the most common.
- **Results in progressive flattening of the longitudinal arch of the foot**
- **Associated with frequent ankle sprains**
- **Restriction of subtalar motion** is often present.
- Look for the C-sign on a lateral foot radiograph (Figure 3.26)
  - The C-sign is formed superiorly by the medial talar dome and inferiorly by the sustentaculum tali.
- CT is the gold-standard imaging for tarsal coalitions.
- Nonoperative management with casting is always attempted to resolve symptoms.
- If less than 50% of the joint is involved in the coalition, treatment involves resection of the coalition with interposition of muscle or fat.
- *If greater than 50% of the joint is involved or if arthritic changes are already present, treatment is a triple arthrodesis.*

Accessory Navicular

- Classified by shape with type I accessory naviculars having a small pellet-shaped ossicle, type IIs having a bullet-shaped ossicle joined by a synchondrosis, and type IIIs having a fully fused ossicle in the shape of a horn (Figure 3.27).
- Type II accessory naviculars are usually the most symptomatic.
- Surgery is only indicated after nonoperative treatment has failed.
  - The Kidner procedure is classically described as removal of the accessory navicular with distal advancement of the tibialis posterior tendon.

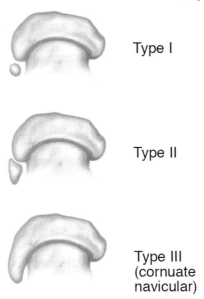

Type I

Type II

Type III
(cornuate
navicular)

Figure 3.27 Three types of accessory navicular. Type I, round and separated; type II, triangular with fibrous attachment; and type III, prominent medial tubercle or cornuate navicular. Type II is most often associated with posterior tibial tendon dysfunction. From Berquist TH. Anatomy, normal variants, and basic biomechanics. In: *Imaging of the Foot and Ankle*. 3rd ed. Philadelphia, PA: Wolters Kluwer; 2011:1-46.

Kohler Disease

- **Self-limited** condition of the tarsal navicular
- Classic features on a lateral a radiograph are sclerosis, fragmentation, and flattening of the navicular bone (Figure 3.28).
- Treatment is nonsurgical.
- Casting (for 8 weeks) affects only the duration of symptoms, but it does not affect the overall outcome, which is resolution of symptoms of radiographic changes.

Toe Disorders

- Juvenile hallux valgus
  - Most are asymptomatic
  - Many patients have **bilateral hallux valgus.**
  - **Surgical management should be avoided** while they are skeletally immature due to the high rate of recurrence.
- Polydactyly
  - More common in black patients
  - Classified as preaxial if the great toe is duplicated, central if the second through fourth toes are involved, and postaxial if the small toe is involved.
  - Resection of a central ray polydactyly does not appreciably narrow the foot.
- Syndactyly
  - Failure of segmentation of adjacent toes
  - Possible etiology lies in failure of separation of cells at the apical epidermal ridge.
  - Seen in patients with Apert syndrome, which is characterized primarily by early synostosis of the cranial bones, leading to a sunken midface and wide-set bulging eyes.

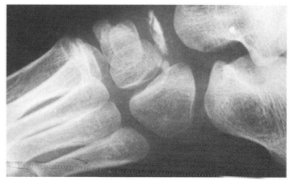

Figure 3.28 Osteochondrosis of the tarsal navicular (Kohler disease) in a 5-year-old boy. The process is in the phase of revascularization with areas of bone deposition and bone resorption. The ossific nucleus is thin, but the cartilage space is thicker than normal, which means that the overall size of the navicular is not diminished. This explains the eventual normal appearance of the navicular at the end of the healing process. From Salter RB. Disorders of epiphyses and epiphyseal growth. In: *Textbook of Disorders and Injuries of the Musculoskeletal System.* 3rd ed. Baltimore, MD: Lippincott Williams & Wilkins; 1999:339-378.

- Curly toe
  - Characterized by one lesser toe deforming to sit underneath the adjacent medial toe
  - Deformity occurs at proximal interphalangeal or distal interphalangeal joints, not MTP joints.
  - Most are asymptomatic and most spontaneously resolve
  - Stretching and taping have not been proven to be effective.
  - If surgery is needed, tenotomy of the flexor digitorum longus and/or flexor digitorum brevis is successful in >95% of cases.
  - Normal development until 18 months, then regression with mental retardation, ataxia, and autism
  - Behavioral abnormalities, hand-wringing
  - Neuromuscular scoliosis, PSF
  - Spasticity and contractures
  - Coxa valga

HIP CONDITIONS

Developmental Dysplasia of the Hip

- Definition
  - Decreased or delayed development of the hip joint in the perinatal period, leading to a shallow acetabulum in the least severe form to a completely dislocated hip in the most severe form
  - Children are otherwise normal; not caused by any other condition or genetic syndrome such as spina bifida or arthrogryposis.
- Epidemiology
  - Dislocated hip: 1/1000 live born babies
  - Unstable or poorly developed hip: 1/100
- Etiology
  - Genetic: 4× risk with parental or sibling involvement
  - Racial/Cultural
    - Increased risk—Laplander and Native American
    - Rarely seen in African American

- Hormonal
- Female (4-6×)
- Environmental: uterine crowding
  - Breech (10×)
  - Twins
  - First born
  - Left 3× right (position)
- Environmental: swaddling
- Diagnosis
  - Early (0-3 months)
    - Examination
      - Ortolani: hip out reduces with abduction
      - Barlow: hip subluxes in adduction
      - Hip clicks and asymmetric thigh folds nonspecific
      - **Associated conditions**
        - **Metatarsus adductus**
        - **Torticollis**
        - **Congenital knee dislocation**
  - Imaging—US is modality of choice up to 4 months of age.
    - Indications:
      - Positive physical examination
      - Positive family history
      - Breech presentation/positioning
    - If US performed for risk factors with normal physical examination, wait until 6 weeks of age to avoid false positives.
    - Routine screening with US not recommended
    - Dynamic examination: hip stability
    - Angles:
      - $\alpha > 60°$ (acetabular development)
      - $\beta < 55°$ (position of femoral head)
  - Late (>3 months)
    - Examination
      - Decreased abduction
      - LLD (affected side short Galeazzi sign)
    - Imaging
      - X-ray: AP pelvis
        - Acetabular index <30° by 18 months
        - Center edge angle >25° by age 6 years
  - Late (ambulatory child)
    - Examination
      - Trendelenburg/consistent pelvic obliquity
      - Toe walking/vaulting due to LLD (unilateral)
      - Lumbar lordosis/waddling (bilateral)
- Treatment
  - Reducible
    - **Age: 0 to 3 weeks—observe**
    - **>3 weeks—brace (Pavlik or other)**
      - 100° flexion
      - Block adduction/no forced abduction
      - 2 to 4 weeks follow-up with US to confirm reduction
      - Brace until stable
    - **Pavlik disease**—incompletely reduced hip erodes posterolateral acetabulum
  - Irreducible
    - Closed reduction and casting

- **Age >6 months**
  - **Closed reduction and casting**
    - Arthrogram (goal: <5 mm dye pool)
    - Safe zone (>30° between stable adduction and relaxed abduction)
    - May require adductor tenotomy
    - Excessive abduction (>60°) increases avascular necrosis (AVN).
  - Failure of closed reduction—pathoanatomy
    - **Blocks to reduction**
      - **Psoas tendon**
      - **Capsular contraction**
      - **Inverted labrum/limbus**
      - **Thickened ligamentum teres**
      - **Pulvinar fat**
      - **Transverse acetabular ligament**
  - Open reduction—medial approach
    - If closed reduction unsuccessful
    - At risk: medial femoral circumflex artery
    - Spica cast to hold reduction
- **Treatment: >18 months**
  - **Open reduction: anterior or anteromedial/medial**
  - Femoral shortening for high-riding dislocations or children > 2 years old
  - Pelvic osteotomy for significant acetabular dysplasia
  - Types of pelvic osteotomies
    - Redirectional
      - Salter
      - Steele (triple)
      - Ganz
    - Recontouring (hinge on the triradiate)
      - Dega
      - Pemberton
      - San Diego
    - Salvage (fibrous metaplasia)
    - Chiari
    - Shelf
- **Complications of treatment**
  - **Most prevalent—redislocation (5%)**
  - NV damage (1%)
  - AVN

Legg-Calvé-Perthes Disease

- Definition: idiopathic osteochondrosis of capital femoral epiphysis in a skeletally immature hip
- Etiology
  - Unknown; combination genetic and environmental
  - Possible small vessel coagulopathy
- Self-limited disease course
- Epidemiology
  - 1:1200 kids <15 years
  - Males 4 to 5× more frequently affected
  - 10% to 20% bilateral (asymmetric, different stages)
  - Age range 3 to 11 years
  - Delayed bone age in 89%
- History
  - Limp/abnormal gait
  - Usually intermittent

- May be painless; pain activity related
- No history of trauma
- Mild, sporadic pain: hip, groin, thigh, or knee
- Physical examination
  - Decreased range of motion (ROM), especially internal rotation (IR) and abduction
  - Muscle spasm
  - Positive roll test should invoke guarding or spasm, especially with IR.
  - Trendelenburg gait
- Associated disorders
  - Hypercoagulable disorders (inconsistent/controversial)
- LCP: imaging
  - Plain x-rays: AP pelvis and frog lateral (and bone age) (Figure 3.29)
  - Dynamic arthrography
  - Assesses sphericity and congruence
  - MRI—evolving; may aid in early diagnosis and prognosis
- Radiographic stages (Waldenstrom)
  - Initial
    - Symptoms: irritable hip
    - X-ray: increased medial joint space, small ossific nucleus
  - Fragmentation (duration 1 year)
    - Symptoms: increased pain and limp, decreased ROM
    - X-ray: increased head density, ossific nucleus collapse, fragmentation
  - Reossification (duration 3-5 years)
    - Symptoms: less pain, restricted ROM
    - X-ray: new subchondral bone
  - Residual (remodeling)
    - Symptoms: mild or none
    - X-ray: femoral head reconstituted
- Differential diagnosis: bilaterally symmetric
  - Spondyloepiphyseal dysplasia tarda
  - Multiple epiphyseal dysplasia
  - Meyer dysplasia
  - Hypothyroidism (common with Down syndrome)
  - Steroids (AVN)
  - Genetic syndromes
- Herring classification
  - Integrity of the lateral one-third "pillar" of epiphysis
  - A: no height loss and little density change

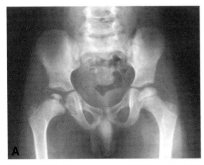 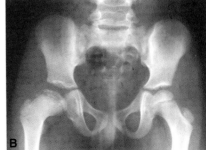

Figure 3.29 Radiographs at different stages of Legg-Calvé-Perthes disease. Flattening and fragmentation of the femoral head with widening of the femoral neck (A) and with reossification 1 year later (B). From Berquist TH. Pelvis, hips, and thigh. In: *MRI of the Musculoskeletal System*. 6th ed. Philadelphia, PA: Wolters Kluwer; 2013:777-869.

- B: lucency and <50% loss of lateral height
- BC border: exactly 50% loss or thin, poorly ossified LC
- C: lucency and >50% loss of height
- Good intra-observer reliability
- **Prognosis**
  - **Inversely related to age**
  - **Directly related to the degree of lateral column involvement and incongruence after remodeling (Stulberg)**
- Treatment: highly controversial
  - Principle of containment during early stages (surgical or nonsurgical)
  - **Indications for containment**
    - **>Age 8 and BC border or B: consider treatment**
  - Methods of containment
    - Petrie casting
    - Salter
    - VDRO
  - Late treatment (late stage 2 or 3)—hinge abduction
    - Extrusion of head—not containable
    - Consider valgus osteotomy and/or shelf or Chiari osteotomy
- Complications
  - Femoral head deformity with possible impingement
  - Labral tears
  - Arthritis
  - LLD

Slipped Capital Femoral Epiphysis

- Demographics
  - Incidence 2:100 000
  - Males 2× > females (possibly equalizing)
  - Age at diagnosis (range 9-16 years)
  - Boys mean age 13.5 years
  - Girls mean age 12.0 years
  - Average 5 months of symptoms prior to diagnosis
  - Pacific Islanders > African Americans > Native Americans and Hispanics > Caucasians > Asians
  - Obesity; most over 95th percentile, earlier onset
  - Bilateral
    - 18% to 63% idiopathic
    - 61% to 100% endocrinopathy
    - >50% bilateral at diagnosis
    - Metachronous bilateral in 18 months
    - 60% unilateral cases: left hip affected
- Slipped capital femoral epiphysis (SCFE): classification
  - **Stable**
    - **Able to weight bear ± crutches**
  - **Unstable**
    - **Unable to tolerate weight bearing**
  - **Acute** (<3 weeks symptoms) versus chronic
- Pathogenesis
  - **Stable**
    - **Widened hypertrophic zone**
  - Unstable
    - Fracture through hypertrophic zone
    - **Accumulation** of proteoglycans and glycoproteins adjacent to cleft

- Metaphysis (femoral neck) externally rotates and slips proximal to the epiphysis (femoral head).
  - Majority produce varus relationship
- Etiology
  - Idiopathic (majority of cases)
  - Endocrine abnormality (7%)—hypothyroidism most common endocrinopathy
  - Down syndrome
  - Hypogonadism
  - Panhypopituitarism
  - Renal osteodystrophy (hyperparathyroidism)
  - Growth hormone supplementation
  - Prior external beam radiotherapy
- Clinical presentation
  - Stable/chronic (85%)
    - Symptoms > 3 weeks (average 5 months)
    - Groin/thigh pain with activity
    - Knee, medial (only c/o in 15%)
    - Able to bear weight, ±Limp
    - ER gait
  - Unstable/acute or acute-on-chronic (15%)
    - Abrupt onset or increase in symptoms
    - Pain at rest
    - Groin/hip
    - Knee (less common complaint)
    - Unable to bear weight (unstable)
    - Presents like subcapital femoral neck fracture
- Physical examination
  - Pain with IR
  - Decreased IR, abduction, and flexion
  - Obligate ER with flexion
  - Gait—foot progression in ER
- Imaging
  - AP: decreased epiphyseal height, physis thin
    - Mild: Klein line lateral to epiphysis
    - Hyperdense: metaepiphyseal overlap
  - Lateral: posterior displacement
    - Rounded, eroded anterior neck (in chronic slips)
  - Radiographic classification (lateral x-ray)
    - Slip severity: degree of displacement
    - Mild: <one-third of neck width
    - Moderate: one-third to one half of neck width
    - Severe: >one half of neck width
- **Treatment**
  - **Indications: any slip with open physis**
    - In situ percutaneous screw fixation (no reduction)
    - 6.5 mm or larger cannulated screw
  - Forceful manipulation increases AVN in unstable hips **(don't do it!)**
    - **Stable—Don't try it!**
  - Unstable:
    - **In situ pinning**
      - Anterior start point
      - Severe slips may need future osteotomy to address impingement.
      - Consider adding second screw
        - Stronger than one screw
        - Higher incidence of intra-articular damage

- Consider capsulotomy to reduce intra-articular pressure
- Serendipitous reduction with gentle operative positioning
  - Controversial
  - Normalizes anatomy
  - No deleterious effect on bone scan
  - Some studies show higher AVN with any reduction.
- Open reduction (surgical hip dislocation)
  - Controversial—only used for severe, unstable slips
  - Normalizes anatomy
  - Some studies show higher rate of AVN than in situ pinning.

- **Contralateral fixation indications**
  - Bilateral disease
  - Contralateral symptoms on examination or abnormal x-ray
  - **Endocrinopathy, metabolic disorder**
  - **Young (age < 10), obese patient**
  - Unstable slip (relative)
- Complications
  - Chondrolysis
    - Loss of >50% joint space or to <3 mm
    - Risk factors:
      - Persistent hardware penetration
      - Increased α angle (impingement)
      - Increased slip severity (impingement)
      - Prolonged pretreatment symptoms
      - Cast immobilization
  - AVN
    - Risk factors
      - Acute, unstable SCFE (50% risk)
      - Reduction of unstable slip (controversial)
      - Use of fracture table
      - Reduction attempts of stable slip
      - Superolateral pin placement
      - Femoral neck osteotomy
  - **Impingement**
    - **32% have clinical impingement 6.1 years after treatment.**
    - **Impingement not correlated with slip angle but instead with α angle.**

Congenital Coxa Vara

- Epidemiology
  - 1/25 000 births
  - 30% to 50% bilateral
  - African American > Caucasian
- Etiology/Pathology
  - Physiologic shear stress
  - Vertically oriented physis
  - Chronic epiphysiolysis without slip
- Presentation
  - Painless, waddling limp
  - LLD in 1- to 6-year-old
  - Lumbar lordosis
- Classification
  - Hilgenreiner epiphyseal angle (HEA)
  - Neck/shaft angle
  - Physeal angle

- Treatment
  - HEA < 45°: no treatment
  - HEA 45° to 60°: observe for progression
  - HEA > 60°: correct
  - Neck shaft (NS) angle < 90°
  - Physeal angle > 45°
  - Goal: correct varus to normal anatomy to eliminate shear
  - Subtrochanteric, valgus derotational osteotomy
  - Goal: create NS angle of 135°, HEA < 40°
  - AVN, recurrent deformity, LLD

SKELETAL DYSPLASIAS
General Characteristics

- Abnormal bone development
- Change be proportionate or disproportionate
- Short limb
  - Rhizomelic—proximal limb
  - Mesomelic—middle limb
  - Acromelic—distal limb

Achondroplasia (Figure 3.30)

- **FGFR3**
- 80% spontaneous mutation, AD
- Clinical findings
  - Frontal bossing, trident hands
  - *Foramen magnum narrowing*—risk of apnea, requires close monitoring, may benefit from decompression
  - Radial subluxation

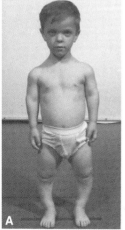
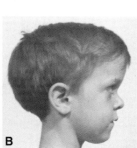
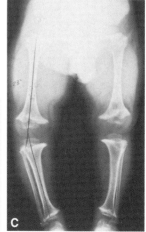

Figure 3.30 Achondroplasia in a 7-year-old boy. A, Rhizomelia. B, Frontal bossing. C, Lower extremity angular deformity. From Wheeler PG, Weaver PD. Skeletal dysplasias. In: McMillan JA, ed. *Oski's Pediatrics: Principles and Practice.* 4th ed. Philadelphia, PA: Lippincott Williams & Wilkins; 2006:2502-2536.

- **Rhizomelic**
- Lower extremity angular deformity, genu varum, ankle varus—arthrogram to visualize epiphysis, for osteotomy planning
- Thoracolumbar kyphosis, which becomes thoracolumbar lordosis at weight bearing. Failure of reversal can cause spinal stenosis
- Lumbar narrowing of interpedicular distance, short pedicles, and lumbar stenosis

Hypochondroplasia

- FGFR3
- AD
- Phenotypically **similar to achondroplasia, but features more mild**, mild short stature, spinal stenosis uncommon, mesomelic, and small portion of mental retardation

Diastrophic Dysplasia

- Diastrophic dysplasia sulfate transporter
- Autosomal recessive
- Rhizomelic
- *Cherub face, cauliflower ear, hitchhiker thumb* (Figure 3.31)
- Cervical kyphosis with bifid lamina, radiographs at 2 years, and monitoring, bracing, and fusion
- Scoliosis, bracing, and PSF
- Hip and knee flexion contracture may require arthroplasty.
- Equinovarus and others deformities, reconstruction

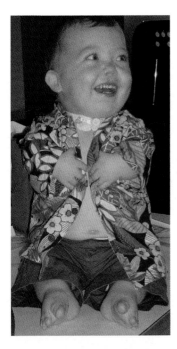

Figure 3.31 Diastrophic dysplasia. From Baum VC, O'Flaherty JE. *Anesthesia for Genetic, Metabolic, and Dysmorphic Syndromes of Childhood.* 3rd ed. Philadelphia, PA: Wolters Kluwer; 2015:117.

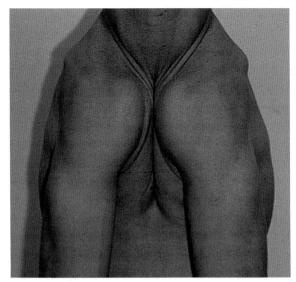

Figure 3.32 Cleidocranial dysplasia: absent clavicles. From Langlais RP, Miller CS, Gehrig JS. Alterations in tooth numbers: hyperdontia. In: *Color Atlas of Common Oral Diseases.* 5th ed. Philadelphia, PA: Wolters Kluwer; 2017:47.

Cleidocranial Dysplasia (Figure 3.32)

- **Runx2/CFBA1 defect**, AD
- Affects membranous bone, cranium, clavicle, and pelvis
- Short stature, front bossing, undeveloped maxilla, cleft palate, and dental abnormalities
- *Clavicle partial or complete absence*
- Narrow pelvis, if mother affected, C-section
- Valgus osteotomy for coxa vara
- Scoliosis, associated with syringomyelia, requiring MRI

Spondyloepiphyseal Dysplasia (Figure 3.33)

- Congenital type, more severe, early manifestations, AD
- Tarda type, manifestations may be minor, present later, X-linked
- Type 2 collagen defect
- Spinal and epiphyseal involvement, delayed ossification
- **Cervical instability**, monitor with flex/ex radiographs
- Scoliosis, sharp apex over few vertebrae, bracing, and PSF
- Hip coxa vara—femoral osteotomies
- Hip subluxation—femoral and iliac osteotomy

Pseudoachondroplasia

- Cartilage oligomeric matrix protein (COMP), AD
- Storage-type disorder, so presents later
- Atypical facies, rhezomelic
- **Cervical instability**, monitor every 2 to 3 years, stabilization, and fusion
- Windswept deformity, early arthritis, osteotomies, or arthroplasty

Multiple Epiphyseal Dysplasia (Figure 3.34)

- COMP, AD
- Cartilage structural deficiency, epiphyseal changes, no spine involvement

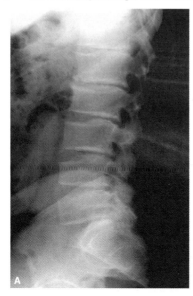
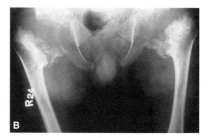

Figure 3.33 Spondyloepiphyseal dysplasia tarda. A, Lateral spine radiograph in an 11-year-old boy showing the vertebral bodies are flattened and wedged anteriorly. The disk spaces are widened anteriorly. B, Pelvic radiograph in another 11-year-old boy showing small inferiorly displaced femoral epiphyses with multiple ossification centers. From Siegel MJ, Coley BD. Musculoskeletal system. In: *The Core Curriculum: Pediatric Imaging.* Philadelphia, PA: Lippincott Williams & Wilkins; 2006:405-554.

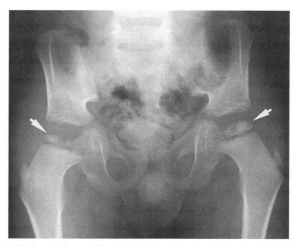

Figure 3.34 Multiple epiphyseal dysplasia, Fairbanks type. Frontal radiograph of the pelvis in a 4-year-old boy shows delayed and irregular proximal femoral epiphyseal ossification (arrows) and epiphyseal flattening. From Siegel MJ, Coley BD. Musculoskeletal system. In: *The Core Curriculum: Pediatric Imaging.* Philadelphia, PA: Lippincott Williams & Wilkins; 2006:405-554.

- Minimal short stature, arthritis
- Early arthritis, in hips in particular—can get superimposed AVN of hips.
- *Differential Perthes, but bilateral and simultaneous*

OTHER MUSCULOSKELETAL DISORDERS

Mucopolysaccharidosis

- Group of genetic disorders, enzyme deficiency, organ deposits, and urine excretion of mucopolysaccharide
- Includes Hurler, Hunter, Sanfilippo, Morquio
- Symptoms appear as patient ages
- Autosomal recessive, except for Hunter that is X-linked
- Thickened facial features, short stature, and joint stiffness
- AVN, spinal cord compression
- **Odontoid hypoplasia with cervical instability requiring monitoring and fusion with cord compression**
- Coxa valgum
- Lower limb malalignment, guided growth, and osteotomies
- *Carpal tunnel* and trigger fingers, requiring releases

Neurofibromatosis (Figure 3.35)

- NF1
- *Neurofibromin gene, AD, 100% penetrance*
- **Café-au-lait spots (coast of California)**, neurofibromas, axillary/inguinal freckling, optic glioma, hamartoma iris, bony lesions that may appear benign or malignant

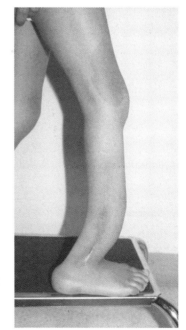

Figure 3.35 Neurofibromatosis. Large café-au-lait spot on the thigh and the anterior bowed tibia typical of pseudarthrosis. From Goldberg MJ. *The Dysmorphic Child: An Orthopedic Perspective.* New York, NY: Raven Press; 1987.

- **Scoliosis, dystrophic** or short, sharp, single thoracic, curves
- Progressive—requires early fusion
- **Pseudarthrosis, tibia with anterolateral bow**, treat with IM rod

Marfan Syndrome

- AD, fibrillin
- Tall, arachnodactyly, long narrow limbs, pectus, scoliosis, cardiovascular (aortic regurgitation, dilatation, aneurysms, mitral valve prolapse), ocular issues
- If suspected, **cardiovascular referral**
- Scoliosis, dural ectasia, early bracing, and later PSF
- Joint laxity

Ehlers-Danlos Syndrome

- Different gene mutations, involving collagen gene or protein processing collagen
- Different manifestations: joint laxity, vascular fragility, kyphoscoliotic
- Joint laxity, subluxation, and dislocation
- Fragile/bruising skin
- Scoliosis, treat like idiopathic

Arthridities—Rheumatoid Arthritis

- Autoimmune disease
- Destructive erosive arthritis
- Joint space narrowing, periarticular erosions osteopenia
- Disease-modifying antirheumatic drugs (DMARDs) mainstay
- Joint arthroplasty

Arthridities—Juvenile Idiopathic Arthritis

- Juvenile idiopathic arthritis is a persistent arthritis lasting more than 6 weeks.
- Soft-tissue swelling, joint space widening, generalized osteoporosis, joint space narrow, and erosion
- **Atlantoaxial instability**—obtain cervical flexion and extension as standard preoperative evaluation
- ANA positive, then referral to **ophthalmologist** for uveitis evaluation
- Nonsteroidal anti-inflammatory drugs, corticosteroids, methotrexate, and other DMARD
- LLD, osteoporosis, and growth retardation
- Subtypes: oligo, poly, systemic

Oligoarthritis

- Most common
- Four or fewer joint involved in the first 6 months.
- Most common single joint, knee
- Morning stiffness, gelling, and pain
- Temporomandibular joint (TMJ), chronic uveitis
- Greatest likelihood of remission with treatment

Polyarthritis

- Five or more joints involved in the first 6 months.
- Large and small joint, and cervical spine and TMJ

- Mild systemic features: low-grade fever, lymphadenopathy, hepatosplenomegaly
- Rheumatoid factor positive, has more destructive joint involvement

Systemic Arthritis

- Least common
- More than one joint, fever more than 2 weeks, and one of the following: rash, lymphadenopathy, hepatosplenomegaly, and serositis
- Can have amyloidosis

Rickets (Figure 3.36)

- Delay in calcification of bone at **zone of provisional calcification** of **physes** of long bones, resulting delayed longitudinal growth and angular deformities
- Rachitic rosary, delayed primary dentition, and kyphoscoliosis
- Short long bones, coxa vara, genu varum or valgum
- *Widened indistinct growth plates*, looser lines
- Multiple etiologies
- Most common X-linked hypophosphatemic rickets, X-linked dominant
- Nutritional rickets due to vitamin D deficiency with prolonged breastfeeding
- **Treatment nutritional first**, may still require osteotomies

Osteogenesis Imperfecta

- Spectrum of abnormal bone fragility diseases
- Collagen 1A
- Type I
  - Mild
  - Nondeforming, normal to short stature, blue sclera, deafness, third decade, fractures of long bones, avulsion fractures of the olecranon, patellar fractures

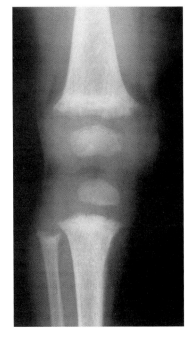

Figure 3.36 Rickets. Anteroposterior radiograph of the knee in a 4-year-old boy shows widening of the growth plates of the distal femur and proximal tibia secondary to lack of mineralization in the provisional zone of calcification. Note also cupping and flaring of the metaphyses. From Greenspan A, Beltran J. Osteoporosis, rickets, and osteomalacia. In: *Orthopedic Imaging: A Practical Approach*. 6th ed. Philadelphia, PA: Wolters Kluwer Health; 2015:986-999.

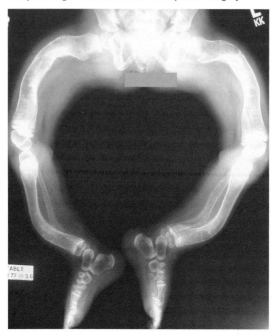

Figure 3.37 Radiograph of a 16-month-old infant with moderately severe osteogenesis imperfecta (OI), with the typical anterolateral bow most severe in the subtrochanteric region. From Esposito PW, Fassier F. Multiple percutaneous osteotomies and Fassier-Duval telescoping nailing of long bones in osteogenesis imperfecta. In: Flynn JM, Sankar WN, eds. *Operative Techniques in Pediatric Orthopaedic Surgery*. 2nd ed. Philadelphia, PA: Wolters Kluwer; 2016:567-579.

- Type II
  - Lethal
- Type III (Figure 3.37)
  - Severe, triangular face, short, limb deformities, coxa vara, scoliosis and kyphosis, rib cage deformity, wheelchair or mobility aid bound, elongated pedicles, codfish vertebrae
- Type IV
  - Moderate
  - Short stature, bowing, and vertebrae fractures, ambulatory
- Treatment
  - **Bisphosphonates, elongating rods** for long bones, PSF with high complication rate for scoliosis

Down Syndrome

- Trisomy 21
- Congenital heart disease, **leukemia**, endocrine abnormalities
- **Increased ADI**, cervical instability, scoliosis, progressive, hip dysplasia
- SCFE, thyroid function testing
- Genu valgum, with patella instability, or asymptomatic patellar dislocation
- Feet, flexible pes planovalgus, orthotics if symptomatic, fusion late if needed

Gaucher Disease

- Type 1 has skeletal manifestations.
- Most common lysosomal storage disorder

- Autosomal recessive
- Splenic involvement: anemia, thrombocytopenia, pancytopenia. Hepatic: clotting disorders
- Bone crisis pain, mimics osteomyelitis, treatment supportive
- Osteomyelitis, osteopenia, pathologic fractures with nonunion risk, osteonecrosis
- Enzyme replacement mainstay of treatment

Caffey Disease
- COL1A1 mutation
- Occurs in infants, resolves by age 2
- Mistaken for child abuse, infection, and neoplasm
- Fever, irritability, periosteal elevation, and bone formation
- Increased erythrocyte sedimentation rate, WBC, alkaline phosphatase, and iron deficiency anemia

Arthrogryposis (Figure 3.38)
- Congenital joint contractures, muscle weakness
- Upper extremity involvement frequent, classic elbow in extension, shoulder IR, forearm pronated, wrist palmar flexion and ulnar deviations, finger flexion deformity with syndactylies
- PT, splinting initially, releases and tendon transfers

Larsen Syndrome
- Facial dysmorphism and hyperelasticity of joints
- **Congenital dislocation** of knees, hips, and elbows

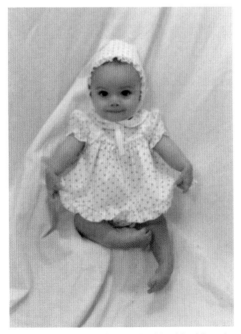

Figure 3.38 The fixed knee deformity is obvious in this girl with arthrogryposis. From Baum VC, O'Flahery JE. *Anesthesia: for Genetic, Metabolic, and Dysmorphic Syndromes of Childhood.* 3rd ed. Philadelphia, PA: Wolters Kluwer; 2015:43.

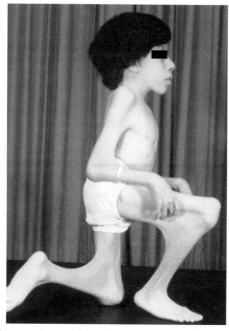

Figure 3.39 Multiple pterygium syndrome in a 12-year-old patient. Antecubital webs fix the elbows, and popliteal webs prevent ambulation. The patient had normal intelligence and became a college graduate. From Goldberg MJ. *The Dysmorphic Child: An Orthopedic Perspective*. New York, NY: Raven Press; 1987.

- Foot deformities
- **Cervical kyphosis** leading to chronic myelopathy and developmental delay—**obtain x-rays**
- Early posterior stabilization

Escobar Syndrome (Multiple Pterygium Syndrome) (Figure 3.39)

- A multiple skin web syndrome
- Webs across flexion creases; most prominent axilla, popliteal, elbow
- Vertical talus, surgically treated
- Knee, physical therapy, surgical releases

PEDIATRIC SPORTS MEDICINE
Female Athlete Triad

- Low-energy availability ($\pm$disordered eating)
- Menstrual dysfunction
- Low bone mineral density
- Not all three required for diagnosis

Little League Shoulder

- Overhead athletes
- **Involves proximal humerus physis**
- Overuse, repetitive microtrauma

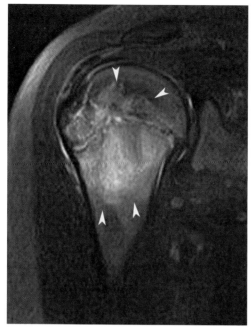

Figure 3.40 A T2 magnetic resonance imaging (MRI) showing periphyseal edema (arrows) associated with Little League shoulder. From Greenspan A, Beltran J. Radiologic evaluation of trauma. In: *Orthopedic Imaging: A Practical Approach*. 6th ed. Philadelphia, PA: Wolters Kluwer Health; 2015:55-106.

- History of pain, altered mechanics, decrease velocity and control
- Tenderness over anterolateral proximal humerus, weakness
- Radiographs early show widening of growth plate, late show fragmentation, sclerosis and cyst formation
  - MRI can be obtained if the diagnosis is in question (Figure 3.40).
- Treatment is cessation of throwing for 2 to 3 months, proper mechanics, pitch count compliance, and gradual return.

Little League Elbow

- Throwing athletes
- **Involves medial epicondyle of the distal humerus**
- Overuse injury
- Kids less commonly have ulnar collateral ligament injury.
- History of pain, altered mechanics, decrease velocity and control
- Tenderness to palpation, pain with valgus stress and milkmaids test
- Radiographs early show widening of growth plate. Late findings are fracture, or avulsion.
- Early treatment is cessation of throwing 2 months, proper mechanics, pitch count compliance, and gradual return.
- Fracture treatment is immobilization for fracture healing and considers reduction and fixation of displaced fractures for restoring valgus stability.

Gymnast Wrist or Distal Radius Epiphysitis

- Upper extremity weight-bearing athletes, such as gymnasts
- Distal radius physis

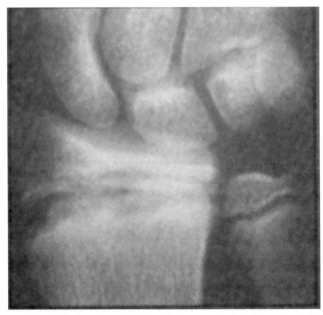

Figure 3.41 Radiograph showing widening of the growth plate. From Willis RB, Kocher MD, Ganley TJ. Sports medicine in the growing child. In: Weinstein SL, Flynn JM, eds. *Lovell and Winter's Pediatric Orthopaedics.* Vol 1. 7th ed. Philadelphia, PA: Lippincott Williams & Wilkins; 2014:1596-1660.

- Repetitive microtrauma
- History of pain with upper extremity weight bearing
- Tenderness to palpation
- Radiographs early show widening of growth plate, late show fragmentation, sclerosis, and cyst formation (Figure 3.41).
- Treatment is rest and immobilization.
- Monitor for future growth disturbance

Panner Disease and Osteochondritis Dissecans of the Elbow

- Throwers and gymnasts
- Disease of the capitellum, controversial if same process
- Both
  - Pain over lateral capitellum
  - Loss of motion, commonly extension
- Panner
  - <10 years old
  - Pain that resolves with rest
  - Radiographic stages: fissuring, irregularity, fragmentation, reossification, and eventual resolution
  - Treatment includes temporary immobilization, rest from offending activity.
  - Resolves
- Osteochondritis dissecans of the elbow
  - >10 years old
  - Pain and can have locking and catching suggestive of loose fragments

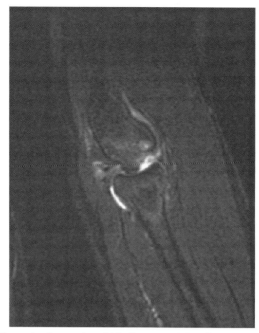

Figure 3.42 Radiograph of osteochondritis dissecans of the elbow showing cartilage and subchondral bone loss, loose body. From Safran M, Kalisvaart M. Arthroscopic treatment of chondral injuries and osteochondritis dissecans. In: Miller MD, ed. *Operative Techniques in Sports Medicine Surgery*. 2nd ed. Philadelphia, PA: Wolters Kluwer; 2016:218-228.

- Radiographs: subchondral lucency early, sclerotic border late, synovial fluid, loose fragment (Figure 3.42)
- Treatment depends on status of lesion. **Intact cartilage can be treated with rest and gradual return to activities.** Unstable cartilage is treated with either drilling, fixation, removal, and microfracture, or cartilage restoration procedure.

Osteochondritis Dissecans of the Knee

- Disease of the bone affecting articular cartilage
- Most commonly *lateral aspect of medial femoral condyle*
- Microtrauma, vascular supply, and genetics
- Pain, possible swelling and locking/catching
- **Better prognosis for healing with open physes**
- Radiographs, include tunnel view
- MRI for further characterization, fluid tracking behind lesion = unstable (Figure 3.43)
- Nonsurgical treatment
  - Open physes, stable lesion
  - **Rest, activity modification, and gradual return to activity when pain free** after 6 to 12 weeks
- Surgical intervention
  - Unresponsive to period of nonsurgical treatment, unstable lesions, or loose bodies
  - Drilling for stable lesions
  - Fixation for unstable lesions that fit into donor site. Be aggressive in fixing.

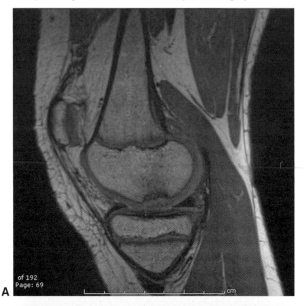

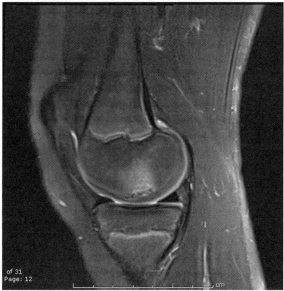

Figure 3.43 Magnetic resonance imaging (MRI) of osteochondritis dissecans (OCD) of the knee. T1 (A) and T2 (B) of a stable OCD lesion, with bone marrow edema, but without chondral breech or fissure, leading to fluid tracking. From Trchan SK, Heyworth BE. Transarticular drilling of osteochondritis dissecans. In: Cordasco FA, Green DW, eds. *Pediatric and Adolescent Knee Surgery*. Philadelphia, PA: Wolters Kluwer; 2015:190-194.

- Removal and microfracture for small loose bodies
- Cartilage restoration for large loose bodies
- Rehab with rest, activity modification, and gradual return to activities based primarily on pain, rather than radiographic appearance

Knee Ligament Injuries

- General
  - MCL injuries most common
  - Tears of any ligament can be treated initially with bracing, rehab, and activity modification.
  - A gradual return to activities is possible with return of motion, strength, and relative stability.
- ACL tear
  - Contact or noncontact injury
  - Pain, swelling, positive Lachman test. Evaluate for concomitant injuries
  - Radiographs to rule out other bony injuries
  - MRI, middle lateral femoral condyle and posterior lateral tibial plateau bone bruise, concomitant intra-articular injuries
  - Potential physeal injury main concern with determining treatment
    - Brace and activity modification may work for select compliant patients.
      - Avoids growth disturbance risk
    - *Physea—protecting reconstruction for active, unstable patients*
      - Estimate growth remaining, Tanner stage, radiographic bone age
      - Delay in reconstruction risks future intra-articular injury.
      - Multiple reconstruction options
        - *Avoid bone plugs or implants across physis*
        - **Tunnel across physis should be central and small.**
  - Rehab for gradual return to sports
    - Neuromuscular training program lowers risk of ACL injury.
    - ACL braces do not lower risk of ACL injury.

Patellofemoral Instability

- Most commonly lateral dislocation
- Risk factors including femoral anteversion, external tibial torsion, genu valgum trochlear and patellar dysplasia, patella alta, high Q-angle, pes planus, and ligamentous laxity
- Contact or noncontact injury
- Pain over medial patellofemeral ligament (MPFL) or medial retinaculum, lateral femoral condyle, swelling, apprehension
- Radiographs can miss osteochondral injuries.
- **MRI with hemarthrosis, for missed osteochondral injury, loose bodies,** medial patellar and lateral femoral condyle bruise
- Treatment
  - **Brace and rehab with first-time dislocators, without osteochondral fracture or loose body**
  - Surgical treatment for loose body or osteochondral fracture, recurrent dislocations
    - Address alignment and rotational issues
    - Soft tissue only, physeal avoiding options for skeletally immature patients
    - MPFL and medial retinacular repair or imbrication, MPFL reconstruction
      - *Schottle point* adjacent to physis
    - Guided growth for alignment or osteotomy for rotation
    - Tibial tubercle osteotomy if tibial tuberosity-trochlear groove distance > 20 with closed physes to avoid recurvatum
  - Rehab and gradual return to sports, with or without a patellar stabilization brace

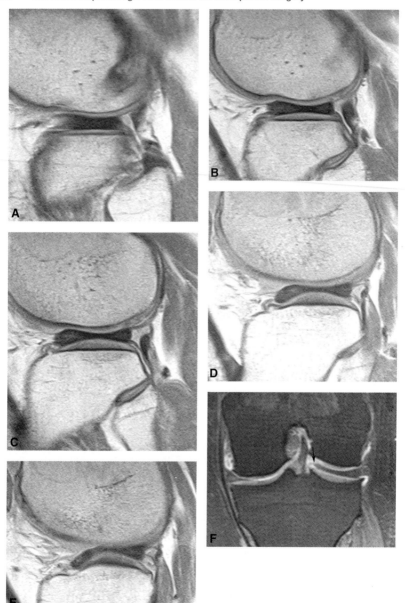

Figure 3.44 Meniscus is visualized on sequential sagittal cuts (A-E) and extends across the joint on a midsagittal coronal cut (F). From Berquist TH. Knee. In: Berquist TH, ed. *MRI of the Musculoskeletal System*. Fig 7-66; 6th ed. Philadelphia, PA: Lippincott Williams & Wilkins; 2013:319-459.

Meniscus Injuries

- <10 year old, commonly discoid meniscus tear
- >10 years old, tear in normal meniscus
- Twisting common, but can be minimal trauma
- Vascularity decreases and becomes adult pattern around age 10
- Pain, catching, clunk/pop, +McMurray
- MRI, **vascularity of meniscus in a young patient can be mistaken for tear, correlate with examination**
- Tears in normal meniscus have higher likelihood of healing when patients <10 years old, otherwise treated as in adults.
- **Discoid meniscus**
  - Most commonly lateral
  - Classified as complete, incomplete, or Wrisberg variant that is unstable due to lack of meniscocapsular attachments
  - Presents with loss of motion and a contracture if long-standing
  - Radiographs may demonstrate squaring of the femoral condyle and symmetric joint widening.
  - MRI demonstrates **bow-tie sign** (Figure 3.44).
  - Treatment
    - **Nonsurgical if asymptomatic**
    - Saucerization, repair, and stabilization if painful, mechanical block
    - Rehab and activity restriction with repair
    - Gradual return to activity with saucerization

4 Hand and Wrist

Clifton G. Meals, Tina Raman, Kenneth R. Means Jr,
Ryan M. Zimmerman, Gregory K. Faucher,
Heather V. Lochner, Lara Atwater, E. Gene Deune,
Thomas J. Kim, and Dawn M. LaPorte

ANATOMY

Bones

- Wrist—eight bones arranged in two rows (Figure 4.1)
  - Proximal row
    - Scaphoid—critical link between proximal and distal rows
      - Tenuous **(retrograde) blood supply** (Figure 4.2)
      - Fractures may not heal or may lead to necrosis.
      - Fracture may cause arthritis.
    - Lunate
    - Triquetrum
  - Distal row
    - Trapezium
    - Trapezoid
    - Hamate
  - Extracapsular
    - Pisiform

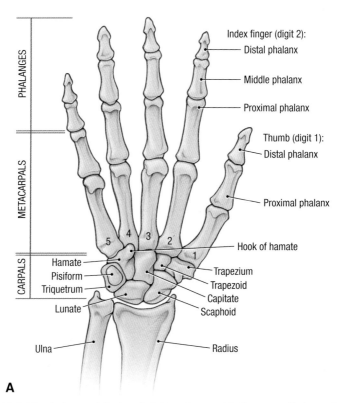

A

Figure 4.1 A, The skeleton of the hand. A: From Detton AK. The upper limb. In: *Grant's Dissector*. 16th ed. Baltimore, MD: Wolters Kluwer; 2017:23-72.

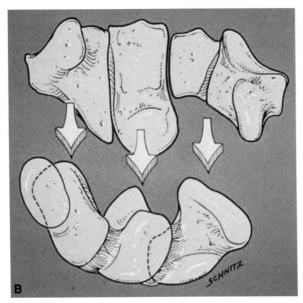

Figure 4.1 (*continued*) B, The proximal and distal carpal rows may be thought of as distinct segments. B: From Rayan G, Akelman E. Osseous anatomy of the hand and wrist biomechanics. In: *The Hand: Anatomy, Examination, and Diagnosis.* 4th ed. Philadelphia, PA: Lippincott Williams & Wilkins; 2011:88-98.

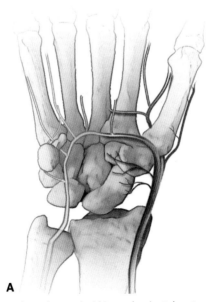

Figure 4.2 The blood supply to the scaphoid is predominately retrograde. Palmar view of blood supply to the scaphoid; superficial palmar branch of the radial artery (A).

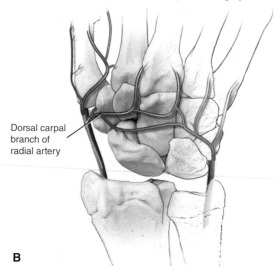

Dorsal carpal branch of radial artery

B

Figure 4.2 (*continued*) Dorsal view of blood supply to the scaphoid; dorsal carpal branch of the radial artery (B). From Diaz-Garcia RJ, Imbriglia FE. Partial scaphoid excision of scaphoid nonunions. In: Hunt TR III. *Operative Techniques in Hand, Wrist, and Elbow Surgery*. 2nd ed. Philadelphia, PA: Wolters Kluwer; 2016:368-379.

- Hand
  - Metacarpals (MCs)
    - Form a transverse and a longitudinal arch
    - Ring and small MCs more mobile
  - Phalanges

Ligaments

- Wrist
  - Extrinsic (connect forearm bones or MCs to wrist bones)
    - Triangular fibrocartilage complex (TFCC)—connects radius, ulna, and ulnar wrist bones (Figure 4.3)
    - Volar ligaments (stronger)—radioscaphocapitate (RSC) ligament prevents ulnar translation of the carpus (Figure 4.4)
    - Dorsal ligaments (weaker)
  - Intrinsic (connect wrist bones to wrist bones)
    - Scapholunate (SL) ligament
      - **Thickest dorsally** (Figure 4.5)
      - Critical link between lunate and scaphoid
      - Rupture may cause deformity, and deformity may result in arthritis.
- Thumb and fingers—metacarpophalangeal (MCP) collateral ligaments
  - Lax in extension
  - Tight in flexion (Figure 4.6)—splinting in flexion prevents ligaments from scarring in contracted position.

Muscle–Tendon Units

- Extrinsic (cross the radiocarpal joint)
  - Dorsal (arranged in six dorsal compartments) (Figure 4.7)
    - First extensor compartment
      - Abductor pollicis longus (APL)
      - Extensor pollicis brevis

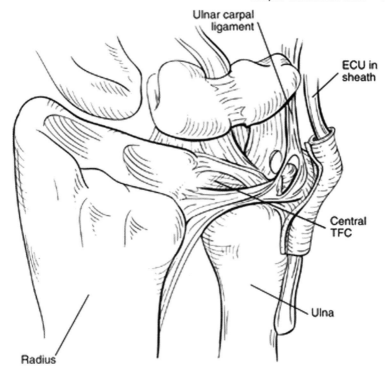

Figure 4.3 The triangular fibrocartilaginous complex. ECU, extensor carpi ulnaris; TFC, triangular fibrocartilage. From Calfee RP, Berger R, Beredjiklian K, et al. Fractures and dislocations: wrist. In: Hammert WC, Calfee RP, Bozenta DJ, Boyer MI, eds. *ASSH Manual of Hand Surgery*. Philadelphia, PA: Lippincott Williams & Wilkins; 2010:216-254.

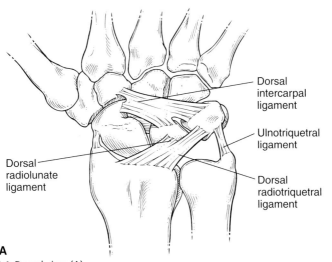

A

Figure 4.4 Dorsal view (A)

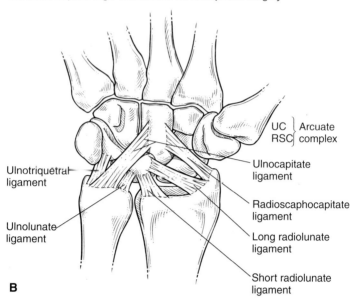

Figure 4.4 (*continued*) palmar view (B) of the extrinsic wrist ligaments, which connect forearm bones or metacarpals to wrist bones. UC, ulnocapitate; RSC, radioscaphocapitate. From Cooney WP III. Fractures of the distal radius: overview of diagnosis, classification, and treatment considerations. In: *The Wrist: Diagnosis and Operative Treatment*. 2nd ed. Philadelphia, PA: Lippincott Williams & Wilkins; 2010:271-310.

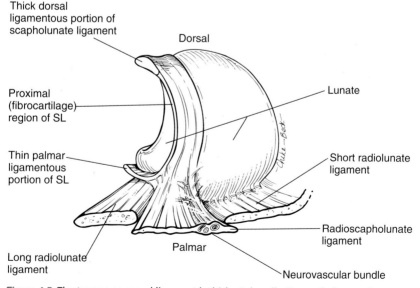

Figure 4.5 The transverse carpal ligament is thickest dorsally. SL, scapholunate. From Berger RA. Wrist anatomy. In: Cooney WP III, ed. *The Wrist: Diagnosis and Operative Treatment*. 2nd ed. Philadelphia, PA: Lippincott Williams & Wilkins; 2010:25-76.

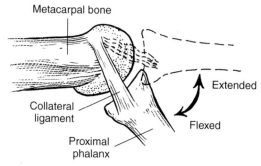

Figure 4.6 The collateral ligaments are stretched in flexion. From Clemente CD. Joints of the upper extremity. In: *Clemente's Anatomy Dissector*. 3rd ed. Baltimore, MD: Lippincott Williams & Wilkins; 2011:65-75.

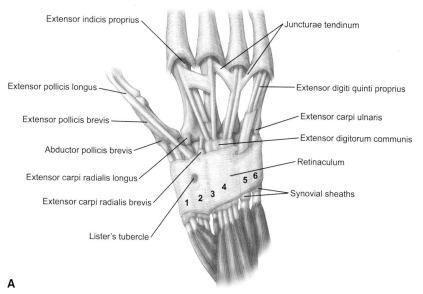

A

Figure 4.7 The extensor tendons are contained in six extensor compartments on the dorsum of the wrist. From Berquist TH. Hand and wrist. In: *MRI of the Musculoskeletal System*. 6th ed. Philadelphia, PA: Wolters Kluwer; 2013:777-869.

- Second extensor compartment
  - Extensor carpi radialis brevis—innervated by posterior interosseous nerve (PIN)
  - Extensor carpi radialis longus (ECRL)—innervated by radial nerve proper (spared in PIN palsy; ie, patient may still extend wrist)
- Third extensor compartment
  - Extensor pollicis longus
- Fourth extensor compartment
  - Extensor indicis proprius—allows independent extension of index finger (IF)
  - Extensor digitorum communis—four interconnected slips
  - Distal branch of PIN lies in base of compartment

- Fifth extensor compartment
    - Extensor digiti minimi (EDM)—allows independent extension of small finger
- Sixth extensor compartment
    - Extensor carpi ulnaris (ECU)
- Volar
    - Flexor carpi radialis (FCR)
    - Flexor carpi ulnaris (FCU)
    - Carpal tunnel contents (10 elements) (Figure 4.8)
        - Median nerve
        - Flexor pollicis longus (FPL)
        - Flexor digitorum superficialis (FDS) and flexor digitorum profundus (FDP) (four slips each)
            - Travel through flexor tendon sheaths in the palm and fingers—sheaths are potential sites of infection.
- Intrinsic (origin and insertion in the hand and wrist)
    - Thumb (Figure 4.9)
        - Abductor pollicis brevis, flexor pollicis brevis, opponens pollicis—innervation is mostly median nerve.
        - Adductor pollicis—innervated by ulnar nerve
    - Fingers
        - Lumbricals
            - Originate from FDP tendons
            - Flex MCP joints, extend interphalangeal (IP) joints
        - Interossei
            - Volar and dorsal
            - Abduct/adduct fingers, flex MCP joints, extend IP joints

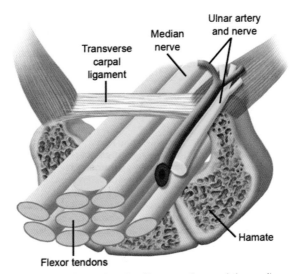

Figure 4.8 The carpal tunnel contains nine flexor tendons and the median nerve. From Diao E. Carpal tunnel release: endoscopic, open, and revision. In: Hunt TR III, ed. *Operative Techniques in Hand, Wrist, and Forearm Surgery.* Philadelphia, PA: Lippincott Williams & Wilkins; 2011:565-573.

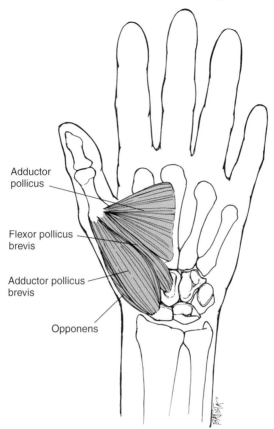

Figure 4.9 Muscles at the base of the thumb. From Oatis CA. Mechanics and pathomechanics of the intrinsic muscles of the hand. In: *Kinesiology: The Mechanics and Pathomechanics of Human Movement*. 2nd ed. Baltimore, MD: Lippincott Williams & Wilkins; 2009:351-369.

Arteries

- Radial artery
  - Passes through "anatomic snuff box"
  - Contributes to deep palmar arch (present in everyone)
- Ulnar artery
  - Passes through Guyon canal
  - Contributes to superficial palmar arch (incomplete in some people) (Figure 4.10)
- Digital arteries
  - **Volar to digital nerves in palm/dorsal to digital nerves in fingers**
  - Volar finger laceration with active bleeding implies digital nerve laceration.

Nerves

- Radial nerve
  - Provides sensory innervation to the dorsum of the hand (Figure 4.11)

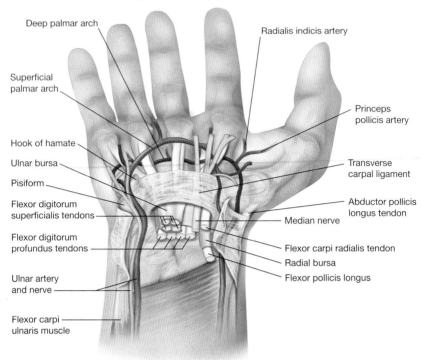

Deep palmar arch

Radialis indicis artery

Superficial palmar arch

Princeps pollicis artery

Hook of hamate

Ulnar bursa

Pisiform

Transverse carpal ligament

Flexor digitorum superficialis tendons

Abductor pollicis longus tendon

Median nerve

Flexor digitorum profundus tendons

Flexor carpi radialis tendon

Radial bursa

Ulnar artery and nerve

Flexor pollicis longus

Flexor carpi ulnaris muscle

Figure 4.10 The ulnar artery is the main contributor to the superficial palmar arch. The radial artery is the main contributor to the deep palmar arch. From Paty PSK, Chang BB. Distal upper extremity revascularization (brachial to radial/ulnar/hand bypass). In: Darling RC III, Ozaki CK, eds. *Master Techniques in Surgery: Vascular Surgery: Arterial Procedures.* Philadelphia, PA: Wolters Kluwer Health; 2016:63-71.

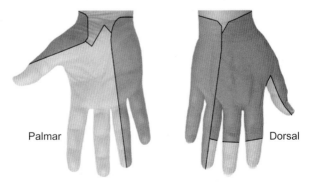

Palmar

Dorsal

Figure 4.11 The median nerve (yellow), ulnar nerve (gray), and radial nerve (pink) provide sensation to different parts of the hand. From Hiro M, Bindra RR. Primary repair and nerve grafting following complete nerve transection in the hand, wrist, and forearm. In: Hunt TR III. *Operative Techniques in Hand, Wrist, and Elbow Surgery.* 2nd ed. Philadelphia, PA: Wolters Kluwer; 2016:824-833.

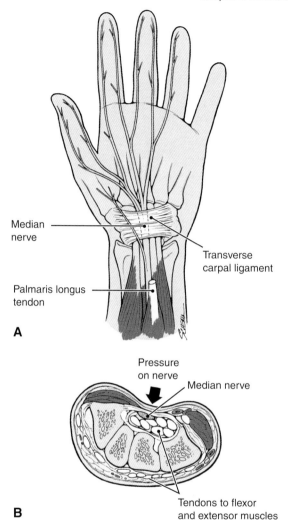

Figure 4.12 The median nerve passes through the carpal tunnel before dividing. A, Anteroposterior view of the hand and carpal tunnel, with median nerve shown in yellow. B, Cross section view of the carpal tunnel, with median nerve shown in yellow. From *Stedman's Medical Dictionary*. 28th ed. Baltimore, MD: Lippincott Williams & Wilkins; 2006.

- Median nerve
  - Passes through and potentially compressed in carpal tunnel (Figure 4.12)
  - Sensory innervation to the palm, thumb, IF, long finger, radial half of ring finger
  - Innervation to adductor, flexor, and opponens (AFO) thenar muscles—wasting may be present in advanced carpal tunnel syndrome (CTS).
- Ulnar nerve
  - Passes through Guyon canal (Figure 4.13)
  - Sensory innervation to ulnar half of ring finger, small finger
  - Innervation to all intrinsic muscles (except AFO muscles)

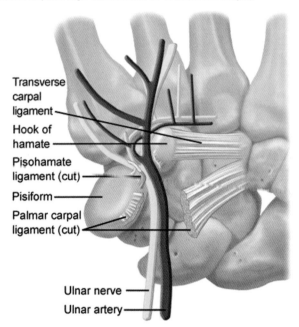

Transverse carpal ligament
Hook of hamate
Pisohamate ligament (cut)
Pisiform
Palmar carpal ligament (cut)
Ulnar nerve
Ulnar artery

Figure 4.13 The ulnar nerve and ulnar artery both pass through (and both branch in) Guyon canal. From Means KR Jr, Graham TJ. Surgical treatment of carpal bone fractures, excluding the scaphoid. In: Hunt TR III. *Operative Techniques in Hand, Wrist, and Elbow Surgery*. 2nd ed. Philadelphia, PA: Wolters Kluwer; 2016:368-379.

FRACTURES AND DISLOCATIONS

Wrist

- Scaphoid fractures
  - Tenuous (retrograde) blood supply—Fractures may not heal or may lead to necrosis.
  - Diagnosis
    - Many nondisplaced fractures are missed on initial radiographs.
      - These fractures may show up on radiographs 2 weeks later after fracture-site bone resorbs.
      - **Magnetic resonance imaging (MRI) may be used to identify fractures earlier.**
  - Natural history
    - Scaphoid is key structural link between proximal and distal carpal rows.
    - Malunion or nonunion disrupts this link and may lead to deformity of wrist bones and arthritis (Figure 4.14).
  - Treatment
    - Acute fractures
      - **Surgery for displaced fractures or any fractures of proximal pole**
        - The proximal pole is dorsal in the wrist, and the distal pole is volar.
          - Fractures may be approached surgically from either the dorsal or volar wrist, depending on their location.
        - Other fractures may be treated in a cast.
    - Malunions and nonunions
      - Correction of deformity with surgery

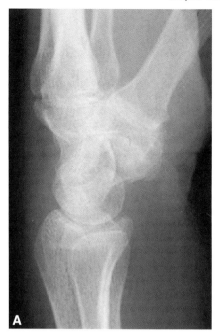

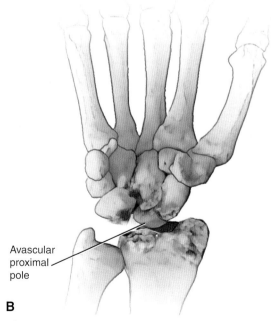

Avascular
proximal
pole

B

Figure 4.14 Scaphoid nonunion advanced collapse (SNAC) wrist describes a predictable pattern of degeneration. Lateral radiograph (A) and illustration (B) showing SNAC wrist. From Diaz-Garcia RJ, Imbriglia FE. Partial scaphoid excision of scaphoid nonunions. In: Hunt TR III. *Operative Techniques in Hand, Wrist, and Elbow Surgery*. 2nd ed. Philadelphia, PA: Wolters Kluwer; 2016:368-379.

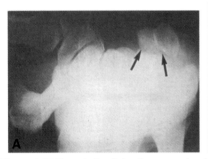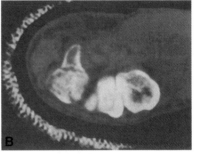

Figure 4.15 Hamate hook fractures may be shown with a carpal tunnel radiograph (A) or computed tomography scan (B). From Topper SM, Wood MB. Athletic injuries of the wrist. In: Cooney WP III, ed. *The Wrist: Diagnosis and Operative Treatment*. 2nd ed. Philadelphia, PA: Lippincott Williams & Wilkins; 2010:1153-1186.

- Difficult malunions and nonunions may be treated with bone graft.
  - **Vascularized bone graft** (bone with arterial inflow) may be used for certain cases (eg, previously operated wrists, in which the scaphoid is less likely to heal).
  - Options—1, 2 intercompartmental supraretinacular artery or medial femoral condyle free graft
- Hook of hamate fractures
  - May be seen on carpal tunnel view or may require computed tomography (CT) (Figure 4.15)
  - May cause ulnar nerve symptoms
  - May cause attritional rupture of flexor to small finger
- Perilunate fracture dislocations
  - Injury pattern
    - Dislocation of bones surrounding the lunate occurs according to a predictable sequence of ligament ruptures (**lesser arc injuries**) (Figure 4.16).
    - Other carpal bones may also be fractured (**greater arc injuries**) (Figure 4.17).
      - Combined perilunate dislocation/scaphoid fracture is typical.

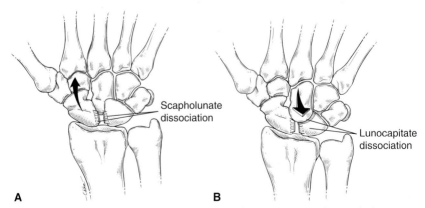

Figure 4.16 Perilunate injuries occur in a predictable sequence according to their severity. Illustrations show scapholunate dissociation (A), lunocapitate dissociation (B), lunotriquetral, midcarpal dissociation.

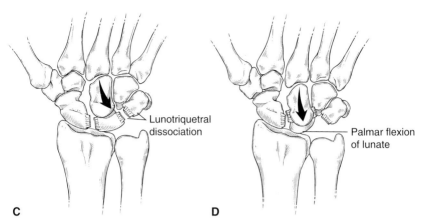

C   **D**

Figure 4.16 (*continued*) Perilunate injuries occur in a predictable sequence according to their severity. Illustrations show scapholunate dissociation (A), lunocapitate dissociation (B), lunotriquetral, midcarpal dissociation (C), and palmar flexion of lunate, lunate dissociation (D). From Kozin SH. Perilunate dislocations. In: Cooney WP III, ed. *The Wrist: Diagnosis and Operative Treatment*. 2nd ed. Philadelphia, PA: Lippincott Williams & Wilkins; 2010:532-549.

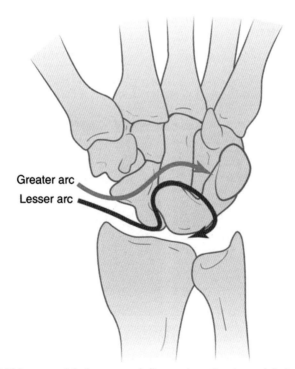

Figure 4.17 Lesser arc injuries are purely ligamentous. Greater arc injuries involve at least one fracture. From Rayan G, Akelman E, eds. *The Hand: Anatomy, Examination, and Diagnosis*. 4th ed. Philadelphia, PA: Lippincott Williams & Wilkins; 2011:205-219.

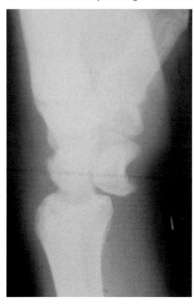

Figure 4.18 The lunate is completely displaced volarly and may compress the median nerve. From D'Addesi LL, Thoder JJ, Matullo KS. Operative treatment of lesser and greater arc injuries. In: Hunt TR III, ed. *Operative Techniques in Hand, Wrist, and Forearm Surgery*. Philadelphia, PA: Lippincott Williams & Wilkins; 2011:421-427.

- Lunate may dislocate completely and compress the median nerve, causing acute median nerve compression (Figure 4.18).
- Diagnosis
  - High-energy injury is typical.
  - Based on radiographs
    - Disruption of normal contour and relationship of proximal and distal row (normal arcs are described by Gilula lines) (Figure 4.19)

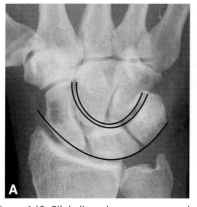
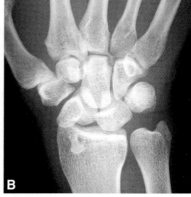

Figure 4.19 Gilula lines drawn on a normal wrist radiograph (A). Disrupted Gilula lines in a wrist with perilunate dislocation (B). From Duckworth AD, Ring D. Carpus fractures and dislocations. In: Court-Brown CM, Heckman JD, McQueen M, et al, eds. *Rockwood and Green's Fractures in Adults*. Vol 1. 8th ed. Philadelphia, PA: Wolters Kluwer Health; 2015:991-1056.

- Natural history
  - Progression to wrist arthritis
- Treatment
  - Surgery (emergency surgery in cases of **acute median nerve compression—** include carpal tunnel release)

Hand

- MC base fractures
  - Thumb
    - **Bennett fracture**
      - Injury pattern
        - Ulnar MC base fragment retains ligamentous attachment to trapezium.
        - MC supinates (pull of adductor pollicis) and moves proximally (pull of APL) (Figure 4.20).
      - Natural history—nonunion or malunion secondary to deforming forces
      - Treatment with surgery
    - Rolando fracture
      - Injury pattern
        - Comminuted, intra-articular MC base fracture
          - MC shaft is completely separated from articular surface (Figure 4.21).
      - Treatment
        - Casting or surgery

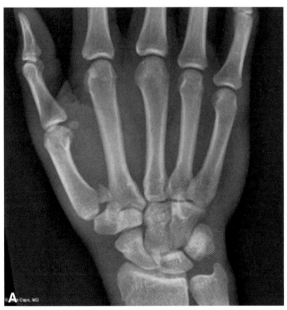

Figure 4.20 A, Bennett fractures are fractures of the ulnar base of the thumb metacarpal. A: From Capo J, Mitgang JT, Harris C. Operative treatment of thumb carpometacarpal joint fractures. In: Hunt TR III. *Operative Techniques in Hand, Wrist, and Elbow Surgery.* 2nd ed. Philadelphia, PA: Wolters Kluwer; 2016:407-417; Tech Fig 43-1A.

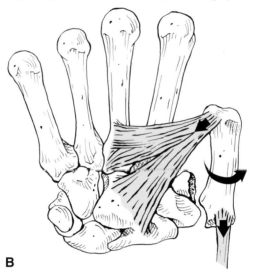

B

Figure 4.20 (*continued*) B, The deforming forces on the thumb metacarpal following Bennett fracture are shown. B: From Henry M. Fractures and dislocations of the hand. In: Bucholz RW, Heckman JD, eds. *Rockwood and Green's Fractures in Adults.* 5th ed. Philadelphia, PA: Lippincott Williams & Wilkins; 2001:655-748.

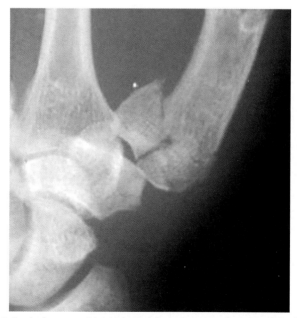

Figure 4.21 Rolando fracture with a Y-shaped three-fragment fracture of the first metacarpal, which extends to the articular surface of the first carpometacarpal (CMC) articulation. From Peterson JJ, Berquist TH. Hand and wrist. In: Peterson JJ, ed. *Berquist's Musculoskeletal Imaging Companion.* 3rd ed. Philadelphia, PA: Wolters Kluwer; 2018:476-529.

- MC shaft fractures
  - Injury pattern
    - Nearly always apex dorsal angulation and/or spiral fracture
    - May cause rotation of MC, which will cause fingers to "scissor" with flexion (Figure 4.22)
  - Natural history
    - Index or small MC—nonunion, malunion
    - Isolated long or ring MC—uneventful healing
  - Treatment
    - Surgery for displaced or unstable index or small MC fractures
    - Surgery for long and ring MC fractures combined with other MC fractures
    - Surgery in cases of rotational deformity

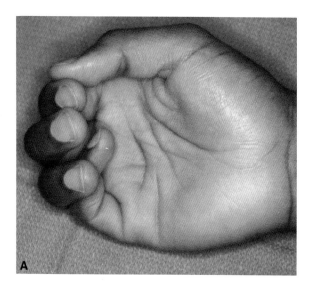

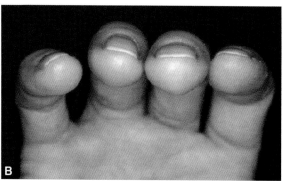

Figure 4.22 Rotational displacement of the small finger metacarpal may cause scissoring. A, Rotation shown with scissoring; small finger crossing palmar to ring and middle fingers. B, Asymmetry seen with rotation of small finger metacarpal. From Uhl RL, Mulligan MT. Operative treatment of extra-articular phalangeal fractures. In: Hunt TR III. *Operative Techniques in Hand, Wrist, and Elbow Surgery.* 2nd ed. Philadelphia, PA: Wolters Kluwer; 2016:471-485.

- MC neck fractures
  - Small finger (boxer fracture)
    - Injury pattern
      - Apex dorsal angulation (Figure 4.23)

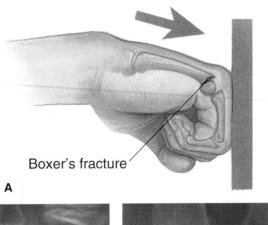

Boxer's fracture

A

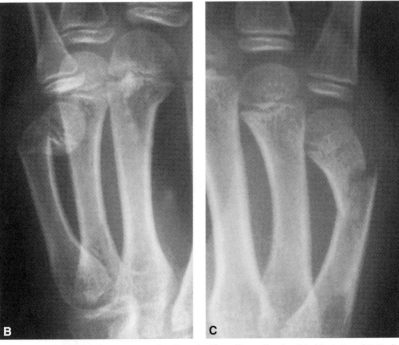

Figure 4.23 A, "Boxer fractures" result when the fist strikes a fixed solid object. B and C, Radiographs showing the apex dorsal angulation in a Boxer fracture. A: Asset provided by Anatomical Chart Company. B and C: From Lightdale-Miric N, Kozin SH. Fractures and dislocations of the hand and carpal bones in children. In: Flynn JM, Skaggs DL, Waters PM, eds. *Rockwood and Wilkins' Fractures in Children*. 8th ed. Philadelphia, PA: Wolters Kluwer Health; 2015:264-347.

- Natural history—asymptomatic malunion in most cases
- Treatment
  - May attempt closed reduction with Jahss maneuver (Figure 4.24)
  - Symptom management only for most fractures
- MCP dislocations/fracture dislocations
  - May attempt reduction with gentle hyperextension and by pushing phalangeal base over MC head
    - Longitudinal traction may entrap volar plate (Figure 4.25).
- Thumb MCP ligament (ulnar collateral ligament) injury
  - Acute—"skier's thumb" (Figure 4.26)
    - Surgery for laxity on examination, or if concern for Stener lesion
      - **Stener lesion:** Ruptured ligament may become trapped behind interposed adductor aponeurosis.
        - Surgery required to return ligament to its anatomic location.
  - Chronic—"gamekeeper's thumb" (Figure 4.27)
    - Surgery for laxity on examination
- Phalanx fractures
  - Natural history
    - Uneventful union for transverse/stable fractures

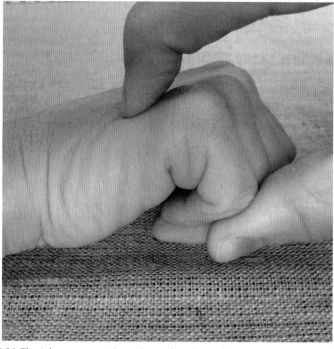

Figure 4.24 The Jahss maneuver is used to reduce boxer fractures. From Noila JM. Operative treatment of metacarpal fractures. In: Wiesel SW, ed. *Operative Techniques in Orthopaedic Surgery*. 2nd ed. Philadelphia, PA: Wolters Kluwer; 2016:2819-2834.

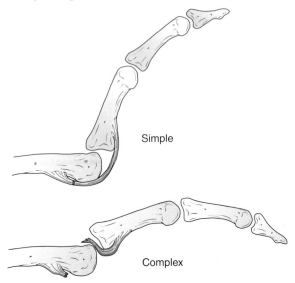

Figure 4.25 Complex metacarpophalangeal joint dislocations involve entrapment of the volar plate and are difficult to reduce. From Bucholz RW, Heckman JD, Court-Brown C, et al., eds. *Rockwood and Green's Fractures in Adults*. 6th ed. Philadelphia, PA: Lippincott Williams & Wilkins; 2006.

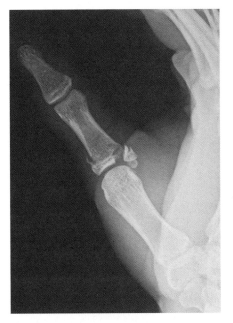

Figure 4.26 A piece of bone may be pulled off the metacarpal base in "skier's thumb." From Lightdale-Miric N, Kozin SH. Fractures and dislocations of the hand and carpal bones in children. In: Flynn JM, Skaggs DL, Waters PM, eds. *Rockwood and Wilkins' Fractures in Children*. 8th ed. Philadelphia, PA: Wolters Kluwer Health; 2015:264-347.

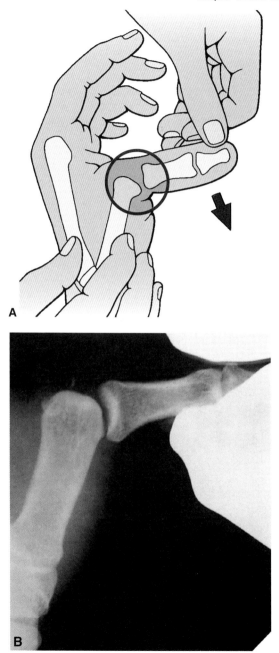

Figure 4.27 Pathologic laxity in "gamekeeper's thumb" may be detected clinically and with radiographs. Illustration of clinical examination (A) and radiograph (B) showing pathologic laxity of thumb ulnar collateral ligament. From Greenspan A, Beltran J. Upper limb III: distal forearm, wrist, and hand. In: *Orthopedic Imaging: A Practical Approach*. 6th ed. Philadelphia, PA: Wolters Kluwer Health; 2015:203-267.

- Treatment
  - Nonoperative for stable fractures
  - Surgery for unstable fractures and/or fractures with rotational deformity
- Proximal interphalangeal (PIP) joint fracture/dislocations
  - Acute
    - Attempt reduction of dislocations (technique similar to MCP dislocations/fracture dislocations)
      - Purely ligamentous injuries and fractures involving less than 20% of middle phalangeal base are likely to be stable once reduced.
        - May be treated nonoperatively
      - Fractures involving 20% to 40% of middle phalangeal base must be tested for stability.
      - Fractures involving more than 40% of middle phalangeal base are likely to be unstable and may be treated surgically (Figure 4.28).
  - Chronic
    - Surgery to recreate joint
      - "Hemi-hamate" graft—moving a piece of the hamate to the deformed middle phalangeal base
- Tuft fractures—nonoperative treatment commonly results in painless, fibrous union.

INFECTION
Infections of the Finger

- **Paronychia**
  - Abscess beneath eponychial fold
  - Risk factors—minor trauma that inoculates nailfold
  - Most common organism, *Staphylococcus aureus*

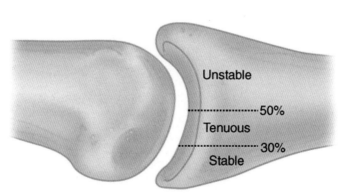

Figure 4.28 Fracture fragment size predicts the stability of proximal interphalangeal joint fracture dislocations. From Kiefhaber TR, Williams RM, Osterman MN. Hemi-hamate autograft reconstruction of unstable dorsal proximal interphalangeal joint fracture-dislocations. In: Hunt TR III. *Operative Techniques in Hand, Wrist, and Elbow Surgery*. 2nd ed. Philadelphia, PA: Wolters Kluwer; 2016:532-540.

- Treatment
  - Acute
    - Incision and drainage (Figure 4.29)—Avoid incision across eponychial fold
    - Warm soaks
    - Partial or complete removal of the nail
  - Chronic
    - Antifungals and topical steroid
    - Nail plate removal, marsupialization
- **Felon**
  - Closed-space infection of the pulp of the distal finger
  - Most common organism, *S. aureus*
  - Treatment
    - No abscess—elevation, warm soaks, antibiotics
    - Abscess present
      - Incision should be lateral to fingernail to prevent injury to volar fat pad, digital artery, and nerve (Figure 4.30).
      - Avoid fishmouth incisions; can compromise digital pulp vascularity
      - Antibiotics
- **Herpetic whitlow**
  - Herpes simplex virus (HSV)-1 or HSV-2
  - Self-limited
  - Physical examination findings
    - Vesicular lesions—initially draining, mature to ulcers
    - Lymphadenitis
  - Diagnosis
    - Clinical/examination
    - **Tzanck smear** of vesicle fluid
  - Treatment—**acyclovir**

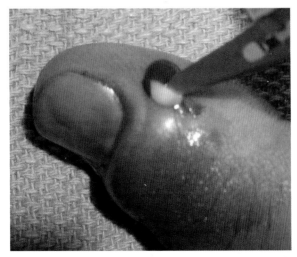

Figure 4.29 Incision to drain a paronychia. From Etcheson J, Yao J. Surgical treatment of acute and chronic paronychia and felons. In: Hunt TR III. *Operative Techniques in Hand, Wrist, and Elbow Surgery.* 2nd ed. Philadelphia, PA: Wolters Kluwer; 2016:1159-1164.

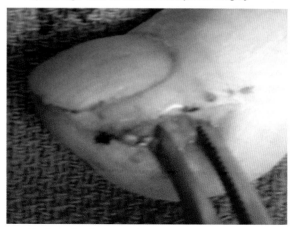

Figure 4.30 Lateral incision for drainage of a felon. From Etcheson J, Yao J. Surgical treatment of acute and chronic paronychia and felons. In: Hunt TR III. *Operative Techniques in Hand, Wrist, and Elbow Surgery*. 2nd ed. Philadelphia, PA: Wolters Kluwer; 2016:1159-1164.

- **Pyogenic flexor tenosynovitis**
  - Bacterial infection of flexor tendon sheath
    - Thumb flexor tendon sheath contiguous with radial bursa
    - Small finger flexor tendon sheath contiguous with ulna bursa
  - Most common organism, *S. aureus*
  - Physical examination findings—**Kanavel four cardinal signs** (Figure 4.31)
    - Tenderness over flexor tendon sheath
    - Semi-flexed position
    - Pain with extension
    - Fusiform swelling
  - Treatment
    - Operative intervention almost always necessary—sparing of the A2 and A4 pulleys

Hand Infections

- Deep spaces
  - Thenar
    - "Pantaloon" abscess; spreads in space between adductor pollicis and first dorsal interosseous
    - Physical examination—patient holds thumb palmarly abducted.
    - Treatment—irrigation and debridement
  - Midpalmar
    - Infection most often from direct penetration
    - Physical examination
      - Loss of normal palmar concavity
      - Painful movement of long and ring fingers
    - Treatment—irrigation and debridement
  - Subfascial web space
    - **Collar button abscess**—spreads peripherally dorsally and volarly
    - Treatment is operative—Incision should not be made through web space, which can cause web contracture.

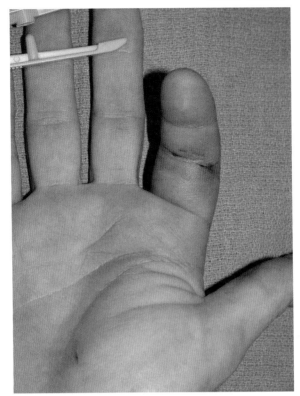

Figure 4.31 Pyogenic flexor tenosynovitis. From Chang B, Kanchwala SH. Treatment of hand infections. In: Thorne CH, ed. *Grabb & Smith's Plastic Surgery*. 7th ed. Philadelphia, PA: Lippincott Williams & Wilkins; 2014:731-736.

- Parona space
  - Physical examination
    - Pain with finger flexion
    - Possible acute CTS
  - Treatment—debridement

Fungal Infections

- Cutaneous
  - Tinea corporis—glabrous skin, nails
  - Tinea manuum—palms
    - Diagnosis—**potassium hydroxide preparations** and fungal cultures
    - Treatment for simple infections—topical antifungal agents
- Subcutaneous
  - **Sporotrichosis** (Figure 4.32)—puncture wounds handling plants, specifically roses
  - Diagnosis—fungal cultures

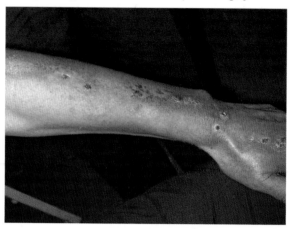

Figure 4.32 Sporotrichosis. From Bravo FG, Mohanna S. Tropical diseases of the skin. In: Hall BJ, Hall JC, eds. *Sauer's Manual of Skin Diseases*. 11th ed. Philadelphia, PA: Wolters Kluwer; 2017:541-559.

Mycobacterial Infections

- Most common organism, *Mycobacterium marinum* (Figure 4.33)
  - Wounds associated with contaminated swimming pools, fish tanks, and fish fin/spine injuries
  - Diagnosis—cultures incubated on **Lowenstein-Jensen media at 30°C** for 6 to 8 weeks
  - Types
    - Cutaneous (verrucal)
    - Subcutaneous (granulomatous)
      - Requires debridement
      - Antibiotic duration 2 to 6 months

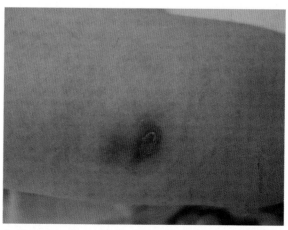

Figure 4.33 Infection of the forearm caused by *Mycobacterium marinum*. Image provided by Stedman's.

- Deep
  - Requires debridement of involved bone or joint
  - Antibiotic duration 4 to 24 months
  - Tetracycline or macrolide and ethambutol; can add rifampin for osteomyelitis

Septic Arthritis

- Infection of joint space
  - Release of bacterial toxins, proteolytic enzymes; cartilage destruction
  - Most common organism is *S. aureus*; should also consider *Neisseria gonococcus*
- Physical examination—swollen, painful, erythematous joint
- Diagnosis
  - Joint aspiration
  - White blood cell counts >50 000, >75% polymorphonuclear lymphocytes, glucose level 40 mg < fasting glucose
- Treatment
  - Incision and drainage
  - Intravenous antibiotics

Osteomyelitis

- Infection involving bone
  - Direct contamination by open fractures or contiguous spread after traumatic event, or hematogenous spread
  - Most common organisms are *S. aureus* and *Streptococcus species.*
- Treatment
  - Parenteral antibiotics after obtaining a bone culture
  - Surgical debridement

Bite Wounds

- Commonly isolated organisms
  - *Eikenella corrodens* unique to human bites
  - *Pasteurella multocida* common in dog bites
- Clenched-fist injuries, "fight bite"—wounds over the MC head (Figure 4.34)

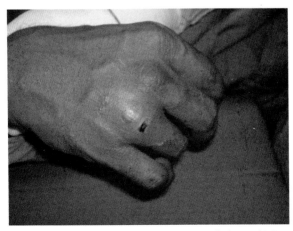

Figure 4.34 Human bite injury over ring finger metacarpophalangeal joint. From Puhaindran ME. Extensor tendon surgery. In: Thorne CH, ed. *Grabb & Smith's Plastic Surgery*. 7th ed. Philadelphia, PA: Lippincott Williams & Wilkins; 2014:792-798.

- True bite wounds—dog bite infection rate 4% versus cat bites 50%
- Treatment
  - Extension of wound, exploration of extensor tendons, joint space debridement
  - Intravenous antibiotics

Other Infections

- Abscess
  - Subcutaneous fluid collection, with central fluctuant area
  - Treatment
    - Incision and drainage
    - Culture-specific antimicrobials
- **Necrotizing fasciitis**
  - Soft tissue infection—true surgical emergency
  - Risk factors
    - Alcohol abuse
  - Physical examination
    - Violaceous bullae
    - Cutaneous hemorrhage
    - Skin sloughing
    - Crepitation (gas in tissue)
  - Can see rapid progression and hemodynamic instability
  - Most often polymicrobial; most common organism, *S. pyogenes*
  - Treatment
    - Resuscitate and initiate empiric intravenous antibiotics
    - Urgent surgical debridement
      - Classic findings of liquefied and gray fat—"dishwater" fluid
  - **Risk factors for poor outcomes**
    - **Delay in treatment**
    - Age > 50 years
    - Diabetes
  - Antibiotic choice
    - Intravenous antibiotics for bone or flexor tendon sheath infections
    - Septic arthritis: 1 to 4 weeks of intravenous antibiotics
    - Osteomyelitis: 4 to 8 weeks of intravenous antibiotics
    - **Trimethoprim-sulfamethoxazole** covers 90% of community-acquired methicillin-resistant *S. aureus*.
    - **Cat or dog bites**—amoxicillin/clavulanic acid or ampicillin/sulbactam

ARTHRITIS

Traumatic Radiocarpal Arthritis

- Following intra-articular fractures
- Rarely treated
- Typical arthritis options: activity modifications, splinting for sleep/activities, oral/topical/injectable medications, pain-coping, surgery
- Surgical options
  - Intra-articular osteotomy; only before advanced degeneration
  - Denervation
  - Radioscapholunate fusion (Figure 4.35); most common/reliable; removing distal scaphoid unlocks midcarpal joint
  - Distal radius arthroplasty; long-term survival concerns
  - Osteochondral transfer; typically from knee; uncommon; only small defects

Scapholunate Advanced Collapse

- Most common wrist arthritis
- Predictable carpal collapse/arthritis

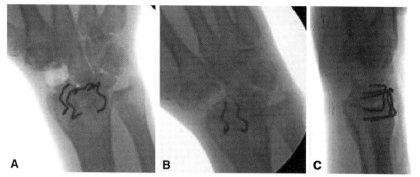

Figure 4.35 Anteroposterior (A), oblique (B), and lateral (C) radiographs of radioscapholunate fusion using bone staples; performed for post-traumatic arthritis following distal radius fracture; removal of the distal scaphoid allows midcarpal range of motion.

- Complete SL injury; secondary stabilizers fail acutely or gradually
- Scaphoid flexes/rotates; lunate follows triquetrum dorsally (dorsal intercalated segment instability [DISI])
- Scaphoid position increases pressures on radius—degeneration at radial styloid/distal scaphoid (stage I scapholunate advanced collapse [SLAC]), then entire radioscaphoid (stage II SLAC)
- Scaphoid-lunate separate (Terry Thomas sign); capitate migrates proximally; degeneration proximal head capitate/distal lunate (stage III SLAC) (Figure 4.36)
- Radiolunate joint spared because lunate extends normally; if radiolunate not spared, consider another diagnosis
- Symptoms do not correlate with radiographs.
- Surgical options
  - Denervation—excising PIN/anterior interosseous nerve (AIN); dorsal incision; test with anesthetic proximal to wrist
    - Few years of symptom relief, often deteriorates; progressive radiographic/motion loss changes; other options may be unavailable later
  - **Proximal row carpectomy**; remove scaphoid, lunate, triquetrum; pisiform retained; capitate sits on radius
    - Need RSC ligament
    - Need quality capitate/radius
    - Lose approximately 50% wrist range of motion (ROM) but better dart-thrower's versus partial fusion
    - Lose approximately 50% grip strength
    - Arthritic changes between capitate and radius do not correlate with outcomes (Figure 4.37)
  - **Partial wrist fusion**; remove scaphoid; fuse capitate-lunate at minimum (two-corner); some fuse capitate-hamate (three-corner); some fuse capitate-hamate and lunate-triquetrum-hamate (four-corner); some remove triquetrum versus fusing
    - Need good radius-lunate
    - Capitate-lunate fused in neutral; correct DISI-lunate
    - Lose approximately 50% wrist ROM/strength (Figure 4.38)
  - Total wrist fusion
    - Plates/screws; long finger MC to radius
    - For very limited ROM preoperatively
    - Reliable pain relief
    - Fused 0° to 30° wrist extension depending on activities

  - Maintain distal radioulnar joint (DRUJ)
  - Avoid if contralateral wrist has or will need also (Figure 4.39)
- Total wrist arthroplasty
  - Only indicated if ROM is not severely limited
  - Avoid unless patient has or will need contralateral total wrist fusion and has low functional demands

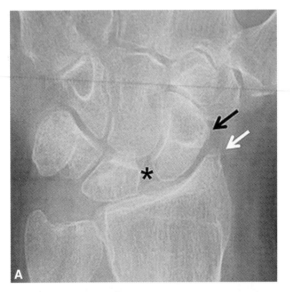

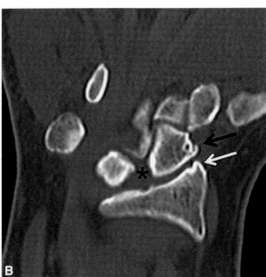

Figure 4.36 Four stages of scapholunate advanced collapse (SLAC). Stage I: Posteroanterior (PA) radiograph of the wrist (A), coronal computed tomography (CT) (B), and coronal proton density fat-suppressed magnetic resonance imaging (MRI)

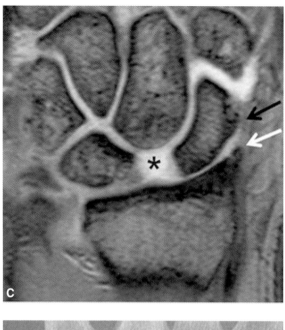

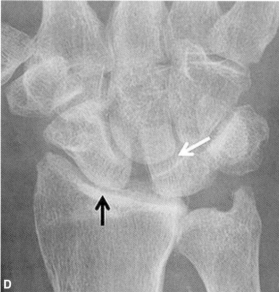

Figure 4.36 (*continued*) (C) showing spurring at the radial side of the scaphoid (black arrows) and at the radial styloid tip (white arrows). Scapholunate diastasis is seen (black asterisks). Stage II: PA radiograph (D),

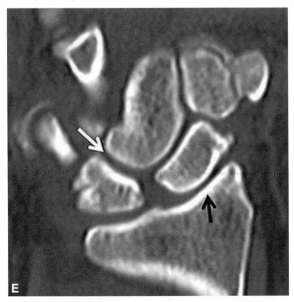

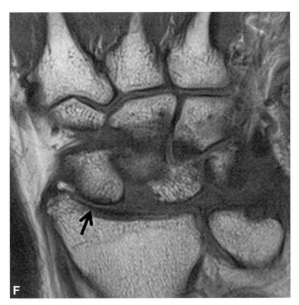

Figure 4.36 (*continued*) coronal CT (E), and coronal T1-weighted MRI (F) showing narrowing of the radioscaphoid (RS) articulation (black arrows) and radial styloid and scaphoid spurring. Note the preservation of the capitolunate (CL) joint at this point (white arrows).

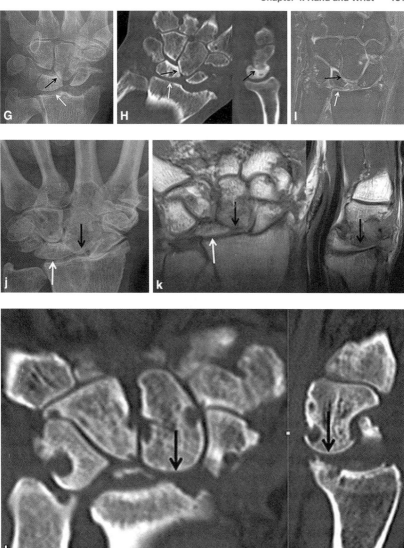

Figure 4.36 (*continued*) Stage III: PA radiograph (G), coronal and sagittal CT (H), and a coronal STIR MRI (I) in a different patient with SLAC wrist arthropathy showing narrowing of the CL joint (black arrow) and involvement of the RS joint. Note preservation of the radiolunate joint (white arrows). There is no significant migration of the capitate at this stage. Stage IV: In a different patient, in addition to extensive osteoarthritic changes, PA radiograph (J), coronal and sagittal T1-weighted MRI (K), and coronal and sagittal CT reformat images (L) demonstrate substantial proximal migration of the capitate (black arrows) with ulnar displacement of the lunate (white arrows). From Tischler BT, Diaz LE, Murakami AM, et al. Scapholunate advanced collapse: a pictorial review. *Insights Imaging*. 2014;5(4):407-417. doi:10.1007/s13244-014-0337-1.

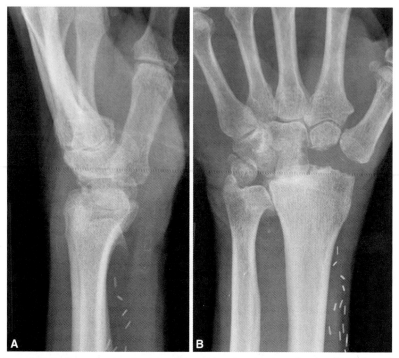

Figure 4.37 Radiographs showing lateral view (A) and posteroanterior view (B) of the wrist after proximal row carpectomy, which consists of removal of the scaphoid, lunate, and triquetrum. This patient also had the trapezium removed; note the distal radioulnar joint arthritis.

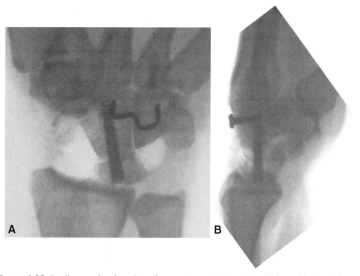

Figure 4.38 Radiographs showing the posteroanterior view (A) and lateral view (B) after partial wrist fusion. The scaphoid is always removed, and the capitolunate joint is always fused (with a screw); in this case, the capitohamate joint was also fused with a staple, and the triquetrum was removed.

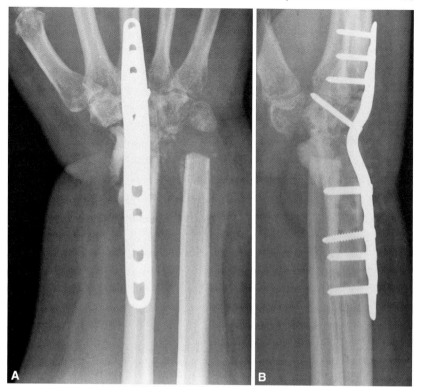

Figure 4.39 Posteroanterior (A) and lateral (B) radiographs of total wrist arthrodesis after severe trauma; in this case, the patient had a proximal row carpectomy first and then the capitate was fused to the radius with additional bone graft around the fusion; the distal ulna was also removed.

Scaphoid Nonunion Advanced Collapse

- Progression similar to SLAC
- Attempt scaphoid healing if reducible and adequate cartilage; confirm SL intact
- Otherwise, same options as SLAC (Figure 4.40)

Wrist Inflammatory Arthropathy

- Symmetric degeneration (radiolunate not spared; destructive bone loss/cysts)
- **Rheumatoid arthritis** (RA) diagnosed by examination/labs; rheumatoid factor non-specific inflammatory marker; anticyclic citrullinated peptide more specific and track treatment response
- **Mannerfelt**—rupture of FPL; synovitis/spurs palmar radiocarpal; tendon transfer if dysfunctional
- **Gout**—crystalline arthropathy; purine metabolism disorder; monosodium urate crystals around joints/tendons; destructive inflammation; **strongly negative birefringent needle-like crystals** under polarizing light microscopy; radiographs **periarticular "punched out" lesions**
- **Pseudogout**—that is, calcium pyrophosphate dihydrate deposition or chondrocalcinosis; crystalline arthropathy; **weakly positive birefringent rhomboidal crystals** under polarizing light microscopy; radiographic calcification of tissues, for example, TFCC

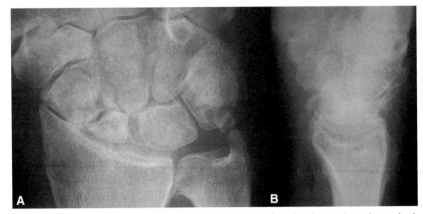

Figure 4.40 Posteroanterior (A) and lateral (B) radiographs of scaphoid nonunion advanced collapse; the scaphoid has a nonunion, there is radial styloid osteophyte with loss of radioscaphoid joint space, and the wrist has progressive dorsal intercalated segment instability deformity.

- Treatment options
  - **Disease-modifying antirheumatic drugs (DMARDs)**—medications that alter natural history
  - Traditional DMARDs: methotrexate, chloroquine, gold salts
  - "Biologic" DMARDs target specific cells, cytokines, or other inflammatory elements; for example, abatacept (Orencia, T-cell inhibitor), adalimumab (Humira, tumor necrosis factor-alpha [TNF-α] inhibitor), etanercept (Enbrel, TNF-α inhibitor), infliximab (Remicade, TNF-α inhibitor), rituximab (Rituxan, B-cell inhibitor/destroyer)
  - Corticosteroids blunt inflammation; do not prevent progression (not DMARDs)
  - Surgical synovectomy if cannot control medically and cartilage is good
  - Avoid partial wrist fusions because all joints affected; total wrist fusion or arthroplasty
  - Total arthroplasty for low-demand patients with contralateral, or likely future, total fusion

DRUJ Arthritis

- Less common than radiocarpal arthritis
- Frequently seen with inflammatory arthropathy
- Caput ulnae—dorsal prominence ulna; DRUJ instability/degeneration
- Along with synovitis, leads to **Vaughan-Jackson syndrome**—finger extensors rupture progressively ulnar to radial
- Differentiate from other causes of ulnar-sided pain (eg, TFCC, ulnocarpal impaction)
  - Tenderness, dorsal DRUJ/pain/crepitus with pronosupination or palmar-dorsal stressing
  - Radiographic joint space loss, spurring inferiorly
  - Scalloping of radius indicates inflammatory arthropathy with impending/concurrent finger extensor tendon rupture (Vaughan-Jackson).
- Extensor tendon debridement/transfer and treat underlying DRUJ synovitis/degeneration to prevent recurrence (Figure 4.41)
  - DRUJ splinting restrict pronosupination
- Surgical options
  - Ulnar matched resection; remove radial side ulnar head; maintain ulnar styloid/TFCC; match radius contour; option if TFCC intact/DRUJ stable; painful convergence between radius and ulna possible (Figure 4.42)

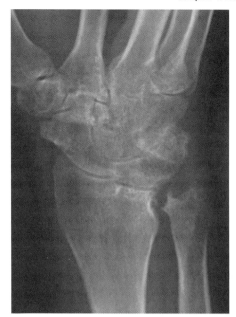

Figure 4.41 Radiograph of scalloping of the distal radius at the distal radioulnar joint (DRUJ); this patient had ruptured finger extensor tendons and was treated with Sauvé-Kapandji arthrodesis and extensor tendon transfers.

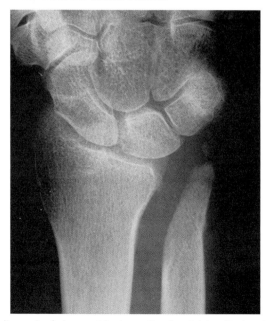

Figure 4.42 Radiograph of ulnar matched resection for distal radioulnar joint (DRUJ) arthritis with well-preserved ulnar styloid/triangular fibrocartilage complex; the contour of the distal ulna was made to closely match that of the radius.

- Hemiresection-interposition arthroplasty; similar to ulnar matched resection; material interposed; attempt to prevent convergence
- Darrach distal ulna resection; remove entire ulnar head; convergence and/or painful/unstable palmar-dorsal translation possible; occurs in patients with deficient distal interosseous membrane
- Sauvé-Kapandji fuse distal radius-ulna, remove approximately 1 cm of bone from ulna proximal to fusion for rotation; convergence and/or palmar-dorsal translation possible; thought better for patients with inflammatory arthropathy who might develop ulnar translocation of carpus; likely does not prevent ulnar translocation of carpus, but if it occurs, there is better support than with distal ulnar resection (Figure 4.43)
- Ulnar head prosthesis; retain ulnar styloid/TFCC insertion versus TFCC attachment to implant; need reasonable radius sigmoid notch
- Complete DRUJ arthroplasty; unconstrained versus constrained; stability concern with unconstrained; implant failure concern with constrained

Scaphotrapezial-Trapezoidal Arthritis

- Not as common as thumb carpometacarpal (CMC)
- Surgical options
  - Remove distal scaphoid (Malerich); dorsal tilt of scaphoid/lunate with carpal degeneration possible
  - Remove trapezium/trapezoid
  - Fuse scaphotrapezial-trapezoidal (STT)

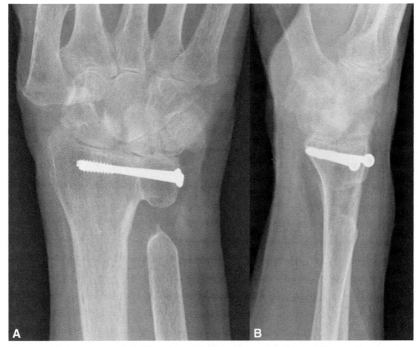

Figure 4.43 Posteroanterior (A) and lateral (B) radiographs of Sauvé-Kapandji arthrodesis of the distal radioulnar joint (DRUJ) in a patient with rheumatoid arthritis; the Sauvé-Kapandji fusion did not prevent ulnar translocation, but as the lunate progressively shifts ulnarly, it has a broader articular support provided by the distal ulna.

Thumb Basilar Joint Arthritis

- Thumb CMC/trapeziometacarpal arthritis
- Most common cause of thumb base pain
- Most cases atraumatic
- Nearly universal radiographically with advancing age; does not correlate with symptoms
- Soft-tissue attenuation; thumb MC base subluxation dorsally/radially
- Most important restraints
  - Dorsal radial joint capsule
  - Palmar oblique ligament, from palmar/ulnar trapezium to thumb MC (ie, beak ligament, anterior oblique ligament, trapeziometacarpal ligament)
- Radiographic progression
  - Stage I—synovitis; increased joint space
  - Stage II—subluxation of thumb MC base, joint space narrowing, early osteophytes
  - Stage III—more subluxation/joint space narrowing, spurs >2 mm
  - Stage IV—arthritis surrounding entire trapezium (thumb CMC/STT) (Figure 4.44)
- Surgical options
  - All decrease pain/increase strength
  - Thumb CMC stabilization (Littler-Eaton); half-slip of FCR reconstructs soft tissues; only early stage (I/II)
  - Complete trapeziectomy; regained favor; most studies show equal outcomes with fewer complications; additional temporary pinning thumb MC termed hematoma distraction arthroplasty
  - Hemitrapeziectomy/interposition; remove distal half of trapezium, interpose biologic or artificial material; only for early stages; few studies
  - Trapeziectomy with ligament reconstruction (suspensionplasty); use biologic or artificial material to "suspend" thumb MC from index; FCR and ECRL first/second most common; or APL through FCR or suture to FCR; when with interposition between thumb MC and scaphoid termed ligament reconstruction tendon interposition

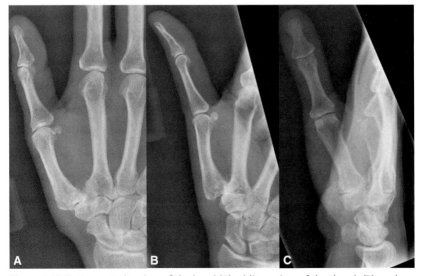

Figure 4.44 Posteroanterior view of the hand (A), oblique view of the thumb (B), and posteroanterior view of the thumb (C) showing stage III thumb carpometacarpal osteoarthritis with advanced joint subluxation, near-complete loss of joint space, and large spurs but maintained scaphotrapezial-trapezoidal joint space.

- **Address thumb MCP hyperextension**/degeneration
  - <10° of hyperextension with firm endpoint—splinting/retraining after CMC procedure
  - 10° to 30° of MCP hyperextension—temporary pinning, extensor pollicis brevis release/transfer, volar capsulodesis if good cartilage/flexion, or fusion
  - >30° to 40° of hyperextension with poor flexion or MCP arthritis fusion (Figure 4.45)

Finger MCP Arthritis

- Long finger most common
- If >1 MCP and/or joint/tendon synovitis or ulnar deviation, consider inflammatory disease/rheumatologist
  - It cannot control medically, typical progression is corticosteroid injection, synovectomy, joint replacement.
  - MCP synovitis attenuates soft tissues, leading to extensor ulnar subluxation/dislocation.
    - Extensor subluxation—unable to actively extend MCP joint from flexion; can hold after passive extension
    - Extensor rupture—unable to actively hold extension after passive extension
    - MCP dislocation—unable to passively extend
    - MCP good—synovectomy and centralize extensors; release ulnar sagittal band for centralization; use portion of extensor or other reconstruction to maintain centralization; radial sagittal band attenuated
    - MCP poor—silicone arthroplasty and extensor centralization (Figure 4.46A)
- Silicone arthroplasty best record; arthrodesis too limiting except maybe IF (Figure 4.46B)

Finger PIP Arthritis

- Radial/ulnar deviation from asymmetric osteoarthritis (not concerning for rheumatologic diagnosis vs. at MCP)

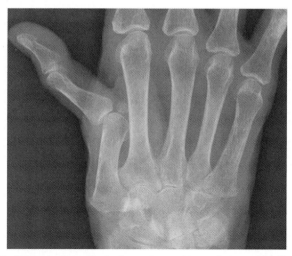

Figure 4.45 Radiograph of a patient who underwent trapeziectomy with ligament reconstruction tendon interposition but did not have thumb metacarpophalangeal hyperextension addressed; the thumb experienced a Z-collapse deformity with progressive severe metacarpophalangeal hyperextension that now requires arthrodesis.

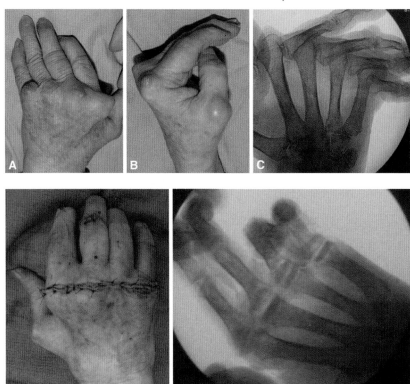

Figure 4.46 A-C, Photographs and radiographs of a patient with rheumatoid arthritis with metacarpophalangeal and extensor tendon dislocations. D and E, The same patient after metacarpophalangeal silicone arthroplasty and extensor centralization of all four fingers.

- Several swan-neck deformities, consider systemic lupus erythematosus
- **Pencil-in-cup** radiograph proximal phalanx into middle phalanx—**psoriatic** arthritis
- Surgical option: arthrodesis, especially IF, or arthroplasty; silicone best record

Finger Distal Interphalangeal Joint Arthritis

- Very common; radial/ulnar deviation; surprisingly maintained ROM
- Ganglion cysts (ie, mucous cysts); pressure on germinal nail matrix causes nail grooves
- Surgical options
  - Open debridement, if good ROM, or arthrodesis
  - Neutral arthrodesis position more cosmetic; flexion for specific activities

TENDON INJURY AND REPAIR

Extensor Tendons

- Anatomy
  - Extensor zones (Figure 4.47)
    - Odd-numbered zones overlie joints
  - Six dorsal compartments at level of wrist (Figure 4.48)

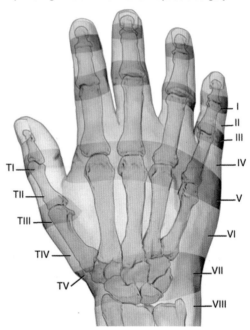

Figure 4.47 Odd-numbered extensor zones overlie joints. From Shapiro DB, Krahe MA, Monaco NA. Repair following traumatic extensor tendon disruption in the hand, wrist, and forearm. In: Hunt TR III, ed. *Operative Techniques in Hand, Wrist, and Forearm Surgery*. 2nd ed. Philadelphia, PA: Wolters Kluwer; 2016:751-761.

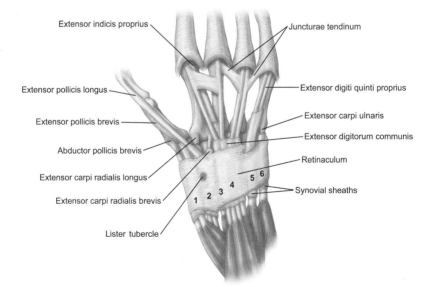

Figure 4.48 The extensor tendons are contained in six extensor compartments on the dorsum of the wrist. From Berquist TH. Hand and wrist. In: *MRI of the Musculoskeletal System*. 6th ed. Philadelphia, PA: Wolters Kluwer; 2013:777-869.

- Extensor indicis proprius and EDM
  - Allow independent extension of IF and small fingers
  - Lie **ulnar to extensor digitorum communis tendons**
- Extensor mechanism (Figure 4.49)
  - Confluence of extrinsic extensor tendons and intrinsic tendons (lumbricals and interossei) on dorsum on IF, long, ring, small fingers
    - Central slip inserts at dorsal base of middle phalanx.
    - Terminal tendon inserts at dorsal base of distal phalanx.
    - Lateral bands flex MCP joints and extend IP joints.
    - Intact extensor mechanism permits physiologic closing of fist.
      - MCP joints contract first followed by IP joints
  - Sagittal bands (Figure 4.50)
    - At level of MCP joint
    - Maintain central location of extensor tendon above joint
  - Triangular ligament/transverse ligament
    - Maintain proper anatomic position of lateral bands (triangular ligament prevents volar subluxation; transverse ligament prevents dorsal subluxation) (Figure 4.51; see also Figure 4.50)
- Injuries and pathology
  - Laceration
    - 50% to 60% of lacerations may be treated nonoperatively.
    - Larger lacerations should be sutured.
  - De Quervain tenosynovitis
    - Irritation of first compartment extensor tendons
    - Common in new mothers (lifting child)

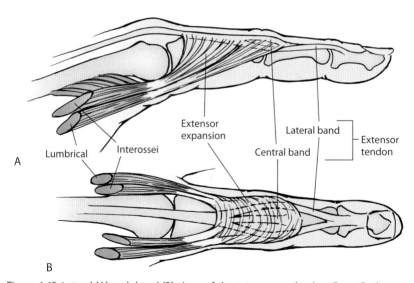

Figure 4.49 Lateral (A) and dorsal (B) views of the extensor mechanism. From Oatis CA. Mechanics and pathomechanics of the special connective tissues in the hand. In: *Kinesiology: The Mechanics and Pathomechanics of Human Movement*. Baltimore, MD: Lippincott Williams & Wilkins; 2004:321-331.

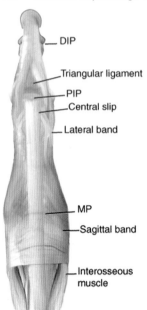

Figure 4.50 The sagittal bands hold the extensor tendon in a central location over the metacarpophalangeal joint. DIP, distal interphalangeal joint; MP, metacarpophalangeal joint; PIP, proximal interphalangeal joint. From Lee BL, Richer RJ, Phillips CS. Extensor tendon centralization following traumatic subluxation at the metacarpophalangeal joint. In: Hunt TR III. *Operative Techniques in Hand, Wrist, and Elbow Surgery.* 2nd ed. Philadelphia, PA: Wolters Kluwer; 2016:770-778.

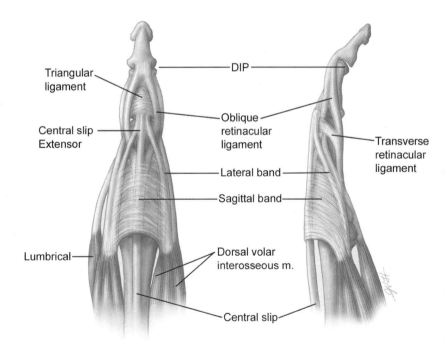

Figure 4.51 The transverse retinacular ligaments prevent dorsal subluxation of the lateral bands. DIP, distal interphalangeal joint. From Berquist TH. Hand and wrist. In: *MRI of the Musculoskeletal System.* 6th ed. Philadelphia, PA: Wolters Kluwer; 2013:777-869.

- Diagnosed with positive Finkelstein test
- Injections, surgery if injections ineffective
- Mallet finger
  - Typically a traumatic lesion of terminal extensor tendon insertion
  - Causes flexion deformity (extensor lag) of finger distal interphalangeal (DIP) joint.
  - Splinting, consider surgery if splinting ineffective (Figure 4.52)

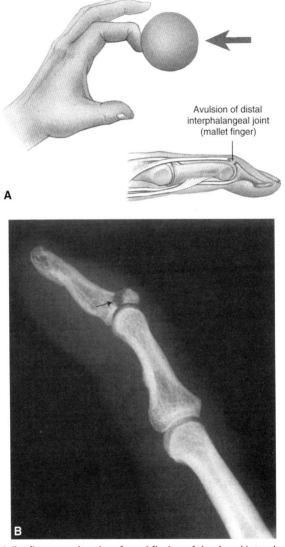

Avulsion of distal
interphalangeal joint
(mallet finger)

A

B

Figure 4.52 Mallet finger results when forced flexion of the dorsal interphalangeal joint (A) causes avulsion of the terminal extensor tendon (B). A: Asset provided by Anatomical Chart Company. B: From Erkonen WE, Boles CA. Musculoskeletal system. In: Erkonen WE, ed. *Radiology 101: The Basics and Fundamentals of Imaging*. 2nd ed. Philadelphia, PA: Lippincott Williams & Wilkins; 2005:175-264.

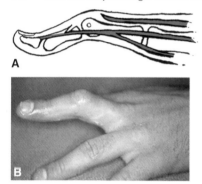

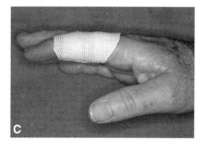

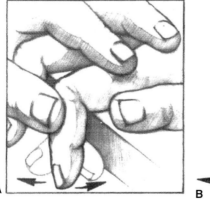

Figure 4.53 Boutonniere deformity involves flexion of the proximal interphalangeal joint and extension of the distal interphalangeal joint. A, Illustration of disruption of the central slip and resulting boutonniere deformity. B, Photograph of boutonniere deformity. C, Immobilization of the proximal interphalangeal joint in neutral may be effective. From Schultz K, Jacobs ML. Stiffness. In: Jacobs ML, Austin NM, eds. *Orthotic Intervention of the Hand and Upper Extremity: Splinting Principles and Process.* 2nd ed. Baltimore, MD: Lippincott Williams & Wilkins; 2014:391-322.

- **Boutonniere** deformity (Figure 4.53)
  - May be traumatic or atraumatic (eg, RA)
  - Flexion of PIP joint and hyperextension of DIP joint deformity
  - **Essential lesion is to central slip with resulting volar subluxation of lateral bands**
  - Diagnosis with **Elson test** (Figure 4.54)

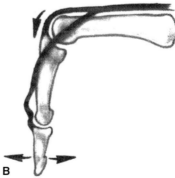

Figure 4.54 The Elson test. A, PIP flexion 90° over the edge of the table and held the family. B, Patient is asked to extend PIP against resistance. Pressure felt by examiner over middle phalanx can only be exerted by intact central slip. DIP joint remains flail since the competent central slip prevents the lateral bands from acting distally. C and D, In the presence of a complete rupture of the central slip, any extension felt by the examiner will be accompanied by rigidity at the DIP joint with a tendency to extension—produced by the lateral bands. From Doyle JR, Botte MJ. *Surgical Anatomy of the Hand and Upper Extremity.* Philadelphia, PA: Lippincott Williams & Wilkins; 2002.

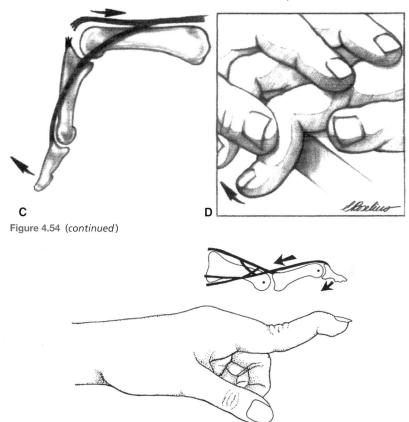

C   **D**

Figure 4.54 (*continued*)

Figure 4.55 Swan-neck deformity involves hyperextension (proximal arrow) of the proximal interphalangeal joint and compensatory flexion (distal arrow) of the distal interphalangeal joint. The volar plate (not shown), spanning the proximal interphalangeal joint, may be stretched. From Rayan G, Akelman E, eds. *The Hand: Anatomy, Examination, and Diagnosis.* 4th ed. Philadelphia, PA: Lippincott Williams & Wilkins; 2011:197-204.

- Treat with PIP splinting and active DIP flexion exercises, surgery if nonoperative treatment ineffective
- **Swan-neck** deformity (Figure 4.55)
  - Typically atraumatic (eg, RA)
  - Hyperextension of PIP joint and flexion of DIP joint deformity
  - Essential lesion is to flexor digitorum brevis insertion/volar plate at volar base of middle phalanx
  - Treat with surgery
- **Sagittal band rupture**
  - May be traumatic—"boxer knuckle" or atraumatic (eg, RA)
  - Allows ulnar subluxation of extensor tendon
  - Patients cannot actively extend MCP joint, but if joint is placed in extension, they can hold it there (Figure 4.56).
  - Treatment
    - Acute injuries may be splinted in extension.
    - Chronic injuries treated with surgical sagittal band repair or extensor centralization if repair impossible

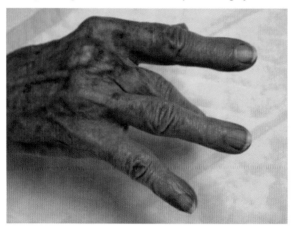

Figure 4.56 Sagittal band rupture allows the extensor tendon to drift ulnarly off the metacarpophalangeal joint. The patient cannot actively extend the finger but may be able to hold it extended if the finger is passively extended. From Rayan G, Akelman E, eds. *The Hand: Anatomy, Examination, and Diagnosis*. 4th ed. Philadelphia, PA: Lippincott Williams & Wilkins; 2011:197-204.

- **Vaughn-Jackson syndrome**
  - Sequential rupture of extensor tendons (occurs in ulnar to radial sequence) over prominent ulnar head
  - Occurs with RA
  - Treat with excision of distal ulna (Darrach procedure), tenosynovectomy, tendon transfers
- **Extensor pollicis longus rupture**
  - May occur after nonoperative treatment of **nondisplaced distal radius fracture**
  - Treat with extensor indicis proprius to extensor pollicis longus transfer

Flexor Tendons

- Anatomy
  - Flexor zones
    - Zone 2
      - Contains flexor sheaths
        - **A2 and A4 pulleys most important** to prevent "bowstringing of tendons" (Figure 4.57)
        - Tendon nutrition derived from synovial fluid in sheath and blood flow from vincula
- Injuries and pathology
  - Trigger finger
    - Stenosing tenosynovitis of flexor tendons
    - Nodule on tendon prevents it from passing smoothly beneath A1 pulley.
    - Treat with injections, surgical release of A1 pulley if injections fail
    - Pediatric trigger finger
      - Common in the thumb
      - Release of trigger must **avoid radial digital nerve**, which lies directly in surgical field
      - Triggers in other digits rare and associated with other abnormalities

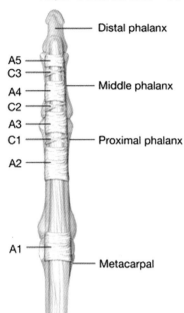

Figure 4.57 The annular A2 and A4 pulleys are most important to prevent bowstringing of the flexor tendons. From Tosti R, Machol JA IV, Chen N. Staged flexor tendon grafting and pulley reconstruction. In: Chung KC, ed. *Operative Techniques in Plastic Surgery*. Philadelphia, PA: Wolters Kluwer; 2019:2065-2072.

- Lacerations
  - 50% to 60% of lacerations may be treated nonoperatively.
  - Larger lacerations should be sutured.
    - **Gold-standard surgical technique** involves **at least four core sutures and a running epitendinous suture.**
    - **Number of core suture strands crossing repair site** is the most important factor in repair strength.
  - Zone 2 flexor tendon lacerations
    - Often involves FDS and FDP tendons
    - Zone 2 is formerly referred to as "no man's land" because of historically poor outcomes after repair in this area.
      - Modern techniques achieve excellent results.
  - Many rehabilitation protocols; all involve early controlled finger motion
    - **Motion improves tendon gliding and prevents adhesion formation.**
  - **Quadriga** effect (Figure 4.58)
    - Because FDP has common muscle belly, overtightening of one slip prevents full contraction of other slips.
  - **Lumbrical-plus** finger (Figure 4.59)
    - Amputations just proximal to FDP insertion allow tendon to retract.
    - Retracted tendon causes retraction of lumbrical muscle insertion on tendon.
    - Results in paradoxical extension of IP joints when patient attempts to make a fist
- Ruptures
  - **Jersey finger** (Figure 4.60)
    - FDP avulsion from insertion at volar base of distal phalanx
    - Tendon may remain in place or retract to level of the palm.

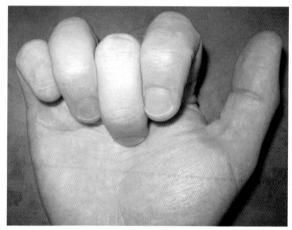

Figure 4.58 Quadriga effect. The long finger, in which the flexor digitorum profundus has been repaired with too much tension, is maximally flexed into the palm, and the adjacent fingers cannot be actively flexed further. From Peers SC, Malone KJ. Staged digital flexor tendon reconstruction. In: Hunt TR III. *Operative Techniques in Hand, Wrist, and Elbow Surgery.* 2nd ed. Philadelphia, PA: Wolters Kluwer; 2016:743-750.

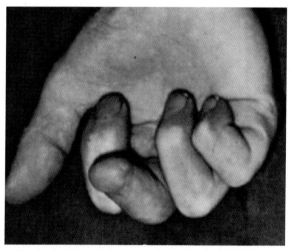

Figure 4.59 Lumbrical-plus deformity. With the metacarpophalangeal (MCP) joint in extension and the proximal interphalangeal (PIP) joint in flexion, active flexion of the MCP joint will cause paradoxical extension of the PIP joint. From Medhoff TL, Crouch CC, Bennett JB. Injuries of the hand. In: Brinker MR, ed. *Review of Orthopaedic Trauma.* 2nd ed. Philadelphia, PA: Lippincott Williams & Wilkins; 2013:253-286.

- Treat with surgical repair for retracted tendons
- Classification of FDP avulsion
  - I: Tendon retracts to the palm; vincula ruptured, necessitating early repair.
  - II: Tendon retracts to PIP; vincula intact, permitting delayed repair.
  - III: Tendon attached to large bony fragment that catches on distal sheath (minimal retraction).
  - IV: Tendon separates from bony fragment, retracts to the palm (subtype I) or PIP (subtype II).

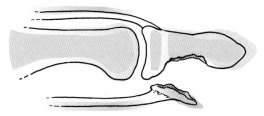

Figure 4.60 Jersey finger may or may not involve avulsion of a piece of bone from the distal phalanx. From Lightdale-Miric N, Kozin SH. Fractures and dislocations of the hand and carpal bones in children. In: Flynn JM, Skaggs DL, Waters PM, eds. *Rockwood and Wilkins' Fractures in Children.* 8th ed. Philadelphia, PA: Wolters Kluwer Health; 2015:264-347.

COMPRESSION NEUROPATHIES
Median Nerve

- CTS
  - Most common compression neuropathy in the upper limb
  - Anatomy (Figure 4.61)
    - **Carpal canal contents**—median nerve, four FDPs, four FDS, FPL (most radial)
    - Borders—radially, scaphoid tubercle; ulnarly, hook of hamate; dorsally, proximal carpal row; volarly, transverse carpal ligament
    - Thenar motor branch of the median nerve has numerous anatomic variants.

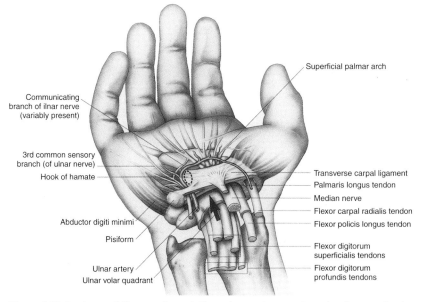

Superficial palmar arch

Communicating branch of ilnar nerve (variably present)

3rd common sensory branch (of ulnar nerve)

Hook of hamate

Abductor digiti minimi

Pisiform

Ulnar artery

Ulnar volar quadrant

Transverse carpal ligament
Palmaris longus tendon
Median nerve
Flexor carpal radialis tendon
Flexor policis longus tendon

Flexor digitorum superficialis tendons
Flexor digitorum profundis tendons

Figure 4.61 Anatomy of the carpal canal. The palmar cutaneous branch arises proximal to the carpal tunnel, and the thenar motor branch arises postligamentously. From Putnam M, Adams JE. Nonacute elbow, wrist, and hand conditions. In: Swiontkowski MC, ed. *Manual of Orthopaedics.* 7th ed. Philadelphia, PA: Lippincott Williams & Wilkins; 2013:369-400.

- Postligamentous (nerve emerges from median nerve distal to carpal tunnel) is most common.
- Preligamentous or transligamentous variants also exist.
- Pathophysiology
  - Compression of the median nerve in the carpal canal with resultant sensory and motor dysfunction (Figure 4.62)
  - Most cases are idiopathic.
  - Associated with systemic conditions—diabetes, thyroid disease, RA, obesity
  - Some high-level evidence supports relationship between repetitive activities and CTS, although remains controversial.
- Symptoms
  - Paresthesias in radial 3.5 digits (but may be nonspecific)
    - Night-time awakening is classic.
  - Thenar atrophy—late finding
    - **Abductor pollicis brevis** is main muscle clinically deficient—purely median innervated
- Diagnosis
  - History and physical examination
  - Physical examination—thenar atrophy
  - Provocative maneuvers—Durkan compression test (pressure over carpal canal); Phalen wrist flexion test; Tinel test (percussion over canal)
  - Electromyography (EMG)/nerve conduction study (NCS)—not needed for diagnosis or surgery, but commonly performed
    - Limited evidence supports NCS per recent clinical practice guideline
    - Normal values—motor latency <4.5 ms; sensory latency <3.5 ms
- Treatment
  - Night-time splinting
  - Steroid injection—favorable response associated with successful surgery

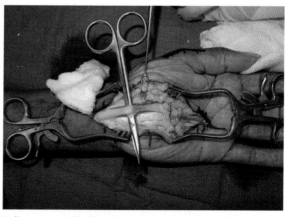

Figure 4.62 Median nerve with chronic, severe compression at the transverse carpal ligament (just distal to the scissors) after open carpal tunnel release. Note superficial arch at the distal end of the incision. The patient subsequently underwent opponensplasty to restore thumb abduction. From Means KR, Segalman KA. Carpal tunnel syndrome. In: Trumble TE, Budoff JE, eds. *Hand Surgery Update IV.* Rosemont, IL: American Society for Surgery of the Hand; 2007:299-407.

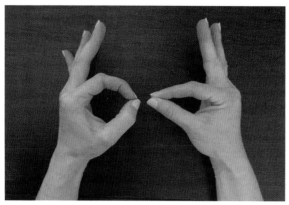

Figure 4.63 Classically, dysfunction of the anterior interosseous nerve (AIN) manifests as the inability to make an "OK sign" because of flexor digitorum profundus and flexor pollicis longus weakness. The normal hand is on the left, and the hand on the right shows the pathognomonic finding of AIN palsy. Copyright © Ryan M. Zimmerman, MD, 2017.

- Surgical release—endoscopic or open
    - Outcomes generally equivalent
    - Limited data—endoscopic has faster return to work but higher frequency of incomplete release.
    - In most circumstances, it can be assumed that the two techniques are the same.
    - Be wary of a **double crush**, especially with history of cervical spine disease, abnormal Spurling maneuver, or atypical symptoms
- **Acute CTS**
  - Pathophysiology—pressure on median nerve or in carpal canal from acute injury (distal radius fracture, perilunate fracture dislocation, crushing injury)
  - Treatment—**urgent surgical decompression**
  - Acute onset of median nerve dysfunction should almost always be treated with surgical decompression.
- **Pronator syndrome**
  - Anatomy—more proximal compression of median nerve by **supracondylar process and ligament of Struthers**
  - Symptoms—CTS symptoms plus forearm pain and palmar cutaneous branch paresthesias
- **AIN syndrome** (Figure 4.63)
  - Same pathophysiology as pronator syndrome, but painless muscle **weakness (FPL, FDP, IF/middle finger [MF])**
  - Often a transient neuritis, similar to Parsonage-Turner syndrome
  - Treatment—**observation for 6 months**; decompress if unimproved

Ulnar Nerve

- Neuropathy at the elbow (cubital tunnel syndrome)
  - Most common neuropathy of ulnar nerve
  - Seven possible sources of compression, but cubital tunnel is most common (Table 4.1)
  - Pathophysiology
    - Similar to CTS but may be associated with trauma or malunion

Table 4.1 Possible Sources of Compression of the Ulnar Nerve

Source of Compression	Description
Anconeus epitrochlearis	Anomalous muscle in cubital tunnel
Arcade of Struthers	Runs from triceps to medial septum
Cubital tunnel	By far the most common
FDS arch	
Flexor carpi ulnaris aponeurosis	Release flexor carpi ulnaris to first motor branch
Medial intermuscular septum	
Medial epicondyle	

FDS, flexor digitorum superficialis.

- Symptoms
  - Paresthesias of ulnar 1.5 digits
  - Intrinsic atrophy/weakness
- Diagnosis
  - Elbow flexion test—flexion reproduces symptoms.
  - Tinel sign—percussion at the elbow produces symptoms.
  - **Froment sign**—adductor pollicis weakness requires flexion of thumb IP joint during key pinch.
  - **Wartenberg sign**—small finger abduction because extensor digiti quinti (radial nerve) overpowers weak intrinsics abductor digiti minimi muscle—first sign to present
  - EMG/NCS—motor conduction velocity <50 m/s with drop-off across the elbow
- Treatment
  - Night-time elbow extension splinting
  - Decompression with or without transposition
    - In situ decompression—currently favored by most
    - Transposition—needed if nerve subluxating preoperatively or intraoperatively or following in situ decompression
  - TEST TIP—In situ decompression is reasonable surgical option unless nerve is unstable.
  - TEST TIP—Decompression typically not needed in acute trauma setting unless patient is having ulnar nerve symptoms.
  - TEST TIP—If shown an MRI or photo of ulnar nerve with a muscle running with it at the elbow, think **anconeus epitrochlearis (anomalous muscle—can cause ulnar compression).**
- Neuropathy at the wrist **(ulnar tunnel syndrome)**
  - Anatomy—Guyon canal bordered by hook of hamate radially, pisiform medially, transverse carpal ligament dorsally, and volar carpal ligament palmarly
  - Much less common than cubital tunnel syndrome and more likely caused by a mass (ganglion is most common)
  - Diagnosis—**MRI to look for a mass (ganglion most common)**

Radial Nerve

- Compression of the radial nerve is rare compared with median and ulnar nerves.
- **PIN syndrome**
  - Symptoms—**weakness** of PIN innervated muscles; pain is absent or relatively minor
  - Pathophysiology—typically compression at leading edge of supinator (arcade of Frohse)
  - May be associated with mass, so consider MRI
  - Treatment—observation initially unless caused by a mass

- **Radial tunnel syndrome**
  - Symptoms—primarily lateral arm **pain**, similar to lateral epicondylitis; no weakness
    - Provocative maneuvers—resisted supination or long finger extension
    - Can **confirm diagnosis with lidocaine injection**
  - Pathophysiology and treatment—same as PIN syndrome
- **Wartenberg syndrome**
  - Symptoms—pain and numbness in distribution of superficial radial nerve
  - Pathophysiology—compression of **superficial branch of radial nerve between brachioradialis and ECRL**
    - May have history of handcuffs, tight watchband, splint/cast
  - May appear similar to De Quervain tenosynovitis
    - Both have positive Finkelstein maneuver.
    - Wartenberg syndrome will have **positive Tinel over sensory radial nerve**, be exacerbated by pronation.
  - Treatment—observation with or without injection initially; decompress after 6 months

Suprascapular Nerve

- Anatomy—arises from C5 to C6 and courses posteriorly, passes through the suprascapular notch, under the suprascapular ligament, innervating supraspinatus, then around the spine of the scapula, through the spinoglenoid notch, to innervate the infraspinatus
- Pathophysiology—compression can occur at the **suprascapular notch or the spinoglenoid notch** (Figure 4.64).
  - Suprascapular notch compression—affects supraspinatus and infraspinatus
  - Compression can occur via tight or calcified suprascapular ligament; traction injury can occur via a retracted rotator cuff tear.
    - Treatment—arthroscopic or open decompression, rotator cuff repair
  - Spinoglenoid notch compression—affects only infraspinatus; note weakness in external rotation primarily; typically caused by spinoglenoid notch cyst secondary to labral tear
    - Treatment—cyst decompression and labral repair

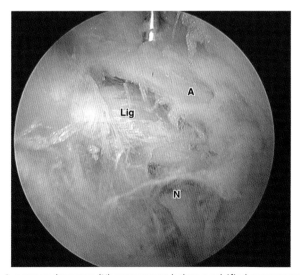

Figure 4.64 Suprascapular nerve (N) entrapment below a calcified suprascapular ligament (Lig). The artery (A) courses above the ligament, and the nerve passes below it. The ligament was subsequently resected with resolution of the patient's symptoms. Copyright © The Curtis National Hand Center, 2017.

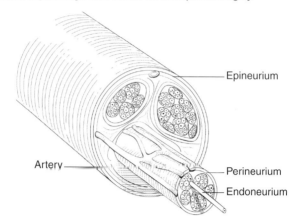

Figure 4.65 Cross section of a peripheral nerve showing internal neuroanatomy. From Elfar J, Petrungaro JM, Braun RM, et al. Nerve. In: Hammert WC, Calfee RP, Bozenta DJ, Boyer MI, eds. *ASSH Manual of Hand Surgery*. Philadelphia, PA: Lippincott Williams & Wilkins; 2010:294-342.

NERVE INJURIES

Neuroanatomy (Figure 4.65)

- Each axon covered by endoneurium.
- Many axons make a fascicle, which is covered by perineurium.
- Fascicles form a nerve, which is encompassed by epineurium.

Types and Classification

- Types of injury—penetrating or blunt trauma, compression, stretch, metabolic, genetic, autoimmune
- Two common classifications (Table 4.2)
  - Seddon (I-III)
  - Sunderland (I-V)

Table 4.2 Classifications of Nerve Injury

Seddon Grade	Sunderland Grade	Common Term	Definition	Prognosis	Treatment
I	I	Neurapraxia	All nerve structures intact	Good	Observation
II	II	Axonotmesis	Myelin disrupted	Fair	Surgery only after nerve fails to recover, often because of scar
NA	III	NA	Epineurium disrupted	Fair	Surgery if spontaneous recovery does not occur
NA	IV	NA	Perineurium disrupted	Poor without surgery	Surgery
III	V	Neurotmesis	Nerve is completely transected	Impossible without surgery	Surgery

NA, not applicable.

- In both classifications, **grade I (neurapraxia) and grade II (axonotmesis)** are the same; the highest/worst grade in each classification (neurotmesis) is also the same; the Sunderland classification inserts two additional grades between axonotmesis and neurotmesis.

Physiology

- In **axonotmesis** (Seddon and Sunderland II and above), **Wallerian degeneration** occurs—degeneration of axons distal to site of injury all the way to neuromuscular junction.
- Nerve regenerates from the site of injury distal, replacing tissue lost via Wallerian degeneration at **approximately 1 mm/d or 1 in/mo.**
  - Faster in children
  - Slower in smokers
- Budding axons are attracted to distal targets by neurotrophic factors and can successfully regrow if epineurium remains intact to provide structural framework and concentrated setting for neurotrophic factors.
- **Motor endplates degenerate after 18 months**, so consider nerve repairs or transfers during that window.
  - After endplates have degenerated, tendon transfers are the only option.

Diagnosis

- Explore penetrating injuries, lacerations immediately.
- EMG/NCS
  - Order 6 weeks after injury if no improvement
  - TEST TIP—No hard rule on when to order EMG/NCS, but need to wait at least 3 to 4 weeks for changes to occur; be wary of ordering EMG/NCS during acute period after nerve injury.
  - **Neurapraxia**—nerve will still conduct proximal and distal to injury because there is **no Wallerian degeneration**, but there may be slowing or conduction loss at injury site; EMGs will be essentially normal.
  - Axonotmesis and worse—no conduction at injury site or distal because of Wallerian degeneration distally; EMG—positive sharp waves and fibrillations
  - TEST TIP—EMG/NCS cannot differentiate between axonotmesis (Seddon II/Sunderland II) and worse injuries because Wallerian degeneration occurs in all such injury patterns; only advanced imaging or surgical exploration can differentiate.

Treatment

- Penetrating injuries/lacerations—explore, repair acutely
- Closed injuries
  - Observation initially
  - EMG/NCS at 6 weeks if no/minimal improvement
  - Continue observation with or without serial EMG/NCS if clinical or electrical improvement is occurring
  - Consider exploring closed injuries at approximately 6 months if no improvement
- Surgical treatment
  - Neuroma-in-continuity—controversial situation unlikely to appear on test; do not resect unless no hope for recovery
  - Complete transection
    - Primary **tension-free repair** when possible (Figure 4.66)
    - TEST TIP—All nerve repairs must be tension free; correct answer will never include a repair on tension or one in which a joint is bent to allow primary repair; transposition can be performed, but repair must still be tension free with joint fully extended.

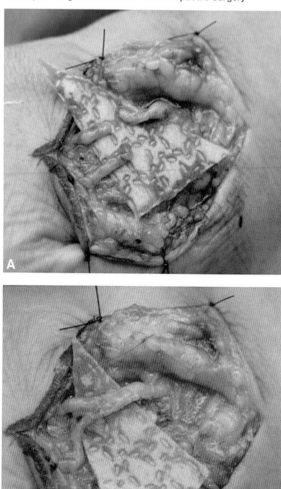

Figure 4.66 Laceration of the dorsal radial sensory nerve (A) and primary tension-free repair (B) (proximal is to the right in both images). Copyright © Ryan M. Zimmerman, MD, 2017.

- Fascicular matching for major nerves
- Deficits (Figure 4.67)
  - Nerve conduits for deficits ≤2 cm
  - Allograft for deficits ≤5 cm
  - Autograft for deficits >5 cm

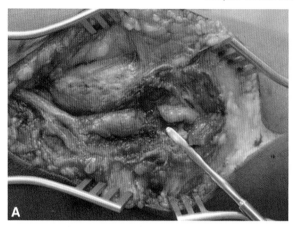

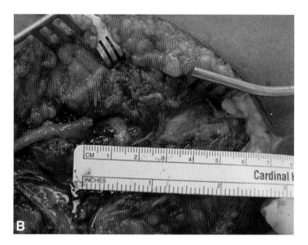

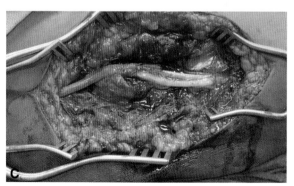

Figure 4.67 High ulnar nerve lesion at the level of the flexor carpi ulnaris motor branch in situ (A) and after neuroma resection and transposition (B). Autograft sural nerve cable grafting used to reconstruct the 5-cm deficit (C). Left is proximal in all images. Copyright © Ryan M. Zimmerman, MD, 2017.

NERVE TRANSFERS
General Considerations

- Nerve transfers—newer technique (Table 4.3)
- Many transfer options exist; only commonly accepted procedures are discussed below.
- Theory—use expendable nerve branches or expendable fascicles from within a nerve to provide source of healthy axons for injured nerve that has failed to regenerate or has low likelihood of regeneration (ie, high ulnar nerve laceration)
  - Fascicles should be identified intraoperatively using nerve stimulator before harvest.
- Transfers can be performed:
  - End to end
    - Involves cutting donor and recipient nerves, should be performed only when minimal chance of spontaneous recovery
    - Most transfers are performed end to end, especially for brachial plexus lesions that have not recovered spontaneously.
  - End to side
    - Donor nerve is cut distally and transplanted into an epineurotomy made along intact recipient nerve; this allows donor nerve to provide new axons while maintaining possibility of spontaneous recovery.
- Transfers can be performed instead of or in addition to primary repair.
- **Motor nerve transfers must be performed before motor endplates degenerate** (~18 months); after this period, only tendon transfers should be considered.
- All transfers follow the principle of donor distal, recipient proximal.
  - Obtain maximum length on the donor nerve
  - Transfer it to the recipient in a slightly proximal, tension-free manner

Shoulder Function Transfers

- Abduction—spinal accessory (cranial nerve XI) to suprascapular nerve, innervating supraspinatus and infraspinatus
- Abduction—triceps branch of radial nerve to anterior division of axillary nerve, innervating deltoid
- External rotation—triceps branch of radial nerve to axillary nerve branch to teres minor

Table 4.3 High-Yield Nerve Transfers

Purpose	Donor	Recipient	Note
Shoulder stabilization, abduction	Spinal accessory (CN XI)	Suprascapular	NA
Shoulder abduction	Triceps branch of radial	Axillary (anterior division)	NA
Elbow flexion	Ulnar FCU fascicle	Biceps branch of musculocutaneous	Oberlin transfer
Elbow flexion	Median FCR or FDS fascicle	Brachialis motor branch	Added to above to yield modified or dual Oberlin transfer
Intrinsic hand function	Anterior interosseous nerve	Ulnar nerve motor fascicle	Typically end-to-side

CN, cranial nerve; FCU, flexor carpi ulnaris; FCR, flexor carpi radialis; FDS, flexor digitorum superficialis; NA, not applicable.

Elbow Flexion Transfers

- Oberlin transfer—ulnar nerve FCU fascicle transferred to biceps motor branch of musculocutaneous nerve
- Modified Oberlin/dual transfer (Figure 4.68)
  - Ulnar nerve FCU fascicle to biceps motor branch
  - Median nerve FCR or FDS fascicle to brachialis motor branch
- Intrinsic hand function—pronator quadratus branch of the AIN to the ulnar nerve motor branch (Figure 4.69)
  - Typically performed end to side for a high ulnar nerve lesion

Sensory Nerve Transfers

- Typically performed in the hand to regain sensation in critical sensory zones, such as ulnar thumb and radial IF, to create a sensate pinch
- Less critical digital nerves (ie, those to ring or small finger) or branches of the radial sensory nerve are transferred to critical areas, typically median nerve sensory deficits following high median nerve injuries.

ULNAR-SIDED WRIST PAIN

TFCC Tears

- Anatomy and function
  - **TFCC**
    - Triangular fibrocartilage proper (articular disc)
      - Deep and superficial fibers

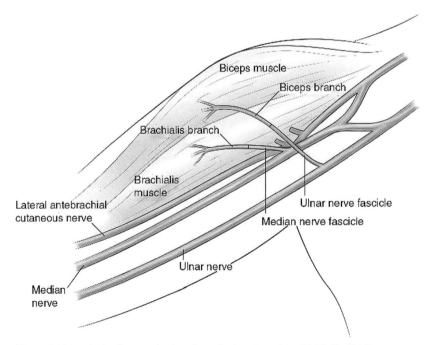

Figure 4.68 Dual Oberlin transfer for elbow flexion. From Lee SK, Wolfe SW. Nerve transfers for the upper extremity: new horizons in nerve reconstruction. *J Am Acad Orthop Surg.* 2012;20(8):506-517.

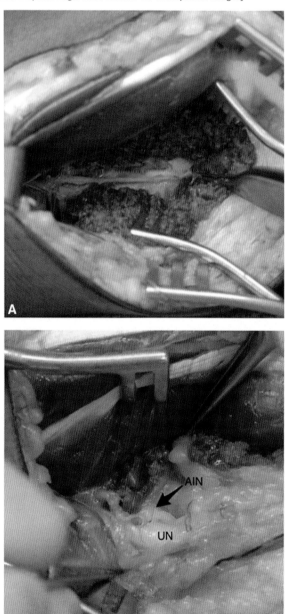

Figure 4.69 Anterior interosseous nerve (AIN) being dissected from the pronator qua-dratus (A) for end-to-side transfer to the ulnar motor branch (B). This nerve transfer was performed for the same patient in Figure 4.67 during the same operation as the nerve grafting. Proximal is left in both images. UN, ulnar nerve. Copyright © Ryan M. Zimmer-man, MD, 2017.

- Meniscus homolog
- Ulnar collateral ligament
- Dorsal radioulnar ligament
  - Tightens during pronation
- Volar radioulnar ligament
  - Tightens during supination
- ECU subsheath
- Blood supply
  - **Red zone**—peripheral 10% to 40% rich blood supply; good healing
  - **White zone**—central, avascular; poor healing response
- Function
  - Cushions ulnar carpus
  - DRUJ stabilizer
- Evaluation
  - Symptoms
    - Ulnar-sided wrist pain
    - Mechanism—hyperpronation and axial loading
    - Pain with terminal forearm/wrist ROM, often with associated "clicking"
  - Examination
    - Inspection
    - Palpation
    - ROM; pronation, supination, flexion, and extension of the wrist; reproducible "clicking"
    - **Provocative maneuvers**
      - Fovea sign—foveal tenderness between ulnar styloid and FCU tendon
      - "Shucking" test—dorsal-volar force applied to ulnar head in neutral, pronation, and supination
      - Press test—ulnar-sided pain while pushing off of table with affected wrist
  - Imaging
    - Radiography—often negative
    - **MRI/MR arthrography most sensitive/specific** for TFCC tears (Figure 4.70)
    - **Arthroscopy; gold standard**
- **Classification** (Table 4.4)

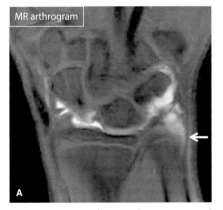
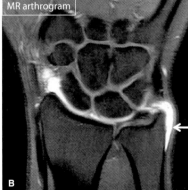

Figure 4.70 Coronal magnetic resonance arthrography (A) with dye extravasation (B) medial to ulna indicating a peripheral triangular fibrocartilage complex tear. Arrows show dye at ulnocarpal joint. MR, magnetic resonance. From Chhabra A, Demehri S, Soldatos T. The wrist. In: Chhabra A, Soldatos T, eds. *MRI Structured Evaluation: How to Practically Fill the Reporting Checklist*. Philadelphia, PA: Wolters Kluwer Health; 2015:245-294.

Table 4.4 Palmer Classification

Type	Class I: Traumatic	Class II: Degenerative (Ulnocarpal Abutment Syndrome)
A	Central perforation	TFCC wear
B	Ulnar avulsion with or without distal ulnar fracture	TFCC wear and lunate and/or ulnar chondromalacia
C	Distal avulsion	TFCC perforation and lunate and/or ulnar chondromalacia
D	Radial avulsion with or without sigmoid notch fracture	TFCC perforation and lunate and/or ulnar chondro-malacia and lunotriquetral ligament perforation
E	NA	TFCC perforation and lunate and/or ulnar chondro-malacia and lunotriquetral ligament perforation and ulnocarpal arthritis

NA, not applicable; TFCC, triangular fibrocartilage complex.

- Treatment
  - Nonoperative—splinting, nonsteroidal anti-inflammatory drugs, steroid injections, therapy
  - Arthroscopic debridement—type 1A and some 1D tears
  - Arthroscopic repair
    - Outside-in versus inside-out
    - Types 1B and 1C in "red zone," some 1D

Ulnocarpal Impaction

- Anatomy and function
  - Neutral variance—18% to 20% of axial load transmitted through the ulnocarpal joint; 42% with +2.5-mm variance and 4.3% to 6% with −2.5-mm variance
  - Inverse relationship between ulnar variance and TFCC thickness
- Evaluation
  - Symptoms
    - Chronic, progressive presentation
    - Ulnar-sided wrist pain
  - Examination
    - Ulnocarpal stress test—wrist pronation and supination with maximum ulnar deviation and axial loading reproduces ulnar-sided pain
    - Tenderness distal to ulnar head and volar to ulnar styloid
  - Imaging
    - Radiography
      - Ulnar variance: posteroanterior radiograph of the wrist in neutral
      - Pronated grip view: dynamic ulnar-positive variance
      - Cystic change in ulnar head or lunate (Figure 4.71)
    - MRI
      - Increased signal intensity in ulnar head or lunate on T2
  - Classification
    - Palmer class II injuries (see Table 4.4)
- Treatment
  - Nonoperative initially
  - **Ulnar shortening osteotomy**
    - Can shorten ulna >2 mm
    - Junction of middle and distal third ulna

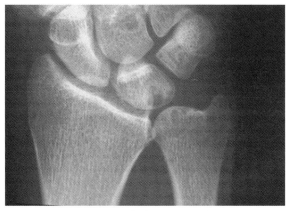

Figure 4.71 Posteroanterior wrist radiograph showing cystic lesions in the lunate and ulnar head that can be seen in ulnocarpal abutment syndrome. From Rayhack JM. Ulnar carpal abutment—ulnar shortening osteotomy. In: Cooney WP III, ed. *The Wrist: Diagnosis and Operative Treatment.* 2nd ed. Philadelphia, PA: Lippincott Williams & Wilkins; 2010:908-919.

- Tensions and stabilizes ulnar-sided wrist ligaments; prevents dorsal ulnar subluxation
- Limited by potential for DRUJ incongruity
  - Peak loads increase proportionally to the degree of shortening.
  - Complications
    - **Nonunion—smoking and diabetes**
    - Plate prominence
- **Wafer resection**
  - Open or arthroscopic
  - Limited to 2 to 3 mm of the distal ulnar dome

ECU Subluxation and Tendonitis

- ECU anatomy and function
  - Sixth extensor compartment
  - Wrist ulnar deviator and extensor, as well as static and dynamic stabilizers
- Evaluation
  - Tendonitis: chronic overuse or idiopathic injury
  - Subluxation: acute trauma or chronic attenuation of the sheath
  - Subluxation typically volar and ulnar
  - Symptoms
    - Ulnar-sided wrist pain
    - Numbness in the distribution of the dorsal ulnar sensory nerve
  - Examination
    - Pain or crepitation with palpation/rolling of the tendon
    - Pain with resisted ulnar deviation
    - **ECU synergy test**—distinguish tendon versus Intra-articular pathology
    - ECU subluxation—visible or palpable
  - Imaging
    - Radiography—rule out other pathology
    - MRI—tendinopathic changes
    - Ultrasonography—subluxation of ECU tendon
- Treatment
  - Nonoperative
  - ECU tendonitis; sixth dorsal compartment release

- ECU subluxation
  - Primary subsheath repair; acute cases
  - Subsheath reconstruction; extensor retinaculum sling

Lunotriquetral Ligament Injuries

- Anatomy and function
  - **Lunotriquetral interosseous ligament (LTIL)**
    - Dorsal
    - Membranous
    - **Volar (strongest)**
  - LTIL deficiency—**volar intercalated segment instability (VISI)** pattern
- Evaluation
  - Mechanism—dorsal force to a palmar-flexed wrist
  - Can occur with perilunate injury
  - Examination
    - Painful snap with ulnar deviation, pronation, and axial compression
    - Triquetrum ballottement
    - Kleinman shear test
  - **Imaging**
    - Radiography—**VISI** deformity (SL angle <30°) in dissociative injuries (ie, direct LTIL tear, as well as tear of secondary stabilizers); decreased SL angle; increased capitolunate angle (Figure 4.72)

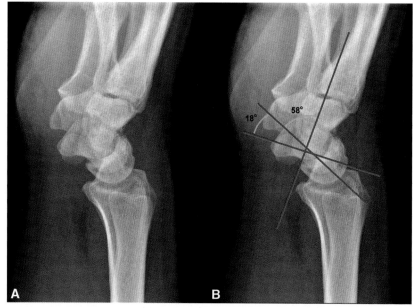

Figure 4.72 A, Lateral wrist radiograph showing a decreased scapholunate angle and increased capitolunate angle. Volar intercalated segment instability deformity involves excessive extension of the scaphoid and excessive flexion of the lunate (this is opposite the deformity seen in more common dorsal intercalated segment instability deformity). B, Lines drawn to measure scapholunate and capitolunate angles. From Greenspan A, Beltran J. Upper limb III: distal forearm, wrist, and hand. In: *Orthopedic Imaging: A Practical Approach*. 6th ed. Philadelphia, PA: Wolters Kluwer Health; 2015:203-267.

- Dynamic radiography—ulnar deviation and clenched-fist views show dynamic deformity in nondissociative (ie, LTIL only) injury.
  - MRI—unreliable
  - Arthroscopy—gold standard
- Viegas classification
  - 1: Partial or incomplete tear without VISI deformity
  - 2: Complete tear with palmar ligament injury and dynamic VISI
  - 3: Complete tear with palmar and dorsal ligament injury and static VISI
- Treatment
  - Nonoperative
  - Arthroscopic debridement—partial tear without instability
  - Ulnar shortening osteotomy: chronic tear with ulnar-positive variance
  - Reduction and pinning with or without ligament repair or reconstruction—acute complete tears with instability
  - Lunotriquetral (LT) fusion—chronic tears

CONGENITAL CONDITIONS

Genetics and Embryology of Hand Formation

- **4th to 8th week**—early upper limb development
  - Limb bud outgrowth
    - *HOX* gene
    - **Fibroblast growth factor (FGF)** determines mesoderm outgrowth.
    - *TBX5*
  - Patterning in three axes
    - Proximodistal, **apical ectodermal ridge (AER)**—laboratory removal of AER or FGF results in limb truncation.
    - Anteroposterior (radioulnar), **zone of polarizing activity (ZPA)**—relies on *SHH*
    - Dorsoventral, *WNT7A*
  - Increased growth and cell differentiation

Classifications

- Swanson
  - International Federation of Societies for Surgery of the Hand, 1976
  - Limited understanding of limb development
- Oberg, Manske, and Tonkin, 2013—embryology-based classification system

Syndactyly

- Failure of apoptosis
- Classification
  - Incomplete
  - Complete
  - Simple
  - Complex
  - Complicated
    - Transverse phalanges
    - Symphalangism
    - Apert—craniosynostosis
- Treatment
  - Surgery
    - Skin separation
    - Web reconstruction with full-thickness skin grafts (FTSGs)
    - Nail separation

- Early release of border digits
- Staged release of central digits
- Complications
  - Creep
  - Graft loss
  - Keloids
  - Nail deformity

Polydactyly

- Postaxial
  - Most common in African Americans
  - Often autosomal dominant (AD)
  - Classification
    - Type A—well-formed with bony articulation
    - Type B—rudimentary digit
  - Treatment
    - Type A—excision and reconstruction
    - Type B—ligation or excision
- Preaxial
  - **Wassel classification**
    - **Type 4, duplicated proximal phalanx—most common** (Figure 4.73)
  - Surgery
    - Excise smaller digit
    - Reconstruct
      - Stabilize collateral ligament
      - Centralize tendons
      - Corrective osteotomy
    - Complication—zigzag deformity

Radial Dysplasia

- Classification—Bayne and Klug (Table 4.5)
- Associations
  - **VACTERL**
    - **V**ertebral anomalies, **a**nal atresia, **c**ardiac abnormalities, **t**rache**o**esophageal fistula, **r**enal anomalies, and **l**imb anomalies
    - Autosomal recessive (AR)/complex inheritance
  - Holt-Oram
    - AD inheritance

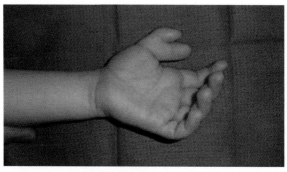

Figure 4.73 Wassel type 4 preaxial polydactyly.

Table 4.5 Bayne and Klug Classification of Radial Longitudinal Deficiency

Type	Definition	Description
I	Short distal radius	Distal radial epiphysis present but delayed; little radial deviation; thumb hypoplasia almost always present
II	Hypoplastic radius	Growth defective in proximal and distal radial epiphyses; radius in miniature
III	Partial absence of the radius	Defect can be proximal, middle, or distal third, but most frequently proximal; hand is radially displaced; wrist is unsupported
IV	Total absence of the radius	Most common type; hand is often severely radially displaced

Data from Bayne LG, Klug MS. Long-term review of the surgical treatment of radial deficiencies. *J Hand Surg.* 1987;12(2):169-179.

- Fanconi anemia
  - AR/X-linked inheritance
- Thrombocytopenia-absent radius syndrome
  - AR inheritance
- Other syndromes
- Treatment
  - None
  - Stretching and splinting
  - Surgery
    - Indications
      - Failed nonoperative treatment
      - Marked wrist angulation
    - Types 0, I, II
      - Tendon transfers and rebalancing
    - Types III, IV—most common
      - Centralization
      - Radialization
      - Preoperative soft-tissue distraction
      - Microvascular procedures

Thumb Hypoplasia

- Classification
  - Blauth (Figure 4.74)
    - I: Minor hypoplasia; all elements present
    - II: Normal skeleton, although there may be narrowness of MC shaft; first web space adduction contracture with adducted MC; MCP joint collateral ligament laxity; thenar muscle hypoplasia/aplasia
      - Lister modification
        - IIA: uniaxial instability
        - IIB: multiaxial instability
    - III: Skeletal hypoplasia with aplasia of the proximal MC and aplasia of the CMC joint; variable absence of radial carpal bones; significant hypoplasia; thenar muscle aplasia; extrinsic tendon abnormalities
      - IIIA: up to proximal one-third of MC is missing.
      - IIIB: up to proximal two-thirds of MC is missing.
      - IIIC: less than distal one-third of MC is present.
    - IV: Absent MC with rudimentary phalanges; pouce flottant (floating thumb)
    - V: Total absence of thumb

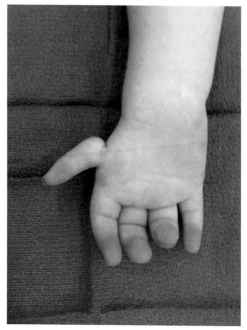

Figure 4.74 Type 4 thumb hypoplasia—pouce flottant.

- Treatment
  - Nonoperative
  - Types II to IIIA
    - MCP joint stabilization
    - First web deepening
    - Opposition tendon transfers
  - **Types IIIB to V**
    - **Pollicization**
    - Contraindicated
      - Stiff IF
      - Ulnar grasp pattern

Ulnar Dysplasia

- Rare
- Sonic hedgehog (*SHH*) deficiency
- Lower limb deficiencies
- Oligodactyly, syndactyly, first web deficiency, poor elbow function
- Classification—Bayne (see Table 4.5)
- Treatment
  - None
  - Excision of ulnar anlage
  - Radial osteotomy
  - First web reconstruction
  - Syndactyly reconstruction

Madelung Deformity

- *SHOX* **gene deletion**
  - Often idiopathic
  - **Short stature**
  - Leri-Weill dyschondrosteosis
- X chromosome
  - Sex-linked dominant
- Treatment
  - Vicker ligament resection
  - Corrective osteotomy

Symbrachydactyly

- Subclavian artery insult
- Distal ectoderm preserved
- Unilateral
- Classification
  - Short finger
  - Atypical cleft
  - Monodactylous
  - Peromelic
- **Associations—Poland anomaly**
- Treatment
  - Syndactyly reconstruction
  - Web space deepening
  - Lengthening
  - Nonvascularized toe phalanx transfer
  - Microvascular toe transfer

Constriction Band Syndrome

- Variable
- **Acrosyndactyly**
- Associations
  - Clubfoot
  - Leg length discrepancy
  - Cleft lip and palate
- Treatment
  - Nonoperative
  - Operative
    - Constriction band excision
    - Syndactyly reconstruction
    - Toe-to-hand transfer

Camptodactyly

- PIP joint contracture
- Most common—small finger
- **Abnormal attachments of lumbrical or flexor tendons**
- Treatment
  - Stretching and splinting
  - Surgery

Clinodactyly

- Coronal plane deviation (Figure 4.75)
- Most common—small finger middle phalanx
- Surgery

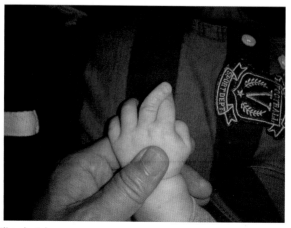

Figure 4.75 Clinodactyly.

Trigger Finger

- **Abnormal relationship between flexors**
- Treatment
  - Stretching and splinting
  - Excise FDS slip, A1 pulley release

Trigger Thumb

- Flexed IP joint
- Bilateral 25%
- Notta node
- **Treatment—A1 pulley release**

REPLANTATION

- Evaluation
  - Mechanism
  - Patient factors
    - Age
    - Comorbidities
    - Tobacco
  - **Ischemia time**—Digits tolerate longer ischemia time because of absence of muscle.
    - Warm ischemia
      - Digits (distal to carpus): 8 to 12 hours
      - Limb (proximal to carpus): 4 to 6 hours
    - Cold ischemia
      - Digits (distal to carpus): 24 to 30 hours
      - Limb (proximal to carpus): <12 hours
    - Amputated parts—wrap in moistened saline gauze, then place in ice
- **Indications**
  - Single digit distal to FDS insertion
  - Thumb, any level
  - Multiple digits
  - Midpalm
  - Wrist or proximal

- Child any level
- Mechanism—sharp associated with better outcomes
- **Contraindications**
  - Single digit proximal to FDS insertion
  - Patient factors
    - Elderly
    - Vascular disease
    - Medically unstable
    - Active psychosis
  - Crush, avulsive, contaminated, or segmental mechanism
- Technique
  - **Structure-by-structure** technique for multiple digits
  - Priority—thumb > long > ring > small > index
  - Order of structures **macro before micro**
    - Debridement of parts
    - Identification of structures
    - Bones
    - Extensors
    - Flexors
    - Nerves (before or after vessels)
    - Arteries—reverse vein graft if tension-free repair not possible
    - Veins
    - Closure—loose with no constrictive dressings
- Postoperative period
  - Warm environment
    - Warming blanket
    - Ambient temperature >27°C
  - Avoid vasoconstriction
    - Pain control
    - Anxiolytics
    - No caffeine
  - Monitoring
    - Appearance—color, turgor, capillary refill
    - Doppler pulses
    - Fingerstick
      - Brisk red—well-perfused digit
      - Sluggish purple—congestion
      - No return—arterial insufficiency
    - Thermometry
    - Oxygen saturation monitoring
    - Laser Doppler flowmetry
  - Anticoagulation (controversial)
- Complications
  - Acute
    - Arterial insufficiency, 0 to 24 hours
      - Release constrictive dressings
      - Consider intravenous heparin
      - Sympathetic blockade
      - Operating room for exploration of anastomosis
      - Salvage rare with 4 to 6 hours of secondary ischemia time
        - Causes
          - Thrombus ("zone of injury"; unrecognized intimal injury)
          - Technical error
          - Repair under tension
    - Venous insufficiency, 24 to 72 hours

- **Leeches**
  - **Hirudin:** potent anticoagulant—continued venous egress after leech removed
  - Complications
    - Blood loss; monitor hemoglobin/hematocrit
    - Infection; *Aeromonas hydrophila*
      - ◆ Prophylaxis with fluoroquinolones
      - ◆ Children; sulfamethoxazole/trimethoprim, or ceftriaxone
  - Heparin pledgets
- Chronic
  - Cold intolerance
  - Myonecrosis—limb replantations proximal to carpus
  - Adhesions—**tenolysis** most common secondary procedure
  - Malunion
  - Infection

RING AVULSION

- Evaluation
  - Mechanism—digital degloving by catching of a ring by immovable object
  - Doppler pulses
  - Circumferential skin compromise: inadequate venous circulation
  - Injury typically more severe than appearance of the digit (Figure 4.76)
- Classification (Tables 4.6 and 4.7)
- Treatment
  - Revascularization/replantation
    - Indications—Kay I to IV (see Table 4.7)
    - Technique
      - Similar to replantation
      - Two veins repaired: better outcomes

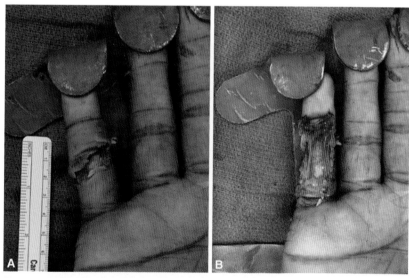

Figure 4.76 Ring avulsion injury with severe internal degloving (B) despite small superficial laceration (A).

Table 4.6 Urbaniak Classification of Ring Avulsion Injuries

Class	Injury	Treatment
I	Avulsion injury with adequate circulation	Standard bone and soft-tissue treatment
II	Incomplete avulsion with inadequate circulation	Revascularization
III	Avulsion injury with complete avulsion or amputation	Replantation or revision amputation

Table 4.7 Modified Kay Classification of Ring Avulsion Injuries

Class	Description
I	Circulation adequate, with or without skeletal injury
II	Arterial and venous circulation inadequate; no skeletal injury
II-A	Only arterial circulation inadequate
II-V	Only venous circulation inadequate
III	Arterial and venous circulation inadequate; fracture or joint injury present
III-A	Only arterial circulation inadequate
III-V	Only venous circulation inadequate
IV	Complete amputation
IV-P	Complete avulsion with amputation proximal to FDS insertion
IV-D	Complete avulsion with amputation distal to FDS insertion

FDS, flexor digitorum superficialis.
Data from Kay S, Werntz J, Wolff TW. Ring avulsion injuries: classification and prognosis. *J Hand Surg.* 1989;14(2 pt 1):204-213.

- Vein graft if large zone of injury
- Consider DIP joint fusion
  - Outcomes/complications
    - Survival rate: up to 66% reported in complete avulsion injuries
    - Success rate: without skeletal injury 91%, with skeletal injury 76%
    - Cold intolerance
- Revision amputation
  - Indications
    - Kay IV—proximal/distal injuries
    - Complete and severe degloving
  - Complications—Stump hypersensitivity

COMPARTMENT SYNDROME

- Anatomy
  - Ten compartments
    - Thenar
    - Hypothenar
    - Adductor pollicis
    - Four dorsal interossei
    - Three volar interossei
  - Carpal tunnel
  - Digital compartments
- Evaluation
  - Mechanism
    - Fracture
    - Bleeding disorder

- Reperfusion injury
- Constrictive dressing/casting
- Examination
  - Five Ps (pain, pallor, pulselessness, paralysis, paresthesia)
  - Pain out of proportion and pain with passive stretch most important
  - Pulselessness, paralysis are late findings
  - Tense, swollen compartments
  - Intrinsic minus
  - Pressure monitoring
    - $\Delta P > 30$ mm Hg (diastolic pressure − compartment pressure) diagnostic
    - Measurement taken from compartments that appear to be most involved
- Treatment
  - Serial examinations
    - $\Delta P < 30$
    - Concerning but nondiagnostic examination
  - Fasciotomy
    - High clinical suspicion or $\Delta P > 30$ mm Hg
    - Technique (Figure 4.77)
      - Release all involved compartments
      - Volar and dorsal interossei: released through longitudinal dorsal incisions over second and fourth MCs

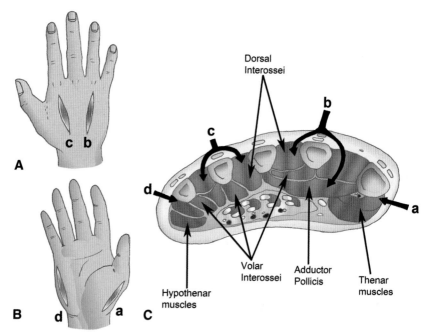

Figure 4.77 Fasciotomy technique for compartment syndrome of the hand. Dorsal hand incisions, centered over the second (c) and fourth (b) metacarpals, to release interossei (A), incisions to release the thenar (a) and hypothenar (d) compartments (B), and cross section illustrating hand compartment release (C). From Galez MG, Chang J. Upper extremity arterial reconstruction and revascularization distal to the wrist. In: Mulholland M, ed. *Operative Techniques in Surgery*. Vol 2. Philadelphia, PA: Wolters Kluwer Health; 2015:1894-1901.

- Thenar and hypothenar: longitudinal incisions at junction of glabrous and nonglabrous skin
- Open carpal tunnel release
- Complications
  - Ischemic contracture
    - **Intrinsic minus**
    - MCP joints extended, IP joints flexed (Figure 4.78)
  - Loss of function

SOFT-TISSUE COVERAGE

- Indicated for structures that require overlying vascularized tissue—bone, nerve, tendon, ligament, joint capsule

Reconstructive Ladder

- Primary closure
- Secondary intention
  - Consider if no exposed bone, tendon, nerve
  - **Defect $\leq$1 cm^2**
  - Skin grafts
    - Nutrition derived via diffusion (no exposed tendon, nerve, bone, vessel—paratenon acceptable)
    - Fail via shear stress and hematoma
      - Split-thickness skin graft (STSG)—contraindicated over joints and web spaces because of contracture
      - FTSG
        - Superior sensation
        - Less contraction
  - Random flaps
    - Fed by microcirculation and anomalous vessels
    - Length-to-width ratio 1:1
      - Random local flap—mobile donor tissue adjacent to defect
      - Distant random flap—if local tissue cannot support local flap
    - Parasitic manner: cross-finger flap, groin flap, chest/abdominal flaps
  - Axial pattern flaps
    - Single named arteriovenous pedicle running along flap axis
    - Predictable blood supply
    - Length-to-width ratio >2:1
      - Axial pattern local flaps (Figure 4.79)
      - Distant axial pattern flaps

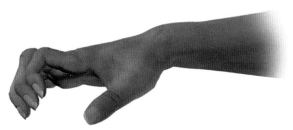

Figure 4.78 Intrinsic minus hand with metacarpophalangeal extension and interphalangeal joint flexion. From Cannada LK. Forearm injuries. In: Brinker MR, ed. *Review of Orthopaedic Trauma*. 2nd ed. Philadelphia, PA: Lippincott Williams & Wilkins; 2013:314-322.

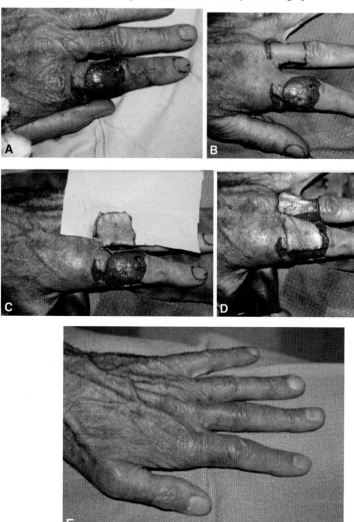

Figure 4.79 A, Wound with exposed tendon. B, Axial flag fasciocutaneous flap. Pedicle: dorsal branches of palmar proper digital artery with flap elevated (C) and flap rotated to cover the deficit (D). E, Donor site covered with full-thickness skin graft.

- · Groin, hypogastric artery (Figure 4.80)
  · "Island flap"
- Free tissue transfer or "free flap" (Figure 4.81, Table 4.8)
  - Pedicle transected and re-anastomosed
    - Fasciocutaneous
    - Fascia
    - Muscle
- Perforator flaps—Perforating musculocutaneous vessel dissected until adequate pedicle length or size.

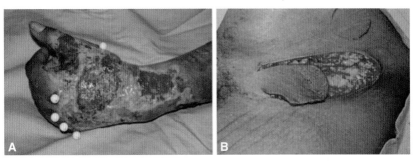

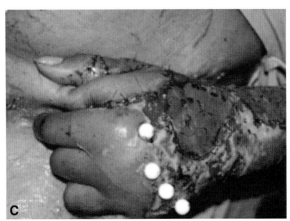

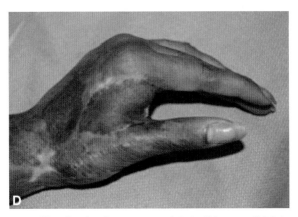

Figure 4.80 A, Dorsal hand and web space wound. B, Pedicle: superficial circumflex iliac artery. C, Postoperative photograph. D, Five months after separation.

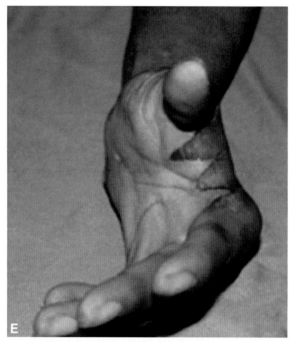

Figure 4.80 (*continued*) E, Four-flap Z-plasty with 90° cuts widens web space by 100%.

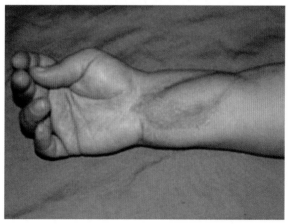

Figure 4.81 Distal forearm wound after coverage with free ipsilateral lateral arm flap and split-thickness skin graft (STSG). Pedicle: posterior radial collateral artery.

Table 4.8 Commonly Tested Vascular Pedicles

Flap	Vascular Supply	Coverage Indication
Flag	Anastomosis between dorsal metacarpal artery and proper digital artery	Volar aspect of adjacent or ipsilateral digit; dorsal aspect of adjacent digit
First dorsal metacarpal artery	First metacarpal artery	Dorsal thumb coverage
Posterior interosseous artery	Posterior interosseous artery	Wrist, dorsal hand/thumb
Radial forearm	Radial artery	Arm, dorsal hand, head/neck
Lateral arm	Posterior branch of radial collateral artery	Arm, dorsal hand
Latissimus	Thoracodorsal artery	Shoulder/arm/elbow
Serratus	Subscapular artery	Shoulder/upper arm
Gracilis	Medial femoral circumflex artery	Most common free muscle transfer, used at many sites
Groin	Superficial iliac circumflex artery	Hand/arm (as axial flap)
Anterolateral thigh	Descending branch of lateral femoral circumflex artery	Forearm and elbow (as free flap)
Medial gastrocnemius	Medial sural artery	Medial/midline proximal one-third tibia
Soleus	Posterior tibial artery medially, peroneal artery laterally	Middle one-third tibia

Hand Coverage

- Fingertip coverage
  - Homodigital
    - V-Y: creates sensate tissue coverage in transverse or volar fingertip defects
      - Atasoy (V-Y)
      - Kutler (lateral V-Y)
    - **Moberg (thumb):** indicated for volar soft-tissue defects or transverse amputations distal to the thumb IP joint; replaces distal defect with sensate, glabrous skin
  - Heterodigital: indicated for volar defects of the middle and distal phalanges
    - Cross-finger
    - Reverse cross-finger
  - **Thenar flap:** indicated for fingertip injuries with exposed bone or extensive pulp loss; **risk of contracture** in patients aged >30 years
  - Axial regional flaps
    - Dorsal MC artery: used for dorsal thumb coverage, including exposed bone (nerve can be mobilized with the artery)
    - Reverse dorsal MC artery
  - Defects proximal to the MCP joint
    - Radial forearm flap (Figure 4.82)
    - Reverse posterior interosseous artery flap
  - Addressing contractures in the hand
    - Z-plasty—two 60° flaps **lengthen approximately 75%**
    - FTSG preferable to STSG.
- Dorsal and palmar finger coverage (middle or proximal phalangeal level)
  - Cross-finger flap
  - Reverse cross-finger flap
  - Flag flap

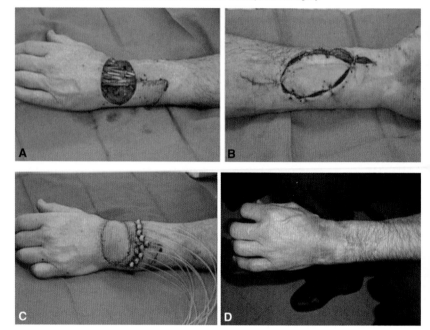

Figure 4.82 A, Sarcoma incision. B, Radial forearm flap raised, but not yet rotated/inset. Pedicle: distally based radial artery. C, After rotation of flap into defect with brachytherapy tubes. D, Twenty-two months postoperatively.

- Dorsal hand coverage
  - Primary closure
  - FTSG
  - Rotational flap (rhomboid fasciocutaneous)
  - Regional rotational flap (radial artery free, posterior interosseous)
  - Free flap (lateral arm, radial artery, groin)
  - Parasitic random flap (groin or abdominal)

VASCULAR DISEASE

- Glomus tumor (Figure 4.83)
  - Temperature-sensitive benign tumor at tip of digit or under the nail
  - Diagnosis—bluish color, pain; consider MRI
  - Treatment—marginal excision
- Hypothenar hammer syndrome (Figure 4.84)
  - Traumatic thrombosis of superficial palmar arch of ulnar artery
  - **Repetitive use** injury; mechanics, construction workers
  - *Treatment for thrombosis with aneurysm—excision and reconstruction with or without vein graft*
  - Treatment for thrombosis without aneurysm—endovascular fibrinolysis
- Raynaud syndrome (Figure 4.85)
  - Vasospastic disease with a underlying associated cause
  - Associated with scleroderma; lupus; dermatomyositis; RA; and **c**alcinosis, **R**aynaud phenomenon, **e**sophageal dysmotility, **s**clerodactyly, and **t**elangiectasia syndrome
  - **Triphasic color change**—white to blue to red

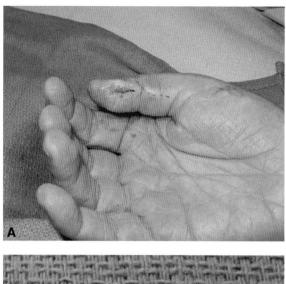

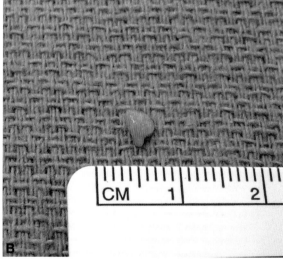

Figure 4.83 Glomus tumor (A) that was excised from the thumb (B).

- Treatment
  - Medical—calcium channel blockers, **botulinum injections**, biofeedback techniques
  - Surgical—digital sympathectomy
- Thromboangiitis obliterans **(Buerger disease)**
  - Small/medium vessel inflammatory disease
  - Prevalent in **smokers**
  - Imaging—*arteriography*

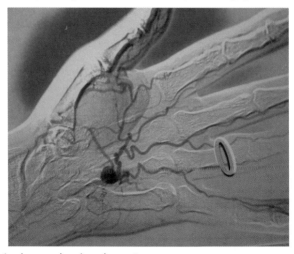

Figure 4.84 Angiogram showing ulnar artery aneurysm.

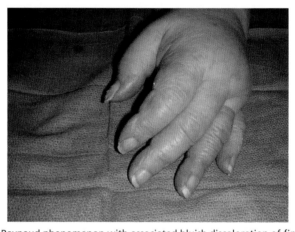

Figure 4.85 Raynaud phenomenon with associated bluish discoloration of fingers.

- Treatment
  - Medical—smoking cessation, vasodilators, aspirin
  - Surgical—sympathectomy, amputation
- Digital artery aneurysm (Figure 4.86)
  - False/pseudoaneurysms
    - Occur after traumatic penetration of vessel wall and replaced by organized hematoma and fibrous tissue
    - Sac-like appearance

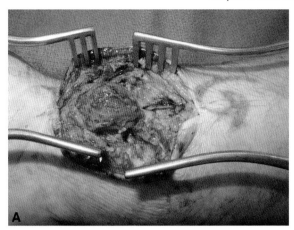

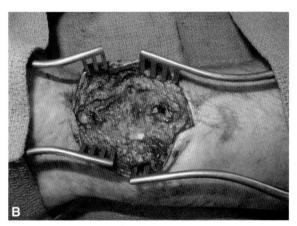

Figure 4.86 Radial artery aneurysm before (A) and after (B) excision.

- True aneurysm—blunt trauma to vessel that causes weakness in vessel wall and dilation
- Examination
  - Pulsatile mass
  - Most common in the thumb
- Treatment—surgical exploration and ligation versus repair with interpositional grafting

5 Trauma

POLYTRAUMA

- Cause of death
  - **50% central nervous system (CNS), most occur in the field**
  - 30% CNS within days
  - 20% **infection** and multisystem organ failure
- **Injury Severity Score (ISS)**
  - Sum of **square** of **highest** three Abbreviated Injury Scale scores for patient (Table 5.1)
  - ISS > 15 is polytrauma
  - Correlated with mortality and length of stay
- Glasgow Coma Scale (GCS)
  - See Table 5.2.
  - **Intubate if GCS is less than 8.**
- Shock
  - Blood loss
    - **Systolic pressure decreases after loss of 30% blood volume (class III blood loss) from 1500 to 2000 mL.**
    - **Tachycardia** occurs with class III blood loss.
    - Most common cause of shock in trauma patients is **hypovolemic shock.**
  - Lactate
    - Patient is in shock if **serum lactate is more than 2.5.**
    - **Elevated lactate correlates with mortality.**
  - Compensated shock: normal BP, urine output, improved with resuscitation by other measures, **but lactate more than 2.5**
- **FAST (focused assessment with sonography in trauma) examination**
  - **Accurate for intraperitoneal fluid, pericardial fluid, right upper quadrant, left upper quadrant, and pelvis**

Table 5.1 Abbreviated Injury Scale

Score	Description
0	None
1	Minor
2	Moderate
3	Serious
4	Severe
5	Critical
6	Maximal, possibly fatal

Table 5.2 Glasgow Coma Scale

			Score			
Parameter	**6**	**5**	**4**	**3**	**2**	**1**
Eye opening			Spontaneous	To voice	To pain	None
Verbal response		Oriented	Confused	Inappropriate	Incomprehensible	None
Motor response	Obeys command	Localizes pain	Withdraws from pain	Flexion to pain	Extension to pain	None

- Unreliable for retroperitoneal injury
- May not detect retroperitoneal hemorrhage
- Borderline patients: ISS > 40, ISS > 20 with thoracic trauma, hypothermia, large pulmonary contusion, bilateral femoral fractures, moderate or severe traumatic brain injury
- Damage control—external fixation is stabilization of fractures, and limited incision and drainage (I&D)/wound stabilization to assist in early resuscitation for borderline patients
  - Polytrauma patients have high physiologic inflammatory response 2 to 5 days following trauma.
  - **Nonessential operations should be avoided during this time to prevent "second hit" phenomenon, causing adult respiratory distress syndrome (ARDS) or multiple system organ failure.**
- Early total care
  - **Immediate long-bone surgery in the setting of polytrauma**
  - Fewer intensive care unit (ICU) days
  - Less ARDS for femur fracture patients in polytrauma
- **Elevated IL-6 predicts acute lung injury:** decrease pulmonary complications and ICU days

OPEN FRACTURE

- **Gustilo and Anderson classification**
  - Type I—minimal periosteal stripping; less than 1-cm wound
  - Type II—moderate periosteal stripping; >1cm wound
  - Type III—first generation cephalosporin
    - Type IIIa—significant periosteal stripping; wound closes at time of debridement
    - Type IIIb—significant periosteal stripping; wound does not close and requires free soft-tissue transfer
    - Type IIIc—significant soft-tissue wound with a vascular injury that requires repair
- Infection and nonunion increase with Gustilo grade.
- **Antibiotics based on Gustilo and Anderson classification**
  - **All open wounds warrant tetanus prophylaxis.**
  - **Type I—first-generation cephalosporin**
  - **Type II—first-generation cephalosporin**
  - **Type III—first-generation cephalosporin**
    - Addition of Zosyn is controversial.
    - **Addition of percutaneous nephrostomy for gram-negative exposure and soil contamination**
  - **Timing of antibiotics less than 1 hour after injury is greatest predictor of lack of infection.**
- Timing of surgery
  - There is no absolute rule on when an open fracture must go to the operating room (OR) for I&D.
  - **Consensus is that all open fractures should be irrigated and, more importantly, debrided within 24 hours.**
  - Grossly contaminated open fractures should be brought to the OR urgently, taking into account the patient's overall condition.
- **Best irrigation fluid is low pressure, high volume.**
  - High pressure irrigation is associated with deep penetration of contamination.
  - No additive value of antibiotics or Castile soap in irrigant fluid
  - Amputated part treatment: rinse, moist gauze, plastic bag over ice

BALLISTIC FRACTURE

- **High velocity (>2000 ft/s) versus low velocity (<2000 ft/s)**
- **Implication for injury pattern**

- Low-velocity gunshot wound (GSW) open fractures can be treated with local wound care, I&D in the ED, and closed treatment principles.
- **High-velocity GSW open fractures should be debrided in the OR with possible second-look surgery** to assess progression of normal-appearing tissue to death over 1 to 3 days.
- **Nerve injury/neuropraxia in the setting of GSW is usually caused by traction/ concussive injury and should be observed.**

COMPARTMENT SYNDROME

- **Definition**—high pressure inside closed tissue space leads to tissue necrosis (tissue pressure falls below critical level for perfusion)
- *Diagnosis—pain out of proportion, pain on passive stretch of the compartment*
- **Measurement**—in unreliable, anesthetized, and intoxicated patients, patients with distracting injuries and children
- **Timing of intervention**
  - *Compartment syndrome is a surgical emergency.*
  - Operative intervention should be performed prior to 6 hours of warm ischemia time to prevent nerve and muscle death.
- **Stryker monitoring**
  - ΔP = **diastolic pressure** − **measured pressure**
  - ΔP < **30 mm Hg means the patient has compartment syndrome.**
  - ΔP **more than diastolic pressure means the patient has compartment syndrome.**
- **Intervention**
  - Leg—two incisions, four-compartment fasciotomy
    - Look for superficial peroneal nerve overlying lateral and anterior compartments in distal lateral incision
    - Incomplete deep posterior compartment release is the most common incompletely released compartment.
  - Thigh—two incisions, three-compartment syndrome
  - Forearm
    - Three compartments—volar, dorsal, and mobile wad
    - Volar incision—release volar compartment and carpal tunnel

PELVIS AND ACETABULUM FRACTURE
Pelvic Fracture

- Anatomy
  - Ligaments
    - Pelvic floor ligaments
      - Sacrospinous
      - Sacrotuberous
    - **Posterior sacroiliac (SI) ligaments are the strongest.**
  - **Corona mortis: vascular anastomosis between obturator and external iliac/ femoral/inferior epigastric systems (most frequently venous)**
  - Nerves
    - **L5 nerve root lies on ala of S1 sacrum**
    - Most common (88%) course of sciatic nerve is anterior to piriformis muscle and posterior to obturator internus muscle.
    - Most common variant (11%) is split piriformis and split nerve.
  - Radiographic anatomy (Figure 5.1)
    - L5 nerve root on anterior sacrum axial image
    - **Lateral view of sacrum shows safe zone for iliosacral screws, avoiding L5 nerve root and S1, 2 nerve roots.**
    - Obturator outlet shows teardrop for low anterior external fixation frame.

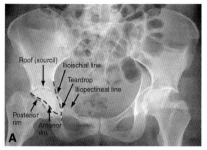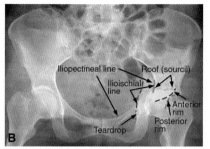

Figure 5.1 Anteroposterior pelvis radiographs showing the six cardinal lines (and their corresponding structures) as dashed lines on the uninjured (A) and fractured (B) sides of the pelvis. Red = ilioischial line (posterior column), dark blue = iliopectineal line (anterior column), purple = anterior rim (anterior wall), orange = posterior rim (posterior wall), green = roof (dome of acetabulum), and circle = teardrop (cotyloid fossa, section of quadrilateral surface and outer wall of obturator canal). From Ahn J, Reilly M, Lorich D, Helfet D. Acetabular fractures: acute evaluation. In: Schmidt A, Teague D, eds. *Orthopaedic Knowledge Update: Trauma 4*. Rosemont, IL: American Academy of Orthopaedic Surgeons; 2010:312.

- Radiographs
  - Anteroposterior (AP, Figure 5.2)
  - Inlet: detects rotational displacement and AP displacement
  - Outlet: detects cephalocaudal displacement
- Early management
  - **Binder**
    - Appropriate for pelvic fracture with other sources of bleeding that require surgery
    - **Any pelvic fracture with shock should have binder applied.**
    - Potential volume into which pelvic ring can bleed is proportional to fourth power of radius of true pelvis.
  - **Pelvic fracture in binder, still hypotensive and refractory to fluid and blood: definitive intervention is warranted**
    - **Laparotomy**
    - **Angiogram and embolization**

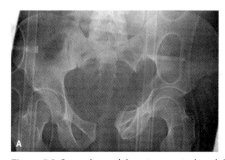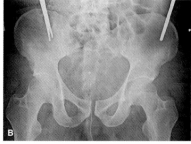

Figure 5.2 Screening pelvic anteroposterior plain radiographs demonstrate an unstable pelvic ring injury. A, The symphysis pubis and left sacroiliac joint are completely disrupted. Manual traction was applied to the left lower extremity and a circumferential pelvic sheet was placed around the patient and clamped. B, The reduction has been achieved. The injury sites mostly are concealed by the reduction. From Rout ML Jr. Pelvic fractures and acute management. In: Ricci WM, Ostrum RF, eds. *Orthopaedic Knowledge Update: Trauma 5*. Rosemont, IL: American Academy of Orthopaedic Surgeons; 2016:375-390.

- Posterior arterial bleed is usually superior gluteal artery.
- Anterior arterial bleed is usually obturator or pudendal artery.

- **Retrograde urethrogram required for:**
  - **Blood at urethral meatus**
  - High-riding prostate on rectal examination
  - Any clinical suspicion of genitourinary injury with pelvic fracture

- Interventions
  - Anterior fixation
    - External fixation
      - Iliac crest pins
      - Anterior inferior iliac spine (AIIS) pins (Hannover frame)
    - Open reduction and internal fixation (ORIF): symphysial plate
    - Anterior percutaneous screws: superior ramus screws
  - Posterior fixation
    - Iliosacral screws
      - Transiliac screws stronger
      - Two screws improve rotational stability
    - Posterior ORIF
      - Posterior transiliac fixation
      - Wound complications in 33% to 50%

- Fracture patterns (Figure 5.3)
  - **Lateral compression (LC)**
    - LC1
      - **Most common pelvic fracture pattern**
      - Almost always **nonoperative**

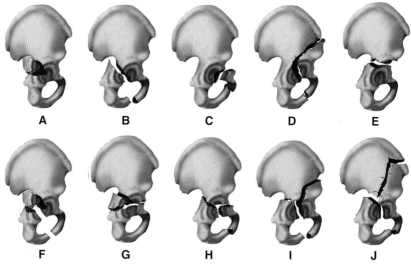

Figure 5.3 Classification of acetabular fractures according to Letournel. A, Posterior wall fracture. B, Posterior column fracture. C, Anterior wall fracture. D, Anterior column fracture. E, Transverse fracture. F, Associated posterior column and posterior wall fracture. G, Associated transverse and posterior wall fracture. H, T-shaped fracture. I, Associated anterior wall or column and posterior hemitransverse fracture. J, Both-column fracture. From Dickson KF. Fractures of the acetabulum. In: Brinker MR, ed. *Review of Orthopaedic Trauma.* 2nd ed. Philadelphia, PA: Lippincott Williams & Wilkins; 2013:224-243.

- Weight bearing as tolerated (WBAT)
- "BAD LC1" fractures: comminution through entire sacral fracture dissociating central sacrum from lateral iliac segment; posterior and anterior fixation indicated
  - LC2
    - Crescent fracture posteriorly
    - Closed treatment (rarely for undisplaced fractures) or anterior and posterior fixation
  - **LC3**
    - **Windswept pelvis**
    - **Anterior and posterior fixation**
    - **Associated head injury and abdominal injury is common.**
- Anterior posterior compression (APC)
  - APC1
    - Nonoperative
    - Less than 2.5-cm anterior symphysis displacement
  - APC2
    - More than 2.5-cm anterior symphysis widening; anterior SI ligaments are torn but posterior SI ligaments are intact
    - Anterior $\pm$ posterior fixation
  - APC3
    - Posterior SI ligamentous disruption; posterior displacement seen on outlet; may have associated vertical displacement
    - Anterior and posterior fixation
- Vertical shear
  - Rotationally and vertically unstable
  - Vertical displacement preset and best seen on outlet view
  - Anterior and posterior internal fixation
- Combined mechanism of injury: anterior and posterior internal fixation

Acetabulum Fracture

- Anatomy: **dome of acetabulum is equivalent to cephalad 10 mm of acetabulum**
- Radiographs
  - AP view
    - **Six acetabular lines**
      - **Ilioischial line**
      - **Iliopectineal line**
      - **Sourcils (eyebrow) = acetabular dome**
      - **Posterior wall line**
      - **Anterior wall line**
      - **Teardrop**
    - Roof arc angle of less than 45° (on AP view) means fracture is in dome of acetabulum.
  - **Obturator oblique**
    - **Anterior column**
    - **Posterior wall**
    - **Best view for spur sign**
  - **Iliac oblique**
    - **Posterior column**
    - **Anterior wall**
- Interventions
  - ORIF
    - Ilioinguinal approach
    - Stoppa approach
    - Posterior Kocher-Langenbeck approach

- Extended iliofemoral and extensile T approaches are associated with significant wound healing and infection complications.
- Percutaneous fixation
  - Indicated when reduction requirements for the individual patient can be achieved percutaneously, given risks of open operative intervention versus potential benefits of this long-duration surgery
  - May be adequate to achieve stabilization of acetabulum fractures to allow earlier mobilization than nonoperative treatment

- Fracture patterns
  - Elementary
    - **Anterior column**
      - **Obturator oblique radiograph shows best**
      - Computed tomography (CT) shows horizontal fracture line on axial view.
    - **Posterior column**
      - **Iliac oblique radiograph shows best**
      - Fracture through greater or lesser sciatic notch, or ischial spine
      - Fracture also through the obturator fossa/ring
      - CT shows horizontal fracture line on axial view.
    - Anterior wall
    - Posterior wall
      - Obturator oblique view
      - Marginal impaction on CT is operative indication
      - Superior wall fragment is more unstable.
      - **Poor outcome is common.**
    - **Transverse**
      - **Fracture through ilioischial and iliopectineal lines**
      - Transtectal (operative), juxtatectal, and infratectal (likely nonop) variants
  - Associated
    - Transverse fracture with a posterior wall component
      - Fracture through **ilioischial and iliopectineal lines**
      - Approach from posterior to address posterior wall fragment and column fractures
    - Posterior column with a posterior wall component
      - Posterior Kocher-Langenbeck approach
      - Femoral head is almost always medial on AP radiograph.
    - T-shaped
      - Fracture through **ilioischial and iliopectineal lines**
      - Fracture line through teardrop
      - Separate moving posterior and anterior segments
      - **May require anterior and posterior approaches if both are displaced**
    - Anterior column posterior hemitransverse: fracture through **ilioischial and iliopectineal lines**
    - Associated both -column
      - Fracture through **ilioischial and iliopectineal lines**
      - All acetabular cartilage is fractured off intact pelvis
      - Spur sign on obturator oblique x-ray
      - Secondary congruence (head is concentric to most acetabular fragments) may allow nonoperative treatment in patients unfit for surgery.

FEMUR FRACTURE
Femoral Head Fracture

- Anatomy
  - **Most blood supply in adult is through retinacular branches of superior gluteal artery (branch of medial femoral circumflex artery).**

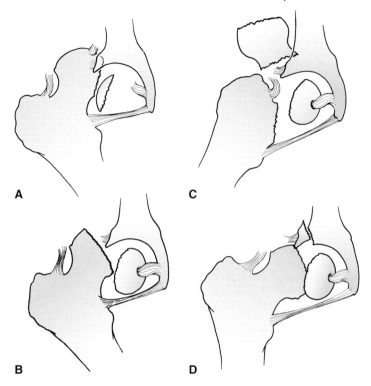

A   **C**

B   **D**

Figure 5.4 The Pipkin classification of dislocation with femoral head fractures: type I (A), type II (B), type III (C), and type IV (D). From Kain MS, Tornetta PT III. Hip dislocations and femoral head fractures. In: Tornetta PT III, Ricci WM, Ostrum RF, et al, eds. *Rockwood and Green's Fractures in Adults*. Vol 2. 9th ed. Philadelphia, PA: Wolters Kluwer; 2019:2181-2230.

- Pipkin classification (Figure 5.4)
  - Type I—fracture inferior to fovea
  - Type II—fracture superior to fovea
  - **Type III—type I or II *plus* femoral neck fracture: anterior surgical approach (high avascular necrosis [AVN] risk)**
  - Type IV—type I or II *plus* acetabulum fracture: posterior or surgical hip dislocation approach
- *Acute reduction of femoral head to prevent AVN*
- Intervention
  - Nonoperative for congruent stable joint with small fragment
  - Smith-Petersen approach
  - Surgical dislocation

Femoral Neck Fracture

- **30% 1-year mortality in elderly**
  - **Anatomy: most blood supply in adult is through retinacular branches of superior gluteal artery (branch of medial femoral circumflex artery).**

- Intervention
  - Subcapital (minimally displaced valgus impacted)
    - Do not attempt improved reduction
    - Percutaneous screw fixation with washers
    - Inverted triangle pattern
      - Inferior screw on calcar
      - Posterior screw on posterior cortex
      - **Screw starting point above lesser trochanter**
      - **Stress riser subtrochanter if below lesser trochanter**
  - Transcervical
    - **Nonunion and AVN are most related to quality of reduction, more than timing of surgery.**
    - Displaced young—ORIF (screws or fixed angle, depending on bone quality and fracture reduction stability)
    - **Displaced in physiologically old—hemiarthroplasty**
    - Displaced in intermediate age—consider total hip arthroplasty (THA) if young patient, especially with preoperative hip pain
      - Improved activity and pain
    - Tension side stress fractures must be fixed.
    - Compression side stress fractures may be nonoperative with toe-touch weight bearing.
  - Basicervical
    - **Low risk of AVN because extracapsular**
    - **Increased risk of rotational malreduction**
    - **May require derotational screw during internal fixation**
  - Vertical pattern/high Pauwels angle fracture
    - Vertical high-energy fracture pattern seen on AP radiograph or internal rotation view.
    - Susceptible to vertical shear and varus displacement
    - Requires perpendicular/fixed-angle fixation resisting fracture shear
  - **Femoral neck nonunion**
    - **Valgus creating intertrochanteric osteotomy and blade-plate fixation in physiologically young**
    - THA in older patient

Intertrochanteric Femoral Fracture

- Anatomy
  - Good blood supply to metaphyseal bone
  - Good fracture interference/stability
- Fracture patterns
  - Stable
    - Fixation with compression hip screw (CHS, lower cost) or cephalomedullary nail (less medialization)
    - **Tip–apex distance (TAD) less than 25 mm has cutout rate of 0%; cutout rate increases with increasing TAD.**
  - Unstable—do not resist postoperative CHS sliding displacement
    - Fixation with cephalomedullary nail—medial calcar fracture/lesser trochanter fracture
    - Reverse obliquity
    - Subtrochanteric extension
    - Lateral greater trochanter comminution

Subtrochanteric Femoral Fracture (Figure 5.5)

- Anatomy
  - **Proximal fragment displacement**
    - Flexion—iliopsoas
    - External rotation—gluteus medius

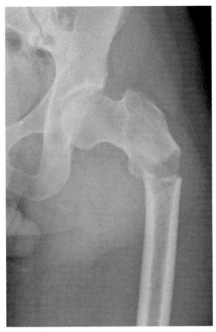

Figure 5.5 Subtrochanteric femoral fracture. From Achor TS. Subtrochanteric femur fractures. In: Mamczak CN, Smith CS, Gardner MJ, eds. *Illustrated Tips and Tricks for Intraoperative Imaging in Fracture Surgery*. Philadelphia, PA: Wolters Kluwer; 2018:187-200.

- • Abduction—gluteus medius
  - • Adduction of distal fragment into varus
  - • Results in apex anterior varus overall fracture deformity
- ● **Intervention**
  - • **Varus malreduction increases nonunion significantly.**
  - • Long fixed-angle internal fixation (blade plate, dynamic condylar screw, locking plate)
  - • Long intramedullary nail
  - • **Not CHS**
- ● Bisphosphonate-related hip fractures
  - • **Most commonly subtrochanteric**
  - • **Lateral cortical beaking on radiograph**
  - • Low-energy fracture
  - • Chronic stress fracture with thigh pain
  - • Bilateral thigh pain common—x-ray contralateral side and consider prophylactic treatment
  - • **Intramedullary (IM) fixation preferred**

Femoral Shaft Fracture

- ● Anatomy
  - • Blood supply through nutrient arteries and periosteal integrity
  - • 9% associated femoral neck fracture
  - • **One-third of associated femoral neck fractures are missed (avoid this through systematic evaluation).**

- Intervention
  - Reamed statically—interlocked intramedullary nail is **gold standard**
  - Plating (small diameter, short femur, excessive bow)
  - **Full weight bearing (WB) of statically locked nails**
  - Rotational malreduction increased by lateral surgical positioning
  - **Damage control external fixation if significant head injury, pulmonary injury, or lactate greater than 2.5 mmol/L**
  - Damage control external fix may be converted to nail within 2 to 3 weeks, otherwise should ORIF
  - Fat embolism and pulmonary embolism may occur during surgery.
  - **Rates of nonunion similar for antegrade and retrograde approaches in modern studies**
  - Rotational deformity
    - External rotation (ER) deformity is tolerated well than internal rotation (IR) deformity.
    - ER deformity common with supine nailing
    - IR deformity common with lateral nailing or fracture table

Distal Femoral Fracture (Figure 5.6)

- Anatomy
  - Trapezoidal shape of distal femur
  - Symptomatic hardware common if distal screws are equal or longer than medial cortex on AP x-ray
  - Apex posterior deformity common due to gastrocnemius origin on posterior distal segment
  - **Varus malreduction common due to fracture comminution and distal insertion of adductor muscles**
  - Hoffa coronal condylar fractures
    - Occur approximately one-third of distal intra-articular fractures
    - More common laterally
    - More common in open fractures
- Intervention
  - Anatomical ORIF of articular surface
  - Stable plate or nail fixation based on ability to provide distal fracture segment stability
  - Use of retrograde femoral nail possible if distal segment allows adequate stability with nail (usually two screws)
  - ORIF with locking screws in distal articular segment when bridge plating across metaphyseal comminution
  - Golf club deformity occurs with plate position too posterior on distal articular fragment
- **Nonunion**
  - **Increased with open fracture, comminution, bone loss, and malreduction (varus)**
  - **Soft-tissue technique and minimal fragment stripping important during ORIF**

PATELLA FRACTURE

- Minimally displaced
  - Nonoperative
    - **Less than 2-mm articular step/gap**
    - Vertical fractures
  - **Extensor mechanism should be intact (straight leg raise)**
  - WBAT with knee straight in cast/brace
  - Gradual progression to range of motion starting 4 to 6 weeks

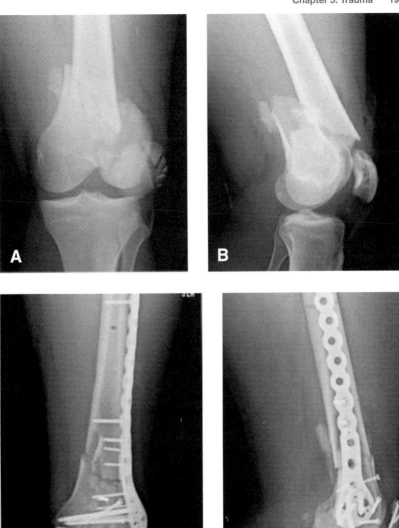

Figure 5.6 Anteroposterior (AP) (A) and lateral (B) radiographs demonstrate a distal femur fracture with articular involvement. Postoperative AP (C) and lateral (D) radiographs. The condylar block was repaired first, followed by plate application. From Avilucea FR, Archdeacon MT. Fractures of the distal femur. In: Ricci WM, Ostrum RF, eds. *Orthopaedic Knowledge Update: Trauma 5*. Rosemont, IL: American Academy of Orthopaedic Surgeons; 2016:493-506.

- Transverse displaced
  - ORIF with tension band technique
  - Cannulated screws may be used for longitudinal fixation with tension band wire (Figure 5.7).

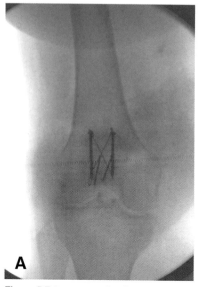 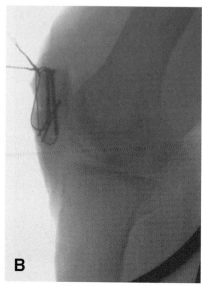

Figure 5.7 Intraoperative fluoroscopic anteroposterior (A) and lateral (B) images show a tension band construct using two cannulated screws with a tensioned wire passing through the cannulae of the screws. Note the intraosseous mini-fragment screws used to address a separate inferior fragment. These screws were placed initially, thus creating a simple transverse fracture pattern amenable to tension band fixation. From Jones T, Tucker MC. Patella fractures and extensor mechanism injuries. In: Ricci WM, Ostrum RF, eds. *Orthopaedic Knowledge Update: Trauma 5*. Rosemont, IL: American Academy of Orthopaedic Surgeons; 2016:5007-5022.

- **Symptomatic hardware common**
- **Less than 20% of inferior pole can be removed in combination with repair of patellar tendon to inferior patella (Figure 5.8).**
- Comminuted: cerclage wire commonly used in addition to other fixation

TIBIA FRACTURE

Tibial Plateau Fractures

- Anatomy
  - **High risk of compartment syndrome**
  - May be associated with knee dislocation
    - Vascular injury is present with ankle brachial index less than 0.9.
    - Document and follow neurovascular examination.
  - **50% risk of intra-articular cartilage/meniscal injury**
- Fracture patterns (Figure 5.9)
  - Schatzker I
    - **Simple split fracture**
    - **Lag screw ORIF**
  - Schatzker II
    - **Risk of associated lateral meniscus injury**
    - **ORIF direct articular visualization**
    - **Lateral buttress plate**
    - **Metaphyseal void filler: calcium phosphate best resistance to axial displacement**

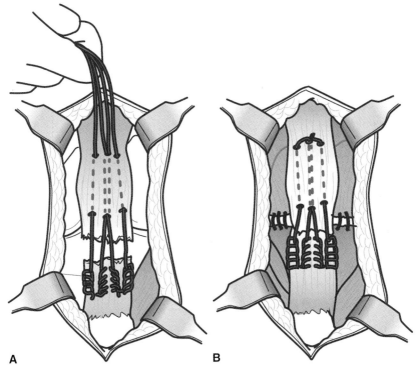

A   **B**

Figure 5.8 Drawings demonstrate the suture technique for a typical patellar tendon repair. A, Krackow style stitch has been placed in distal patellar tendon stump and subsequently passed through vertical drill holes placed in the patella. B, Final construct as sutures are tied securely at the superior pole of the patella. From Jones T, Tucker MC. Patella fractures and extensor mechanism injuries. In: Ricci WM, Ostrum RF, eds. *Orthopaedic Knowledge Update: Trauma 5*. Rosemont, IL: American Academy of Orthopaedic Surgeons; 2016:5007-5022.

- Schatzker III—anatomic joint reduction and stabilization
- Schatzker IV
  - Risk of vascular injury
  - Risk of ligamentous injury
  - Risk of peroneal nerve injury and more complex neurologic injury
  - Risk of compartment syndrome
- Schatzker V
  - Bicondylar fracture
  - High energy
- Schatzker VI
  - High risk of compartment syndrome
  - Temporary external fixation almost always required (Figure 5.10)
  - Lateral plate alone may increase risk of varus malunion or nonunion.
  - Posteromedial plate required for posterior medial coronal fracture patterns
- Intervention
  - Nonoperative if less than 3-mm articular step off and less than 10° of varus/valgus instability in full knee extension
  - Definitive fixation timing when soft tissues appropriate

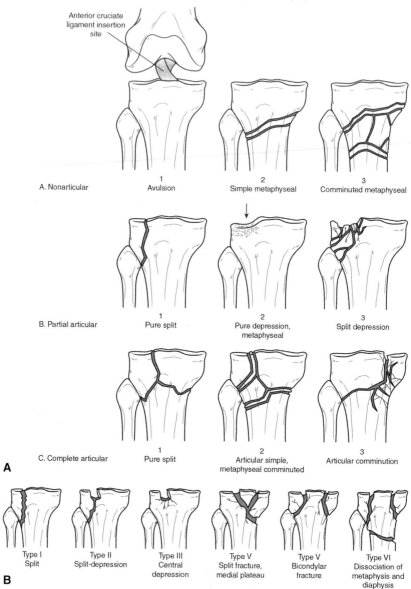

Figure 5.9 Chart demonstrates the two classifications systems that categorize fractures of the tibial plateau—the AO/Orthopaedic Trauma Association classification (A) and the Schatzker classification (B). From Zura R, Kahn M. Fractures of the tibial plateau. In: Ricci WM, Ostrum RF, eds. *Orthopaedic Knowledge Update: Trauma 5*. Rosemont, IL: American Academy of Orthopaedic Surgeons; 2016:533-550.

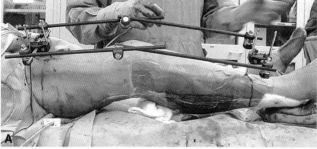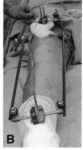

Figure 5.10 Intraoperative photographs of the lower extremity demonstrate a knee-spanning external fixation frame used to stabilize a bicondylar tibial plateau fracture with associated lower leg compartment syndrome. A, Lateral view of a spanning external fixator of the lower extremity. B, Frontal view of a spanning external fixator of the lower extremity.From Tejwani N, Polonet D, Wolinsky PR. External fixation of tibial fractures. *J Am Acad Orthop Surg.* 2015;23:126-130.

- Staged management of axially unstable patterns (Schatzker IV, V, VI)
  - Higher energy fractures
- Separate medial and lateral incisions for ORIF
- Locking screws are not needed for simple patterns (I-IV)

Tibial Shaft Fracture

- Anatomy
  - **Proximal third fracture deformity**
    - **Valgus**
    - **Apex anterior**
    - **Posterior displacement**
  - Distal third fracture varus deformity when fibula is intact
  - High-energy less stable fractures
    - Comminuted
    - Transverse
    - Fibula fracture at same level
- High association with compartment syndrome of the lower leg
- Intervention
  - **Closed management**
    - **2-cm shortening, 5° to 10° sagittal deformity, and 5° varus/valgus may be treated nonsurgically**
    - Varus displacement common if fibula intact
    - Long leg cast for rotational control converted to patellar tendon WB cast at 4 to 6 weeks
  - **Damage control external fixation**
    - Significant head injury, pulmonary injury, or lactate greater than 2.5 mmol/L
    - Damage control external fix may be converted to nail within 2 to 3 weeks, otherwise should ORIF
  - IM nail
    - Starting point immediately anterior to joint on lateral x-ray and just medial to lateral tibial spine on AP
    - There is a possible benefit of reaming in tibial fractures.
    - Interlocking screw breakage increases with screws smaller than 4 mm, and may be decreased with use of larger nails.
  - Plate fixation
    - Periprosthetic fractures
    - Locked plate for short periarticular fractures that do not allow stable rotational fixation with nail

- Blocking screws
  - Placed in short articular segment
  - **Placed on concave side of deformity**
  - Placed near fracture
  - Placed where you do not want the nail to go
  - Shaft should be reamed after blocking screw placement.

Distal/Pilon Fracture

- **Anatomy**
  - **Chaput fragment—reference for anatomic reduction when fibula is fixed first**
  - **Volkman fragment**
  - **Medial fragment**
  - **Articular impaction**
- Intervention
  - **Staged management is gold standard for test**
    - Primary external fixation, with or without fibular fixation
    - Staged ORIF when soft tissues allow
      - Articular ORIF
      - Realignment and stable fixation of articular block to shaft
  - **Tendency to varus displacement**
    - **Intact fibula**
    - **Lack of medial buttressing fixation**
  - Poor outcomes, despite anatomic reduction, common due to articular injury

ANKLE FRACTURE

- Anatomy
  - Bone
    - Medial malleolus
    - Lateral malleolus fibula
    - Posterior malleolus
  - Ligaments
    - Medial deltoid
    - Lateral
      - Anterior inferior tibiofibular ligament
      - Posterior inferior tibiofibular ligament
      - Interosseous ligament
    - Posterior malleolus origin of posteroinferior tibiofibular ligament
- Fracture patterns
  - **Lauge-Hansen classification**
    - **Supination–adduction**
    - **Supination–external rotation**
    - **Pronation–abduction**
    - **Pronation–external rotation**
  - Maisonneuve
    - Medial malleolus fracture
    - Syndesmosis disruption may not be obvious and requires **AP radiograph of tibia/fibula and stress examination.**
  - Bimalleolar and trimalleolar fractures are inherently unstable and require ORIF.
- Intervention
  - **Stress examination** is **required** to demonstrate syndesmosis stability if
    - Isolated medial malleolus fracture
    - Tibiotalar joint appears reduced on injury radiograph
  - ORIF fibula
    - One-third tubular plate is accepted standard
    - Lateral plate more symptomatic postop
    - Posterior plate associated with peroneal tendonitis

TALUS FRACTURE

- Anatomy
  - Blood supply contributions
    - Posterior tibial
    - Anterior tibial
    - Peroneal
  - **Primary blood supply through artery of tarsal canal**
- Fracture patterns
  - Hawkins I—neck minimally displaced
  - Hawkins II—neck fracture and subtalar dislocation
  - Hawkins III—neck fracture and tibiotalar dislocation
  - Hawkins IV—Hawkins II or III plus talonavicular dislocation
- Intervention
  - **Talar neck**
    - **Most biomechanically stable fixation is posterior to anterior lag screws**
    - **Medial and lateral ORIF**
  - Talar body—exposure increased through medial malleolus osteotomy
  - **Body AVN increases with increasing complexity and malreduction**

CALCANEUS FRACTURE

- Anatomy
  - Fracture patterns
    - Tongue type—tuberosity attached to significant articular fragment
    - **Intra-articular (Sanders classification based on semicoronal CT reconstruction at posterior facet)**
  - **Medial sustentaculum is anchor for internal fixation—Constant fragment**
  - Thin, soft tissues with limited blood supply leads to ORIF complications.
- Intervention
  - **Nonoperative**
    - **Böhler angle greater than 0°**
    - **Minimal comminution**
    - **Associated with subtalar arthritis, subfibular impingement, wide heel with poor shoe wear, pain**
  - Percutaneous
  - ORIF
    - **Extended lateral approach**
      - **Follows vascular supply to soft tissues**
      - **Injury to peroneal tendons and sural nerve**
    - **Sinus tarsi approach—fewer soft-tissue complications**
  - ORIF and subtalar arthrodesis are supported for Sanders IV fractures

LISFRANC FRACTURE

- **Anatomy**
  - **Lisfranc ligament on plantar foot between medial cuneiform and base of second metatarsal (MT)**
  - Plantar ecchymosis
  - **2-mm widening of Lisfranc joint**
  - Subtle injury identified on WB foot radiographs or stress views
  - **Injury seen on CT**
    - **Widening of intercuneiform joints**
    - **MT base displacement**
    - **Fleck of avulsed bone off medial second MT base**

- Intervention
  - ORIF
  - Primary arthrodesis supported in pure ligamentous injuries

SCAPULA FRACTURE

- Anatomy
  - Glenopolar angle 30° to 45°
  - **Large muscular coverage leads to union in most fractures**—therefore, most are nonoperatively treated.
- Intervention
  - Nonoperative treatment almost always
  - ORIF
    - Glenopolar angle less than 30°
    - Glenohumeral instability due to fracture
    - Significant joint displacement
    - Significant medialization of glenohumeral joint

CLAVICLE FRACTURE

- Anatomy
  - **Fracture pattern best seen with cephalad tilt**
  - Medial
  - Diaphyseal
  - Lateral (distal clavicle fractures): may be associated with coracoclavicular ligament tears, leading to higher nonunion rate
- Intervention
  - Nonoperative
    - Sling
    - May be associated with decreased strength and more long-term pain
  - **ORIF**
    - **Open fracture**
    - **Floating shoulder**
    - **More than 2-cm shortening**
    - "Z-pattern" deformity secondary to comminution
    - Anterior inferior plates are associated with less hardware prominence.
    - Superior plating higher load to failure, so biomechanically stronger. Use dynamic compression plate (DCP) type (not reconstruction or one-third tubular).
  - IM fixation
    - Only for axially stable fractures with no comminution
    - **Increased rotational malalignment**
    - **Secondary removal of hardware**
- Malunions and nonunions common with more than 2-cm shortening, females, smokers, z-deformity, and elderly

HUMERUS FRACTURE

- Anatomy
  - Primary blood supply to humeral head is ascending branch of anterior humeral circumflex humeral artery.
  - Posterior humeral circumflex humeral artery now shown to have significant contribution

- Fracture patterns
  - Proximal humerus fracture (Figure 5.11)
    - **Greater tuberosity**
      - **Supraspinatus**
      - **Infraspinatus**
      - **Teres minor**
    - **Lesser tuberosity: subscapularis**
    - Articular surface
      - Impacted into valgus most commonly with fracture
      - Varus displacement common during treatment
    - Shaft
    - **"Parts" are displaced greater than 45° or 1 cm (0.5-cm displacement tolerated for greater tuberosity).**
    - **Axillary view is mandatory to show humerus head is reduced.**
    - CT may show head split (double curvature at articular surface on AP radiograph also shows this).
    - **Nonoperative treatment for two-part fractures with minimal displacement, low-demand patients with higher number of parts**
    - **ORIF of displaced two- to four-part fractures in younger patients using locked plates**
    - **Varus malreduction and screw cutout through head is common complication.**
    - **Medial calcar supporting screws are most important.**

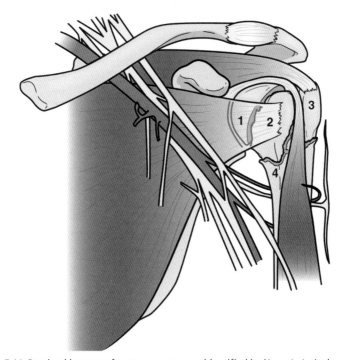

Figure 5.11 Proximal humerus fracture anatomy as identified by Neer. 1, Articular surface. 2, Lesser tuberosity. 3, Greater tuberosity. 4, Humeral shaft. From Simcock X, Seitz WM Jr. Proximal humerus fracture. In: Ricci WM, Ostrum RF, eds. *Orthopaedic Knowledge Update: Trauma 5*. Rosemont, IL: American Academy of Orthopaedic Surgeons; 2016:251-262.

- Tuberosity displacement postoperatively is decreased by suture augmentation of fixation.
  - Most important for function of shoulder
- Disruption of blood supply through periosteum common with fractures having less than 8-mm metadiaphyseal extension
- Total shoulder arthroplasty (TSA) and reverse TSA have good short-term results for three- to four-part fractures.
- Shaft fracture
  - **Nonoperative treatment is mainstay.**
    - **Varus/valgus malalignment up to 30°**
    - **Sagittal malalignment up to 20°**
    - **2-cm shortening**
  - Operative
    - Open fracture
    - Pathologic fracture
    - Floating elbow
    - **Polytrauma (allows arm use and WB in rehabilitation)**
  - *Radial nerve prior to reduction OR after reduction is not indication for surgery.*
  - IM nail
    - Pathologic fracture
    - Segmental fracture
    - Associated with shoulder pain
    - May have increased nonunion rate
    - Intraoperative radial nerve injury may occur at shaft or during distal locking (visualize nerve).
  - ORIF
    - Anterior approach
    - Posterior paratricepital approach
- Distal humerus fracture—most treated operatively to prevent stiffness
  - **ORIF**
    - **Medial and lateral (parallel) plating—biomechanically stronger**
    - **Medial and posterior-lateral (90–90) plating**
    - **Do not fix with one plate.**
    - Olecranon osteotomy for exposure to articular surface may be associated with up to 10% nonunion.
    - Triceps split, triceps peel also indicated for articular visualization
  - **Total elbow arthroplasty—successful in patients with extensive fracture comminution with low postoperative demand and greater than 70 years of age**
  - Radiation therapy not indicated for heterotopic ossification prophylaxis
  - Ulnar nerve transposition should be considered, but is not usually necessary.

ELBOW FRACTURE

- Anatomy
  - Medial collateral ligament resists valgus force.
  - Lateral collateral ligament resists varus and posterolateral instability.
- Fracture patterns
  - Radial head (Figure 5.12)
    - Operative treatment required for Mason II (>50%) with block to motion, comminuted fractures (Mason III), or fracture with dislocation (Mason IV)
    - **All fixations should be placed in "safe zone"—lateral 90° arc with forearm in neutral or arc between Lister tubercle and radial styloid.**
    - Replacement indicated for fractures that cannot be fixed (Figure 5.13)
    - Acute excision is contraindicated due to possibility of Essex-Lopresti lesion (distal radioulnar joint [DRUJ] injury and interosseous membrane injury).

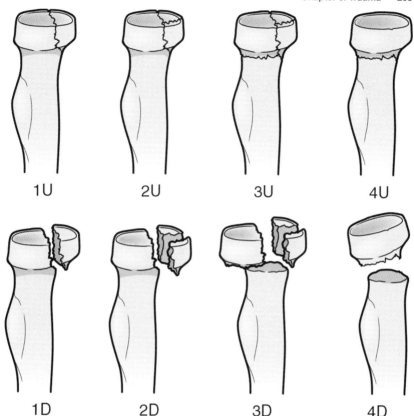

Figure 5.12 Charalambous classification of radial head fractures in which fractures are characterized by the degree of displacement. From Varecka TF. Fractures of the proximal radius and ulna, and dislocations of the elbow. In: Ricci WM, Ostrum RF, eds. *Orthopaedic Knowledge Update: Trauma 5.* Rosemont, IL: American Academy of Orthopaedic Surgeons; 2016:295-308.

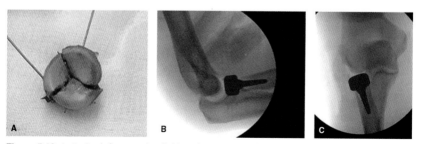

Figure 5.13 A, Excised, fractured radial head consisting of three large articular fragments. Because of the loss of some articular surface material and comminution of the neck portion, reassembly was not indicated. B, Intraoperative image intensifier lateral radiograph shows a noncemented prosthesis with a loose-fitting stem in place. C, Anteroposterior projection from the same patient taken intraoperatively with image intensification shows the noncemented, loose-fitting stem of the radial head prosthesis. Note that the prosthesis is slightly undersized to avoid overstuffing. From Varecka TF. Fractures of the proximal radius and ulna, and dislocations of the elbow. In: Ricci WM, Ostrum RF, eds. *Orthopaedic Knowledge Update: Trauma 5.* Rosemont, IL: American Academy of Orthopaedic Surgeons; 2016:295-308.

- **Metal head arthroplasty—not silicone**
- Posterior interosseous nerve is vulnerable during approaches to radial head and neck.
- Secondary stabilizer to valgus stress
- Coronoid (Figure 5.14)
  - Larger fragments may require ORIF.
  - Larger anterior medial fragments, including the medial collateral ligament (MCL) insertion, often are unstable.
  - Fragments with associated elbow instability require ORIF.
- Monteggia
  - Ulnar shaft fracture with associated radial head dislocation
  - Closed reduction acutely
  - ORIF of ulnar shaft and closed reduction of radial head
  - **Inability to reduce the radial head is usually due to surgeon's malreduction of ulna fracture—revision of ulna ORIF is required.**
- Transolecranon fracture dislocation
- Terrible triad
  - **Fracture of radial head, fracture of coronoid, and dislocation signifying lateral collateral ligament (LCL) injury.**
  - Requires operative treatment due to significant instability
  - **MCL injury in this pattern usually does not require treatment because ORIF coronoid, radial head ORIF, and LCL repair usually result in stable elbow.**
- Olecranon fracture
  - Nonoperative treatment for minimally displaced fractures with intact extensor mechanism

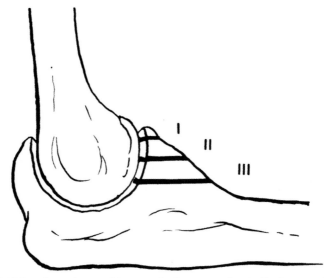

Figure 5.14 Locations of coronoid process fractures according to the Regan and Morrey classification. Type I fractures consist of the tip of the coronoid process. It is important to recognize that these are fractures resulting from a shearing injury to the coronoid, and not avulsion injuries. Type III fractures, and to a lesser extent type II, are associated with elbow dislocation and instability. From Regan W, Morrey BF. Fractures of the coronoid process of the ulna. *J Bone Joint Surg Am.* 1989;71:1348-1354.

- ORIF
  - Tension band wire for simple fractures without comminution; anterior penetration of pins is associated with anterior interosseous nerve injury
  - Dorsal plating associated with symptomatic hardware in majority of patients
  - **May excise up to 50% of olecranon and advance triceps, but this leads to decreased strength**

FOREARM FRACTURE

- **Anatomy**
  - Rotation of radius over ulna during pronation requires anatomic radial bow.
- **Intervention**
  - **Isolated ulna fracture: closed treatment with brace or cast acceptable for up to 50% displacement**
  - Both bone forearm fracture (fracture of both radius and ulna shafts)
    - ORIF required in all but the most unstable patients
      - DCP-type plates required for adequate bending and rotational stability
      - Plate ulna and radius through two incisions, two approaches—prevents synostosis
      - Anatomic reduction required to allow postoperative supination and pronation
      - Acute bone grafting indicated for comminuted fractures
  - Galeazzi fracture dislocation
    - Radial shaft fracture within 8 cm of DRUJ
    - Associated DRUJ instability/dislocation
    - **ORIF of radial shaft and assessment of DRUJ required**
    - **DRUJ is most stable in supination**
      - **Percutaneous fixation is standard treatment of DRUJ.**
      - Closed management of DRUJ in supination also described

SHOULDER INSTABILITY

TUBS—**T**raumatic, **U**nidirectional instability with a **B**ankart lesion often requiring **S**urgery

- **Anterior instability**
  - **Patient age most important factor for recurrence**
  - Trauma (contact sports)
  - **Bankart lesion**
  - Anterior inferior labral lesion
  - **Inferior glenohumeral ligament (IGHL) main restraint to anterior in the abducted and external rotation (ER)**
  - Neurologic examination
    - **Axillary nerve <40 years of age**
    - **Suprascapular nerve**
  - Range of motion (ROM)
  - **Rotator cuff (RTC)—ability to lift arm**
    - **>40 years of age**
    - **30% to 80% RTC injuries in patients aged >60 years**
  - Specialized tests for anterior dislocation (Figure 6.1)
    - **Apprehension**
    - **Relocation maneuver**
  - Imaging
    - Radiographs—three views
      - **Always need axillary**
      - Westpoint view (anterior inferior glenoid)—similar to axillary but prone and beam directed 25° inferiorly and medial
    - Magnetic resonance imaging (MRI) with or without gadolinium (Figure 6.2)
      - 88% sensitivity and 100% specificity for diagnosing IGHL tears
      - Mandatory in chronic dislocations to rule out bony defects
    - Computed tomography (CT) to assess bone loss (Figure 6.3)

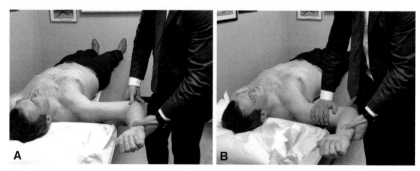

Figure 6.1 Apprehension (A) and relocation (B) tests. From Dugas JR, Ryan MK. Shoulder instability and baseball players. In: Ahmad CS, Romeo AA, eds. *Baseball Sports Medicine*. Philadelphia, PA: Wolters Kluwer; 2019:197-212.

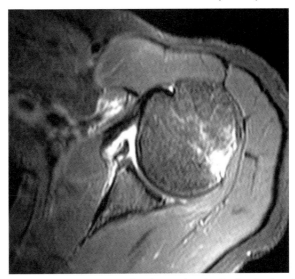

Figure 6.2 Magnetic resonance imaging (MRI) scan showing both a Bankart lesion and a Hill-Sachs lesion.

- Traumatic injuries (Figure 6.4)
  - Humeral avulsion of glenohumeral ligaments
  - Anterior labral periosteal sleeve avulsion
    - Medially displaced labroligamentous complex with absence of the labrum on the glenoid rim
  - Glenolabral articular disruption
    - Represents a partial tear of anterior inferior labrum with adjacent cartilage damage

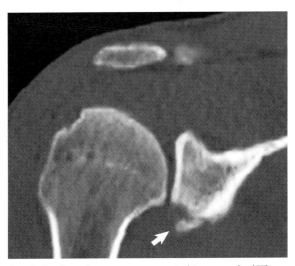

Figure 6.3 Bankart lesion bone loss seen on computed tomography (CT) scan. Arrow: Bony bankart and bone loss. From Greenspan A, Beltran J. Upper limb I: shoulder girdle. In: *Orthopedic Imaging: A Practical Approach*. 6th ed. Philadelphia, PA: Wolters Kluwer Health; 2015:107-163.

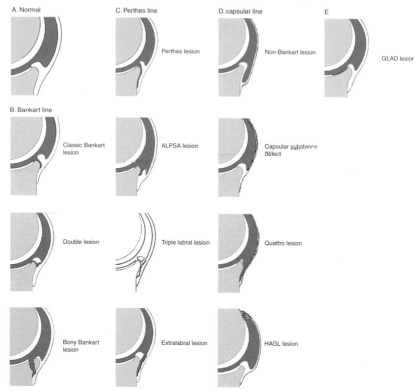

Figure 6.4 Different lesions in anterior inferior shoulder instability. ALPSA, anterior labral periosteal sleeve avulsion; GLAD, glenolabral articular disruption; HAGL, humeral avulsion of glenohumeral ligament. From Lichtenberg S, Habermeyer P. Athroscopic repair of anterior instability. In: Craig EV, ed. *Master Techniques in Orthopaedic Surgery: The Shoulder*. 3rd ed. Philadelphia, PA: Lippincott Williams & Wilkins; 2013:67-88.

- Associated injuries
  - **Bone defects**
    - **Chronic dislocations**
    - **Most common cause of repair failure**
    - **If >25%, may need bone graft or Latarjet-type procedure**
- Nonoperative treatment
  - Closed reduction—first-time dislocation
  - Period of immobilization—Studies show use of small abduction pillow in neutral or ER decreases recurrence.
  - **Supervised rehabilitation**
    - **Cuff strengthening**
    - **Scapular stabilizers**
  - In-season dislocation
    - Consider bone loss after recurrent dislocations
    - May need CT at the end of season
- Operative treatment
  - Repair labrum (Bankart lesion) and tension IGHL complex
  - Randomized studies show equivalent results when arthroscopy compared with open procedure.

- Open—subscapularis tears
- Arthroscopic—ROM might be slightly better (Figure 6.5).
  - **Failure**
    - **Glenoid defects >25%**
    - **Engaging Hill-Sachs**
- Engaging Hill-Sachs lesion (>25%) with recurrent instability—remplissage (Figure 6.6)
  - Infraspinatus (IS) tendon sutured into the Hill-Sachs lesion
  - Arthroscopic
  - Slight loss of ER

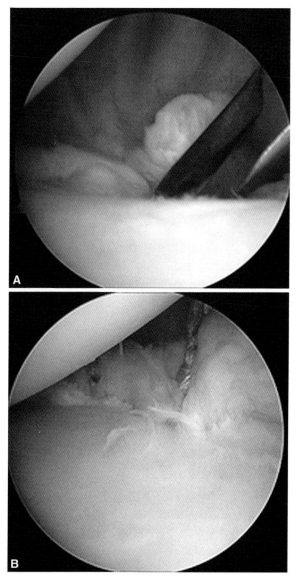

Figure 6.5 A, Bankart lesion off glenoid. B, Repaired lesion.

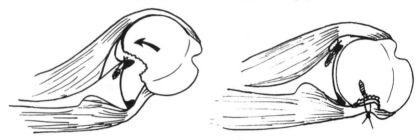

Figure 6.6 Remplissage for Hill-Sachs lesion. From Boileau P, O'Shea K, Vargas P, et al. Anatomical and functional results after arthroscopic Hill-Sachs remplissage. *J Bone Joint Surg Am.* 2012;94(7):618-626.

- Chronic dislocations—Deficiency >25% of the glenoid joint surface treated with soft-tissue repair only is associated with high recurrence rates (Figure 6.7).
  - Latarjet (Figure 6.8)
    - Coracoid transfer—glenoid depth
    - Soft-tissue sling—conjoint tendon
    - Musculocutaneous nerve at risk
- **Posterior instability**
  - Blocking in football—lineman
  - Flexion, adduction, and internal rotation (IR)
  - Posterior instability tests—key in examination
    - **Load and shift**
    - **Jerk test (Figure 6.9)**

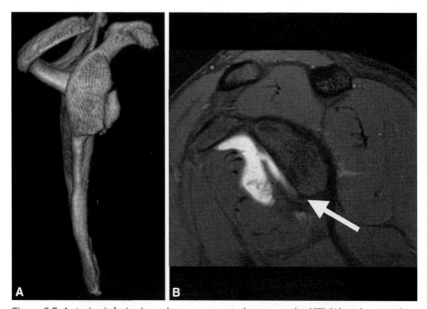

Figure 6.7 Anterior inferior bone loss on computed tomography (CT) (A) and magnetic resonance imaging (MRI) (B). If bone loss is greater than 25%, bony procedure must be undertaken before soft-tissue procedure. From Piasecki DP, Verma NN, Romeo AA, et al. Glenoid bone deficiency in recurrent anterior shoulder instability: diagnosis and management. *J Am Acad Orthop Surg.* 2009;17(8):482-493.

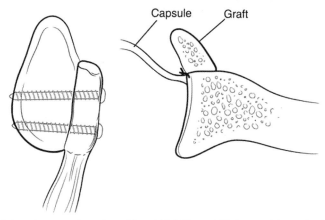

Figure 6.8 Latarjet procedure. From Piasecki DP, Verma NN, Romeo AA, et al. Glenoid bone deficiency in recurrent anterior shoulder instability: diagnosis and management. *J Am Acad Orthop Surg*. 2009;17(8):482-493.

- 90° of abduction and IR, axially loads the humerus in a proximal direction and horizontally across the body
- Positive with "clunk"
- **Kim test (Figure 6.10)**
  - 90° of abduction, axial loading force to arm

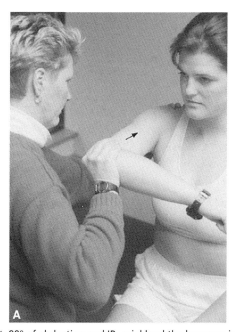

Figure 6.9 Jerk test. 90° of abduction and IR, axial load the humerus in a proximal direction and horizontally across the body. From Palmer ML, Epler ME. *Fundamentals of Musculoskeletal Assessment Techniques*. 2nd ed. Philadelphia, PA: Lippincott Williams & Wilkins; 1998.

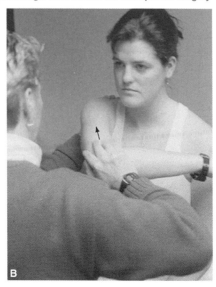

Figure 6.9 (*continued*)

- ∘ With arm elevated 45°, downward and backward force is applied to proximal arm.
  - ∘ Positive with pain
  - • Positive jerk test combined with a positive Kim test—97% sensitivity for posterior instability
- • Primary stabilizers posteriorly
  - ∘ Superior glenohumeral ligament (SGHL)
  - ∘ Coracohumeral ligament
  - ∘ Posterior IGHL
- • Up to 50% misdiagnosed
  - ∘ Always need axillary view
  - ∘ *Key phrases to know for test*—**Any of the phrases or words should lead you to posterior instability.**

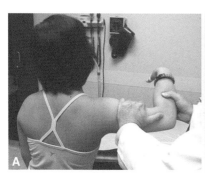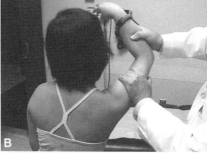

Figure 6.10 Kim test. With arm elevated 45°, downward and backward force is applied to proximal arm. From Leonard JP, Kuhn JE. Natural history of posterior shoulder instability. In: Dodson CC, Dines DM, Dines JS, et al, eds. *Controversies in Shoulder Instability*. Philadelphia, PA: Lippincott Williams & Williams; 2014:197-206.

- Seizures
- Electrical shock
- Offensive lineman
- Push-ups
- Treatment
  - Always treat conservatively first.
  - Posterior Bankart lesion
    - Open or arthroscopic repair
    - Recurrence—most common complication
  - Open capsular plication
  - Chronic locked dislocation
    - <6 months—McLaughlin procedure
      - Subscapularis and lesser tuberosity transfer to reverse Hill-Sachs defect
      - Hill-Sachs >20% but <50%
    - >6 months
      - Hemiarthroplasty
      - Hill-Sachs defect >50%

AMBRI—*A*traumatic, *M*ultidirectional, *B*ilateral instability that Often Responds to *R*ehabilitation First; *I*nferior capsular Shift if Surgery Needed

- Global laxity
- **Two classic lesions**
  - **Patulous inferior capsule**
  - **Functional deficiency of rotator interval**
- Presentation highly variable
  - Shoulder popping, weakness, and paresthesias
  - + Sulcus
  - RTC tendonitis or impingement <20
- Treatment
  - **Exhaustive conservative treatment (6 months)—closed chain physical therapy (PT)**
  - Arthroscopic application or inferior capsular shift—positive drive-through sign
  - Rotator interval
    - Indicated in multidirectional instability
    - Closure of rotator interval decreases ER in shoulder adduction and posterior inferior translation
- Complications of surgery for instability
  - Recurrence
  - Axillary nerve injury
  - Loss of motion
  - Late degenerative disease
  - Open procedures—Subscapularis repair may fail.

SUPERIOR LABRUM ANTERIOR TO POSTERIOR (SLAP) TEARS AND INTERNAL IMPINGEMENT

SLAP Tears
- Mechanism—traction or compression injury related to a fall on outstretched arm
- Most common in throwing athletes—repetitive motion
  - **Pitchers—GIRD >20°**
- Deep pain with catching or locking with overhead activities
- **Contracture of posterior IGHL**
  - **Shifts contact point posterior superior**
  - **Increase shear causes a SLAP tear**

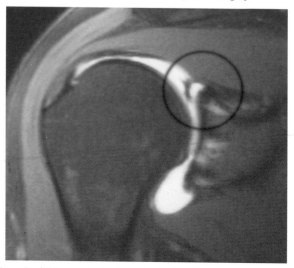

Figure 6.11 Superior labrum anterior to posterior (SLAP) tear on magnetic resonance (MR) arthrography. From Snyder SJ, Karzel RP, Getelman MH, et al. Superior labrum (SLAP) injuries and repair. In: *Shoulder Arthroscopy*. 3rd ed. Philadelphia, PA: Wolters Kluwer Health; 2015:101-118.

- **Testing**
  - **Obrien test**
  - **Crank test**
  - **85% of patients have a positive apprehension or relocation test.**
- MR arthrography—best imaging modality (Figure 6.11)
- Biceps anchor—**Most significant tears are posterior to 12 o'clock position.**
- Arthroscopy test—Evaluate the labrum and determine whether the labrum will "peel back."
  - Abduction and ER
- **Nonoperative treatment—first line**
  - RTC strengthening to stabilize shoulder
  - Scapula stabilizers—dyskinesia
  - GIRD—posterior capsular stretching
- Surgical treatment
  - Incidental finding—no need to repair
  - Treatment based on classification (Figure 6.12)
    - Type I—labral fraying, anchor intact; debridement
    - Type II—detached biceps anchor; repair surgically (Figure 6.13)
    - Type III—bucket-handle, anchor intact; debridement
    - Type IV—bucket-handle into tendon; detached anchor
      - Less than one-third biceps anchor—incise fragment
      - More than one-third biceps anchor—tenotomy versus tenodesis

Internal Impingement

- *Internal versus external impingement*
  - **External impingement**—With cuff fatigue/injury, the bursal cuff is impinged by the coracoacromial arch on abduction.
  - **Internal impingement**—Increased anterior capsular laxity allows increased ER, impinging the articular side of the cuff on the posterior glenoid.

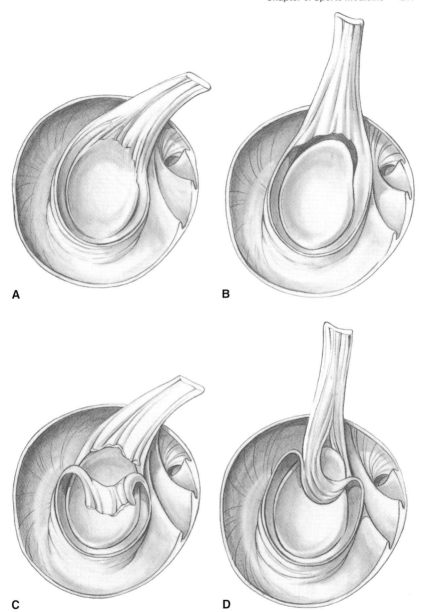

Figure 6.12 A, Type I superior labrum anterior to posterior (SLAP) lesions are characterized by a significant fraying or degeneration of the superior labrum. B, Type II SLAP lesions are characterized by detachment of the superior labrum and biceps tendon from the glenoid rim. C, Type III SLAP lesions are seen as a bucket-handle tearing of the superior labrum. The remaining labral tissue maintains the biceps as anchored to the glenoid rim. D, Type IV SLAP lesions consist of an extension of the bucket-handle labral tear into the substance of the biceps tendon. From Yamaguchi K, Keener J, Galatz LM. Disorders of the biceps tendon. In: Iannotti JP, Williams GR, eds. *Disorders of the Shoulder: Diagnosis and Management*. Vol 1. 2nd ed. Philadelphia, PA: Lippincott Williams & Wilkins; 2007:217-260.

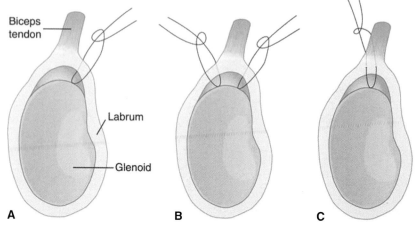

Figure 6.13 Commonly used suture configurations for repair of type II superior labrum anterior to posterior (SLAP) tears. A, Single simple suture. B, Two suture anchors with one simple suture each located anterior and posterior to the biceps origin. C, Single suture anchor with a horizontal mattress suture through the biceps anchor. From Keener JD, Brophy RH. Superior labral tears of the shoulder: pathogenesis, evaluation, and treatment. *J Am Acad Orthop Surg.* 2009;17(10):627-637.

- Mechanism (Figure 6.14)
  - **Mechanical impingement of the articular side of the rotator on the posterior superior aspect of glenoid rim**
  - "Pitcher reports the recent onset of decreased velocity and posterior shoulder pain."
  - Late cocking/early acceleration phase of throwing

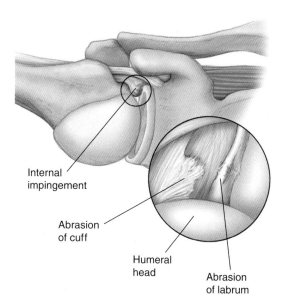

Figure 6.14 Internal impingement: In the throwing motion, as the shoulder goes into external rotation and abduction, the posterior supraspinatus and anterior infraspinatus may experience impingement with the posterosuperior glenoid and labrum, leading to articular-sided tear. From Makhni EC, ElAttrache NS, Ahmad CS. Rotator cuff tears in baseball players. In: Ahmad CS, Romeo AA, eds. *Baseball Sports Medicine.* Philadelphia, PA: Wolters Kluwer; 2019:181-186.

- Examination
  - **GIRD—20°**
  - Bennett lesion—mineralization of posterior inferior glenoid seen on CT or x-ray
  - **Articular-sided RTC tear (Figure 6.15)**
- Treatment—most treated nonoperatively
  - Nonoperative
    - Posterior capsule stretching
    - RTC strengthening
    - Changing mechanics of throwing

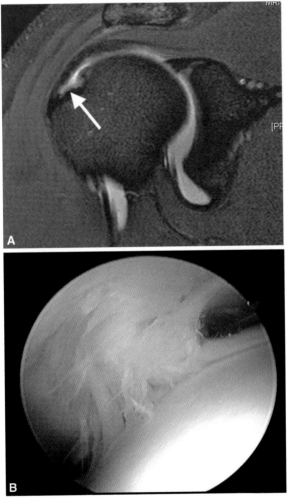

Figure 6.15 Magnetic resonance imaging (MRI) arthrogram (A) and arthroscopic view (B) showing partial articular-sided rotator cuff tear. Arrow: MRI–articular sided rotator cuff tear. From Makhni EC, ElAttrache NS, Ahmad CS. Rotator cuff tears in baseball players. In: Ahmad CS, Romeo AA, eds. *Baseball Sports Medicine*. Philadelphia: PA: Wolters Kluwer; 2019:181-186.

- Surgical
  - Repair of SLAP lesion
  - Debridement of RTC

Scapulothoracic Dyskinesis

- Snapping scapula with overhead activity
- Causes
  - Bursitis
  - Elastofibroma
  - Osteochondroma
- Diagnosis
  - Crepitus
  - Scapula stabilization relieves pain.
- Treatment
  - **Nonoperative—Nonsteroidal anti-inflammatory drugs (NSAIDs), scapular strengthening, and injection of corticosteroid with lidocaine can be diagnostic and therapeutic.**
  - Surgical—bursectomy (open or arthroscopic) or resection of superomedial scapular border

LITTLE LEAGUER SHOULDER

- Overuse of the throwing shoulder
- **Hypertrophic zone of the growth plate**
  - Salter-Harris type I
  - Tension and shear on physis
- Radiographs show widening proximal physis (Figure 6.16).

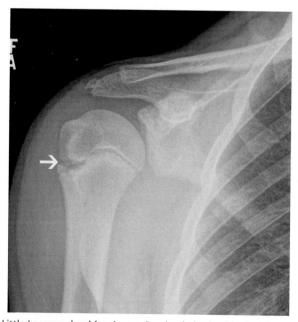

Figure 6.16 Little Leaguer shoulder. Arrow: Proximal physis widening. From Rajiah P, Holden D, Schils J, Polster JM. Imaging of the sports injury: indications and findings. In: Miniaci A, ed. *Disorders of the Shoulder: Diagnosis and Management: Sports Injuries.* Vol 2. 3rd ed. Philadelphia, PA: Lippincott Williams & Wilkins; 2014:31-60.

- Treatment—*nonoperative*
  - Rest and no throwing—3 months
  - Prevention

IMPINGEMENT AND RTC TEARS

- Diagnosis
  - Patient age
    - Instability in young patients (<45 years)—impingement
    - **Increasing age—RTC tear more likely**
      - >60 years old—28%
      - >70 years old—65%
  - Shoulder pain with overhead activity that radiates to arm
  - **Painful arc 60° to 140°**
  - Night pain
  - Impingement test—lidocaine
  - Atrophy
  - Tests for weakness
    - **Jobe sign (empty can; Figure 6.17)—supraspinatus (SS)**
    - **ER at side—IS**
    - **Hornblower—teres minor**
    - **IR—subscapularis**
      - **IR weakness, excessive ER**
      - **Lift-off, cheat, Napoleon test, bear-hug test**
    - *Acute versus chronic RTC tears*
  - **Acute**
    - **Often traumatic in younger patients**
    - **Immediate loss of function**
    - **Lack atrophy**
    - **Usually repair early for examination purposes**
  - **Chronic**
    - **Often atraumatic with insidious onset**
    - **Older, less active patients**

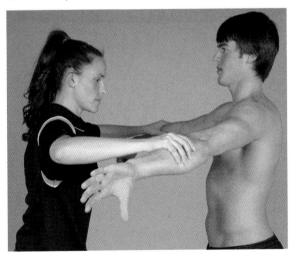

Figure 6.17 Jobe test. From Anderson MK, Parr GP. Injury assessment. In: *Foundations of Athletic Training: Prevention, Assessment, and Management.* 5th ed. Baltimore, MD: Lippincott Williams & Wilkins; 2013:102-150.

- **Muscle atrophy**
- **Weakness, though some retain elevation strength**
- **Generally begin with PT**
- Staging
  - Stage I—impingement
  - Edema, inflammation
    - Younger patients (<30 years)
    - Changes believed to be reversible
  - Stage II—partial RTC tear
    - Middle-aged patients (40s)
    - Incompletely reversible
  - Stage III—full-thickness RTC tear
    - Tendon tear
    - Older patients (50s)
    - Not reversible
- Imaging
  - Radiography (Figure 6.18)
    - **Humeral head elevation**
    - Narrowing of subacromial space
      - <7 mm—consistent with RTC tear
      - <5 mm—massive RTC tear
  - MRI
    - Can assess presence of tear, partial versus full thickness, retraction, atrophy (**Goutallier classification**)

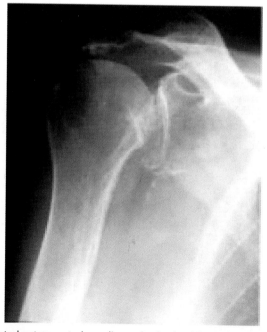

Figure 6.18 Neutral anteroposterior radiograph of a shoulder with a chronic massive rotator cuff tear. Although there is reduction of the acromiohumeral space and the humeral head is elevated relative to the glenoid, there is no glenohumeral arthritis. From Green A. Chronic massive rotator cuff tears: evaluation and management. *J Am Acad Orthop Surg.* 2003;11(5):321-331.

- Can determine status of RTC muscles and size of tear
  - Small—0 to 1 cm
  - Medium—1 to 3 cm
  - Large—3 to 5 cm
  - Massive—>5 cm (involves multiple tendons)
  - 100% sensitivity, 95% specificity for full-thickness RTC tears (Figure 6.19)
  - Coronal oblique—SS retraction and muscle quality
  - Sagittal oblique—AP extent of tear, muscle quality
  - Axial—biceps tendon, subscapularis, and IS tear
- Ultrasonography
  - Increasingly used for diagnosis, assessment of postoperative healing and retearing

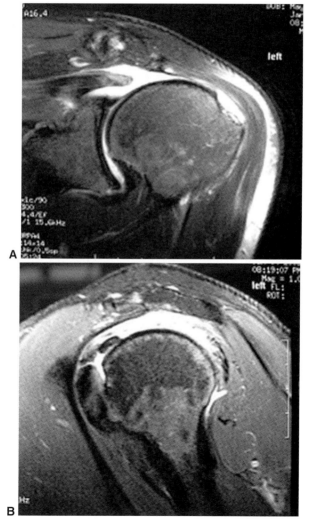

Figure 6.19 A full-thickness rotator cuff tear. Coronal oblique (A) and sagittal (B) MRI for full thickness supraspinatus tear.

- Some centers report high sensitivity and specificity.
  - No difference in detection or accuracy when compared with MRI
  - Highly operator dependent
  - Dynamic
- Treatment
  - Nonoperative—chronic atraumatic tears
    - Rest, activity modification
    - NSAIDs and injections—Lidocaine with cortisone is diagnostic and therapeutic.
      - PT—strengthen RTC and periscapular muscles and deltoid
  - Surgical indications
    - Acute traumatic tears
    - Complete tears in patients aged <50 years within 6 weeks
    - Failure of conservative treatment after 4 to 6 months
    - Pain relief most predictable
  - Surgical techniques
    - Open, arthroscopic, mini-open
    - Anchors, transosseous tunnels
      - Gold standard—open transosseous repair
      - Arthroscopic at least equivalent to open in newer studies
      - Single-row anchors, double-row anchors—no significant difference in clinical outcomes
    - Advantages of arthroscopic versus open repair
      - No deltoid detachment
      - Intra-articular pathology
      - Less soft-tissue dissection
      - Less pain and blood loss
  - Partial tears—surgical indication
    - Failure of conservative management—PT
      - Articular-sided (Figure 6.20A)—more common; repair if >6 mm (50%)
      - Bursal-sided (Figure 6.20B)—less common; repair if >3 mm (25%)
  - Small and medium tears—surgery decreases pain and improves motion.
  - Large tears—high surgical failure rate owing to tissue quality

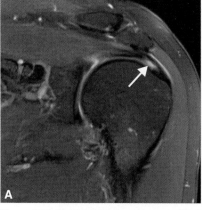 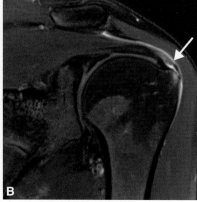

Figure 6.20 Partial-thickness rotator cuff tears. A, Coronal fat saturated T2 (FST2) magnetic resonance (MR) image of a partial-thickness articular-sided rotator cuff tear in the supraspinatus tendon (arrow). B, Coronal FST2 MR image of a partial-thickness bursal-sided rotator cuff tear in the supraspinatus tendon (arrow). From Beltran LS. MRI of shoulder injuries. In: Chew FS, ed. *Musculoskeletal Imaging: The Essentials*. Philadelphia, PA: Wolters Kluwer; 2019:107-133.

- Massive tears
  - Conservative management—older patients
    - Normal motion, strength may be maintained if posterior RTC and subscapularis intact.
    - Preservation of force couples
    - These patients still have progressive migration of humeral head with arm elevation but are asymptomatic.
  - Arthroscopic debridement
  - **Preserve coracoacromial (CA) ligament and arch**
  - Tendon transfers—latissimus combined SS and IS
  - Hemiarthroplasty—able to raise arm
- *Outcomes*
  - **Good function/strength if tendon heals**
    - **Tendon does not heal until approximately 12 weeks.**
    - **Factors for healing—atrophy, retraction, patient age, tendon, quality, and smoking**
    - **Less favorable outcomes after RTC surgery related to:**
      - **Worker's Compensation status**
      - **Tear size**
        - **Fatty degeneration of RTC musculature**
      - **Age at time of intervention**

Subscapularis Tears

- Fall after open shoulder surgery
- Most commonly missed RTC
- Examination
  - Increased ER with arm at side, positive lift-off (Figure 6.21) or positive belly-press sign
  - **Axial MRI—medial subluxation of biceps** (Figure 6.22)
  - **Arthroscopy—SGHL comma**

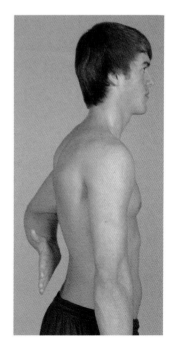

Figure 6.21 Lift-off test. From Anderson MK. Shoulder conditions. In: *Foundations of Athletic Training: Prevention, Assessment, and Management.* 6th ed. Baltimore, MD: Wolters Kluwer; 2017:544-599.

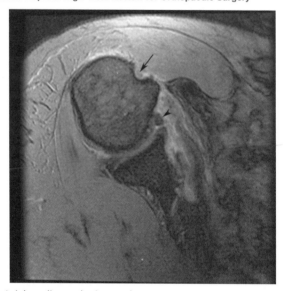

Figure 6.22 Axial gradient-echo image demonstrating an empty biceps groove (arrow) with medial dislocation of the biceps tendon (arrowhead). From Berquist TH, Peterson JJ. Shoulder and arm. In: Berquist TH, ed. *MRI of the Musculoskeletal System*. 6th ed. Philadelphia, PA: Lippincott Williams & Wilkins; 2013:597-705.

- Treatment
  - Repair subscapularis and biceps
  - Tenotomy versus tenodesis
  - Pectoralis tendon transfer (Figure 6.23)

RTC Arthropathy

- Condition resulting from **chronic RTC deficiency (massive tear)**
- Radiographs (Figure 6.24)
  - **Superior migration of humeral head**
  - Erosion and rounding of greater tuberosity (GT)
  - Sclerosis, hypertrophy
  - Visible contact and wear of humeral head on undersurface of acromion (acetabularization)
- Treatment
  - **Total shoulder arthroplasty (TSA) not an option** because of RTC deficiency.
  - Humeral head replacement (hemiarthroplasty) previously best and only option
  - **Reverse TSA** now treatment of choice
    - Biomechanical fulcrum for arm elevation
    - Increases moment arm for deltoid
    - Older patients
    - Instability

CALCIFIC BURSITIS

- Self-limiting
- SS
  - Examination
  - Impingement symptoms
  - Radiographs show calcification.

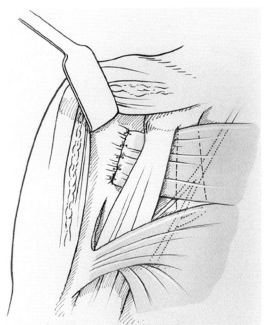

Figure 6.23 Pectoralis transfer. From Resch H, Povacz P, Ritter E, Matschi W. Transfer of the pectoralis major muscle for the treatment of irreparable rupture of the subscapularis tendon. *J Bone Joint Surg Am*. 2000;82(3):372-382.

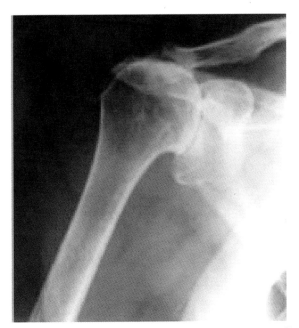

Figure 6.24 Neutral anteroposterior radiograph of a shoulder with rotator cuff tear arthropathy. There is no acromiohumeral space, there are degenerative changes of the glenohumeral joint, and the greater tuberosity is rounded off. From Green A. Chronic massive rotator cuff tears: evaluation and management. *J Am Acad Orthop Surg*. 2003;11(5):321-331.

- Treatment
  - *Always nonoperative first*
    - PT and NSAIDs
    - Open biopsy of the lesion for permanent section
    - Manipulation under anesthesia
    - Injections—needling
  - Shoulder arthroscopy if conservative management fails

BICEPS PATHOLOGY

- Anterior shoulder pain (Figure 6.25)
  - Tenderness to palpation

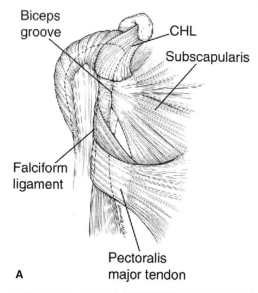

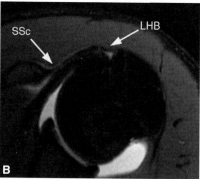

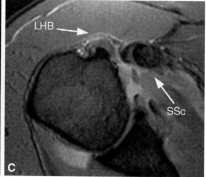

Figure 6.25 A, Anatomic structures around the long head of the biceps. B, T2-weighted axial magnetic resonance arthrogram demonstrating the long head of the biceps (LHB) tendon lying in the bicipital groove. C, T2-weighted axial magnetic resonance image demonstrating a torn subscapularis tendon (SSc) and medial dislocation of the LHB tendon. CHL, coracohumeral ligament. From Nho SJ, Strauss EJ, Lenart BA, et al. Long head of the biceps tendinopathy: diagnosis and management. *J Am Acad Orthop Surg.* 2010;18(11):645-656.

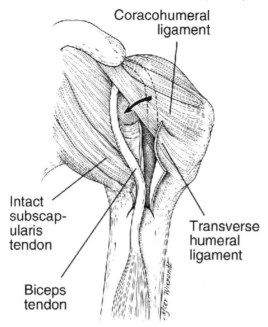

Figure 6.26 Long head of the biceps subluxation and dislocation. From Gambill ML, Mologne TS, Provencher MT. Dislocation of the long head of the biceps tendon with intact subscapularis and supraspinatus tendons. *J Shoulder Elbow Surg*. 2006;15:e20-e22.

- **Key examinations**
  - **Speed test**
  - **Yergason test**
- Nonoperative treatment
  - Initial treatment
  - **Proximal ruptures**
- Surgical indications
  - Partial tears (25%-50%)
  - Medial subluxation (Figure 6.26)
  - Subscapularis tear with medial subluxation
  - Failed SLAP repairs and older patients with SLAP tears
- **No evidence to support tenodesis versus tenotomy**
  - Cosmetic
  - Subjective cramping
  - Subpectoralis tenodesis complication: subpectoral pain of musculocutaneous origin

ACROMIOCLAVICULAR (AC) JOINT INJURIES

Anatomy

- AC ligaments (Figure 6.27)
  - **AP stability—posterior and superior contribute most to horizontal instability**
  - Blood supply—temporal arteries
  - Dual innervation
    - Lateral pectoral
    - Suprascapular

Anterior View of Right Shoulder

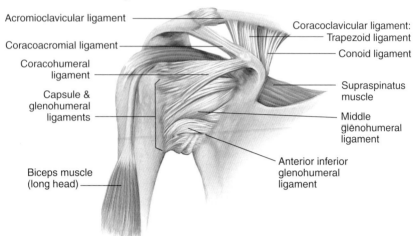

Acromioclavicular ligament

Coracoacromial ligament

Coracohumeral ligament

Capsule & glenohumeral ligaments

Biceps muscle (long head)

Coracoclavicular ligament:
Trapezoid ligament
Conoid ligament

Supraspinatus muscle

Middle glenohumeral ligament

Anterior inferior glenohumeral ligament

Figure 6.27 Acromioclavicular (AC) joint anatomy. Asset provided by Anatomical Chart Company.

- Coracoclavicular (CC) ligaments (Figure 6.28)
  - **Provide vertical stability to AC joint**
  - Two components
    - Trapezoid
      - 2.5 cm
      - Anterolateral
    - Conoid
      - 4.5 cm
      - Posteromedial
      - Stronger

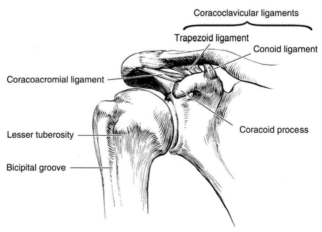

Coracoclavicular ligaments

Trapezoid ligament
Conoid ligament

Coracoacromial ligament

Lesser tuberosity

Bicipital groove

Coracoid process

Figure 6.28 Coracoclavicular ligaments. From Simovitch R, Sanders B, Ozbaydar M, Lavery K, Warner JJ. Acromioclavicular joint injuries: diagnosis and management. *J Am Acad Orthop Surg.* 2009;17(4):207-219.

AC Separation

- Diagnosis
  - Mechanism—fall
  - Tender to palpation
  - 20% intra-articular injuries—SLAP tear
  - **Radiography—Zanca view (Figure 6.29)**
    - **X-ray beam 10° cephalad with 50% penetration**
- Classification (Figure 6.30)
  - Type I—sprain/partial tear of AC ligament; AC joint still aligned
  - Type II—complete tear of AC ligament (arrow) and sprain/partial tear of the CC ligaments, with widening of the AC joint space, normal or slightly widened CC interspace, and 50% superior clavicular displacement
  - Type III—complete tear of AC and CC ligaments, with widening of the AC joint space, increased (25%-100%) CC interspace, and 100% superior clavicular displacement
  - Type IV—complete tear of AC, CC, and CA ligaments, with posterior displacement of distal clavicle
  - Type V—complete tear of AC, CC, and CA ligaments, with marked superior displacement of distal clavicle
  - Type VI—complete tear of AC, CC, and CA ligaments, with inferior displacement of the distal clavicle beneath the coracoid process

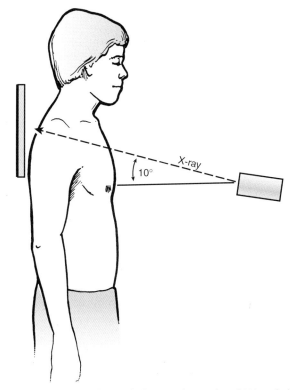

Figure 6.29 Zanca view, which is shot with the x-ray beam placed 10° cephalad to the perpendicular plane. From Edgar C. Acromioclavicular and sternoclavicular joint injuries. In: Tornetta PT III, Ricci WM, Ostrum RF, et al, eds. *Rockwood and Green's Fractures in Adults.* Vol 1. 9th ed. Philadelphia, PA: Wolters Kluwer; 2019:917-975.

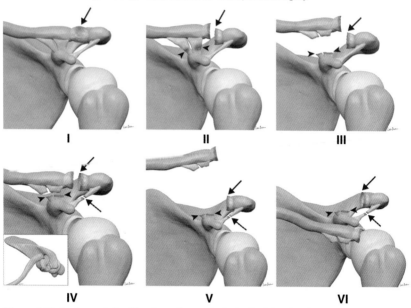

Figure 6.30 Rockwood classification of acromioclavicular joint (ACJ) separation injuries. From Beltran LS. MRI of shoulder injuries. In: Chew FS, ed. *Musculoskeletal Imaging: The Essentials*. Philadelphia, PA: Wolters Kluwer; 2019:107-133.

- Treatment
  - **Types I and II**
    - **Always nonoperative initially**
    - Long-term sequelae
      - **Osteoarthritis (OA)—nearly 50% of patients**
      - Cross-arm adduction and tenderness
      - Radiographs—decreased joint space and osteophytes
    - If nonoperative fails
      - Resection of AC joint (Mumford)
      - 1 cm—preserve CC ligaments (trapezoid)
      - Preserve posterior-superior capsule
  - Type III
    - Trial nonoperative
    - Long-term weakness in bench press
    - **Operative—overhead athletes and laborers**
  - **Type III (chronic symptomatic) to type VI surgical options**
    - Distal clavicle excision with CC ligament reconstruction (Figure 6.31)
    - Needs supplementation with graft: CA ligament alone is 20% as strong
    - **Free tendon graft reconstruction most closely approximates CC ligaments**
    - Complications
      - Pin migration
      - Fractures
      - Hook plate—acromial erosion

Os Acromiale

- Diagnosis—signs of impingement (Figure 6.32)
- Four areas (Figure 6.33)

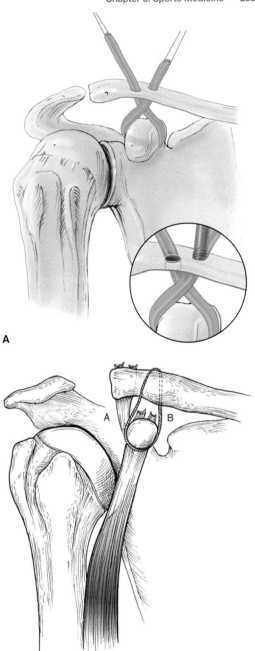

Figure 6.31 A, Anatomic coracoclavicular ligament reconstruction. After the graft is looped around the coracoid, bone tunnels are created, and the free ends of the graft are crossed and passed through the clavicle. The graft is pulled back and forth through the tunnels, and cyclic loading is placed on the graft. A short tail is left superior to the clavicle for the conoid ligament, whereas the remainder of the graft exits the trapezoid tunnel, with one end left longer than the other. From Virk MS, Arciero RA, Mazzocca AD. Repair and reconstruction of acromioclavicular injuries. In: Miller MD, ed. *Operative Techniques in Sports Medicine*. 2nd ed. Philadelphia, PA: Wolters Kluwer; 2016:102-113. B, The modified Weaver-Dunn procedure. The coracoacromial ligament (*A*) is transferred to the clavicle to substitute for the ruptured coracoclavicular ligaments. A suture loop (*B*) can be used for augmentation. From Simovitch R, Sanders B, Ozbaydar M, et al. Acromioclavicular joint injuries: diagnosis and management. *J Am Acad Orthop Surg*. 2009;17(4):207-219.

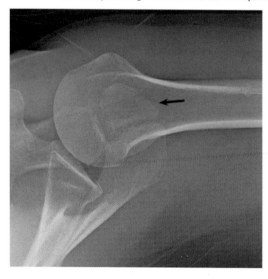

Figure 6.32 Axillary view of os acromiale. Arrow: Os Acromiole. From Greenspan A, Beltran J. Upper limb I: shoulder girdle. In: *Orthopedic Imaging: A Practical Approach*. 6th ed. Philadelphia, PA: Wolters Kluwer Health; 2015:107-163.

- • Preacromion
- • Mesoacromion
- • Meta-acromion
- • Basiacromion
- Most common
  - • Meta-acromion and mesoacromion junction
  - • Best seen on axillary view
- Treatment
  - • Nonoperative
  - • Surgical
    - ∘ Fuse bone graft
    - ∘ Acromioplasty
    - ∘ Complication of large excision—deltoid dysfunction

STERNOCLAVICULAR (SC) DISLOCATION

- Incidence highest in young adult males
  - • Motor vehicles—most common
  - • Contact sports
- Posterior dislocations—25% have complications
- Medial physeal injury
  - • Physes fuse around 23 to 25 years of age
  - • Rarely surgical unless posterior with compression of mediastinal structures
- Imaging
  - • Radiographs with 40° cephalic tilt (serendipity view)
  - • CT best study
- Anatomy (Figure 6.34)
  - • Articular disk—shock absorber and prevents medial translation
  - • Posterior SC ligament/capsule—primary stabilizer of SC joint
  - • Costoclavicular ligament—extracapsular and strongest supporting ligament
- Treatment
  - • Anterior—nonoperative treatment
    - ∘ Analgesics and immobilization
    - ∘ Functional outcome usually good

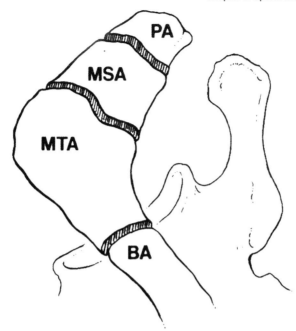

Figure 6.33 Classification of os acromiale. BA, basiacromion; MSA, mesoacromion; MTA, meta-acromion; PA, preacromion. From Ryu RKN, Dopirak RM. The treatment of the symptomatic os acromiale. In: Johnson DH, ed. *Operative Arthroscopy*. 4th ed. Philadelphia, PA: Lippincott Williams & Wilkins; 2013:60-69.

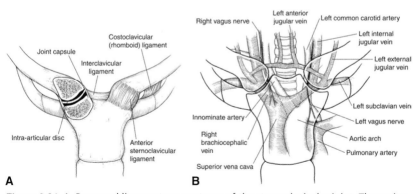

Figure 6.34 A, Bony and ligamentous anatomy of the sternoclavicular joint. The major supporting structures include the anterior capsule, the posterior capsule, the interclavicular ligament, the costoclavicular (rhomboid) ligament, and the intra-articular disk and ligament. B, Retrosternal anatomy. Note the proximity of the sternoclavicular joint to the trachea, aortic arch, and brachiocephalic vein. From Higginbotham TO, Kuhn JE. Atraumatic disorders of the sternoclavicular joint. *J Am Acad Orthop Surg.* 2005;13(2):138-145.

- Posterior
  - **Careful examination of the patient is extremely important to rule out vascular compromise.**
  - Consider CT to rule out mediastinal compression
  - Attempt closed reduction—It is often successful and remains stable.
  - Surgical—thoracic surgeon

DISTAL CLAVICLE OSTEOLYSIS

- **Weight lifters or traumatic injury—repetitive microfracture**
- Radiographs (Figure 6.35)
  - Osteopenia and cystic changes
  - Axillary
- Nonoperative treatment
  - NSAIDs
  - Cortisone injection
  - Activity modification
- Surgical treatment
  - Arthroscopic
  - Distal clavicle excision—0.5 to 1 cm

OTHER SHOULDER PATHOLOGIES

Muscle Injuries

- Pectoralis major
  - Weight lifters—associated with anabolic steroids
  - Eccentric muscle contraction
  - **Axillary webbing and weakness in IR**
  - MRI—identify extent of tear
  - Treatment
    - Incomplete tears—nonoperative
    - **Complete tears**
      - **Sternocostal head more common**
      - Primary repairs do well

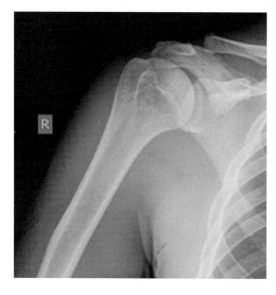

Figure 6.35 Distal clavicle osteolysis.

- Subscapularis
  - Violent ER
  - Shoulder dislocation in older patients or after open procedure
  - Positive lift-off and belly-press
  - Weakness in IR and increase in passive ER
  - Treatment
    - Partial—nonoperative
    - Complete and symptomatic—surgical repair

Nerve Entrapments

- Spinoglenoid cysts
  - Suprascapular nerve (Figure 6.36)
    - Volleyball players
    - **Cysts associated with SLAP tears (Figure 6.37)**
    - Traction injury
    - **Two locations**
      - **Spinoglenoid notch—affects IS only (Figure 6.38)**
      - **Suprascapular notch—affects both SS and IS**
    - Treatment
      - Activity modification with chronic traction injuries
      - Surgery for cysts due to SLAP lesions or labral tears
- Quadrilateral space syndrome (Figure 6.39)
  - **Axillary nerve**
  - **Posterior humeral circumflex**
  - Treatment act modification
  - Surgical—release of space
- Thoracic outlet syndrome (Figure 6.40)
  - More common in women
  - Cervical rib, clavicular nonunions, trauma with resultant fibrosis
  - Adson and Wright tests
  - Nonoperative—activity modification and postural training
  - Surgical—resection of first rib

Adhesive Capsulitis

- More common in women
- Rotator interval—significant thickening and adhesions (Figure 6.41)
- 20% to 30% recurrence in contralateral shoulder
- Associated with:
  - Diabetes mellitus (DM)
  - Thyroid disease
  - Autoimmune disorders
  - Age over 40
- Decreased passive ROM and active ROM
  - Sensitive test—decreased ER at side
  - MRI—axillary recess
  - Fibroblastic proliferation
- Clinical staging
  - Painful—inflammatory
  - Freezing (stiffness)
    - Capsular contracture
    - ROM decreased
  - Thawing—ROM improving
- Treatment
  - **Nonoperative**
    - **NSAIDs, PT, steroids**

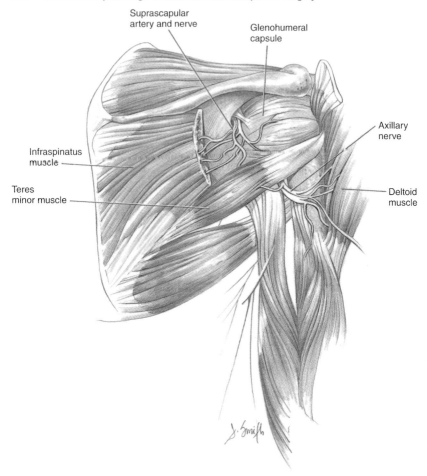

Figure 6.36 Anatomy of the suprascapular nerve as seen from the posterior aspect of the shoulder. Note the nerve traveling under the transverse scapular ligament, whereas the artery travels above the ligament. The nerve and artery then travel under the spinoglenoid ligament at the spinoglenoid notch. From Bragg B, Cheung E, Safran MR. Diagnosis and management of neurovascular disorders about the shoulder in the athlete. In: Miniaci A, ed. *Disorders of the Shoulder: Diagnosis and Management: Sports Injuries*. Vol 2. 3rd ed. Philadelphia, PA: Lippincott Williams & Wilkins; 2014:441-468.

- • **High patient satisfaction**
- • **Decreased ROM versus contralateral side**
- • Surgical
  - • When at least 6 months of conservative measures fail
  - • Arthroscopic capsular release and manipulation under anesthesia

LITTLE LEAGUER ELBOW (MEDIAL EPICONDYLE APOPHYSITIS)

- ● History
  - • Medial pain in cocking
  - • Early or late apophyseal closure
- ● **Treatment—nonoperative**

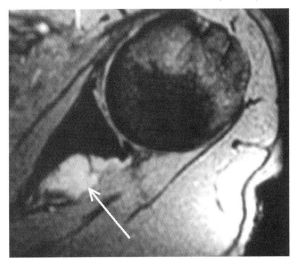

Figure 6.37 Axial T2-weighted magnetic resonance imaging (MRI) scan of a paralabral ganglion cyst. Cysts typically appear loculated with an increased signal on T2-weighted images. An associated labral tear may also be seen. Arrow: Spino glenoid cyst. From Piasecki DP, Romeo AA, Bach BR Jr, Nicholson GP. Suprascapular neuropathy. *J Am Acad Orthop Surg.* 2009;17(11):665-676.

POSTERIOR IMPINGEMENT OF ELBOW

- Diagnosis
  - **Late acceleration to follow-through**
  - Posteromedial spur olecranon—**ulnar collateral ligament (UCL) insufficiency**
  - Catching or locking
  - *Positive valgus extension overload test*
  - Loose bodies

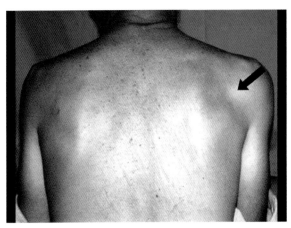

Figure 6.38 Patient with infraspinatus atrophy. The posterior aspect of the scapula demonstrates atrophy in the region of the infraspinatus fossa. Arrow: Infraspinatus atrophy. From Piasecki DP, Romeo AA, Bach BR Jr, Nicholson GP. Suprascapular neuropathy. *J Am Acad Orthop Surg.* 2009;17(11):665-676.

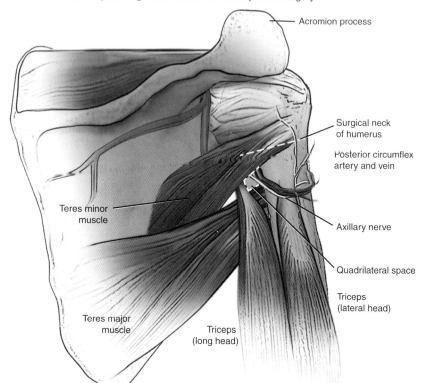

Figure 6.39 Quadrilateral space. From Waldman SD. Ultrasound-guided injection technique for axillary nerve block in the quadrilateral space. In: *Comprehensive Atlas of Ultrasound-Guided Pain Management Injection Techniques*. Philadelphia, PA: Lippincott Williams & Wilkins; 2014:297-303.

- Treatment
  - Nonoperative
  - Surgical
    - Indication—failure of conservative management
    - Arthroscopy
      - UCL insufficiency
      - <3 mm

LOWER EXTREMITY SECTION CRUCIATE LIGAMENTS

Anterior Cruciate Ligament (ACL)

- Overview
  - ACL prevents anterior translation of the tibia relative to the femur.
  - 86% of the total resistance to anterior tibial translation
  - Limit is IR and ER of the knee in extension.
- Anatomy
  - Blood supply—middle geniculate
  - Two bundles (Figure 6.42)
    - Anteromedial—flexion
    - Posterolateral—extension

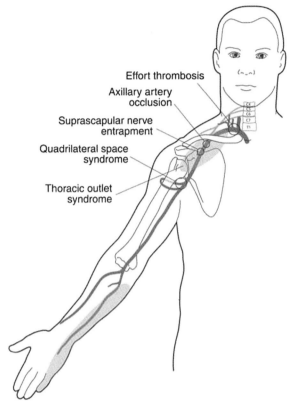

Effort thrombosis

Axillary artery
occlusion

Suprascapular nerve
entrapment

Quadrilateral space
syndrome

Thoracic outlet
syndrome

Figure 6.40 Neurovascular conditions distal to the brachial plexus and their respective areas of involvement, including thoracic outlet syndrome. From Aval SM, Durand P Jr, Shankwiler JA. Neurovascular injuries to the athlete's shoulder: part II. *J Am Acad Orthop Surg.* 2007;15(5):281-289.

- Nerve supply
  - Posterior articular branch of posterior tibial nerve
  - Infrapatellar branch of saphenous nerve—injured during surgery
- Diagnosis
  - "Pop" and effusion
  - Lachman test—sensitive
  - Pivot shift text—most specific and correlates to return to play
- Radiography
  - Segond fracture—lateral capsular avulsion (Figure 6.43)
  - Avulsion fractures
  - Deepened terminal sulcus
- MRI
  - Concomitant injuries
  - Bone bruise (Figure 6.44)
    - Posterolateral tibia
    - Terminal sulcus
- Nonoperative treatment—risk for development of late arthrosis related to meniscal integrity

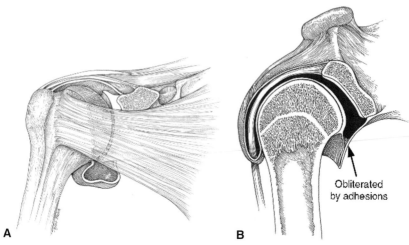

Figure 6.41 Illustrations of the shoulder demonstrating the normal loose axillary fold with the arm dependent (A) and a contracted axillary fold, as is seen in adhesive capsulitis (B). From Neviaser AS, Neviaser RJ. Adhesive capsulitis of the shoulder. *J Am Acad Orthop Surg.* 2011;19(9):536-542.

- Surgical indications
  - Acute tear in young, active individual
  - Functional instability: instability despite activity modification, ±rehab, ±brace
  - Repairable meniscus tear (Figure 6.45)
- Surgical treatment
  - **Regain motion prior to reconstruction**
  - **No superiority of graft choice**
  - **Most important surgical factor is well-performed technique.**
- Complications
  - Graft malposition
    - **Anterior femoral tunnel—reduces flexion and leads to graft rupture (Figure 6.46)**
    - Anterior tibial tunnel—causes graft impingement and loss of extension, leading to graft rupture
  - Loss of stability
    - Early
      - Fixation failure up to 4 to 6 weeks
      - Screw divergence
    - Late—graft failure
  - Loss of motion
    - Arthrofibrosis—timing
    - Loss of ≥10° extension, flexion ≤120°
    - Graft malposition
    - Cyclops lesions may cause loss of extension—MRI is used for diagnosis, which shows soft tissue anteriorly.
    - Infection
      - Deep <1%—aspirate
      - 6 weeks intravenous antibiotics with or without graft
- Rehabilitation and injury prevention
  - Immediate full ROM
  - Hamstring strengthening—agonist
  - Closed chain (foot planted) exercises—primary method of strength training

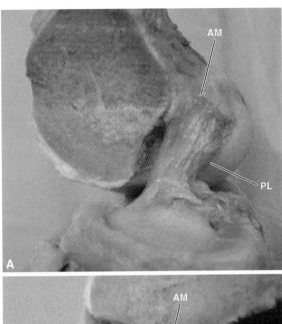

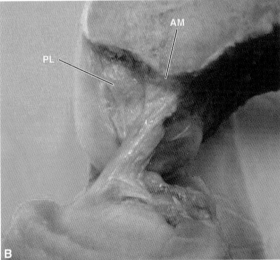

Figure 6.42 The femoral insertion of the anteromedial (AM) and posterolateral (PL) bundles varies based on degree of flexion. At 0°, the femoral insertion is vertical, with the AM bundle superior to the PL bundle (A), whereas at 90°, the femoral insertion is horizontal, with the PL bundle anterior to the AM bundle (B). From Cohen SB, Fu FH. Anatomic double-bundle anterior cruciate ligament reconstruction. In: Miller MD, ed. *Operative Techniques in Sports Medicine Surgery*. Philadelphia, PA: Lippincott Williams & Wilkins; 2011:350-356.

- Return to play
  - 6 months
  - Hop and strength tests—80% to 85% of opposite side
- Prevention (level II)
  - Plyometrics, balance, and technique training reduce risk of serious knee injury in female athletes.

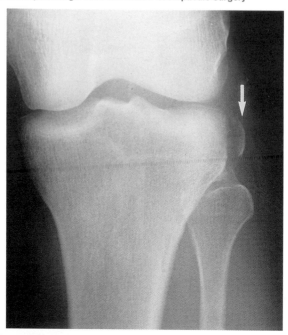

Figure 6.43 Segond fracture. Arrow: Segond fracture. From Greenspan A, Beltran J. Lower limb II: knee. In: *Orthopedic Imaging: A Practical Approach*. 6th ed. Philadelphia, PA: Wolters Kluwer Health; 2015:303-372.

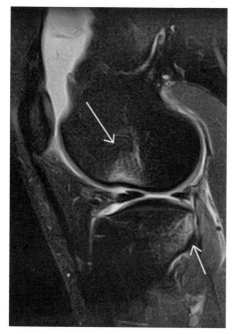

Figure 6.44 Magnetic resonance imaging (MRI) of the knee demonstrating classic bone bruise (arrows) of the midlateral femoral condyle and posterior lateral tibial plateau. From Dempsey IJ, Miller MD. The knee: anterior cruciate ligament. In: *Making the Diagnosis: A Video-Enhanced Guide to Identifying Musculoskeletal Disorders*. Philadelphia, PA: Wolters Kluwer; 2019:13-23.

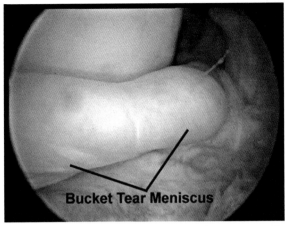

Figure 6.45 Bucket-handle tear. From Lopez-Vidriero E, Johnson DH. Meniscus resection. In: Johnson DH, ed. *Operative Arthoscopy*. 4th ed. Philadelphia, PA: Lippincott Williams & Wilkins; 2013:615-626.

Posterior Cruciate Ligament

- Overview
  - Primary static stabilizer of the knee—location
  - Resists posterior tibial translation
    - At 90° of flexion
    - 95% of force
  - Not isometric during flexion arc
    - Anterolateral bundle tightens in flexion
    - Posteromedial bundle tightens in extension

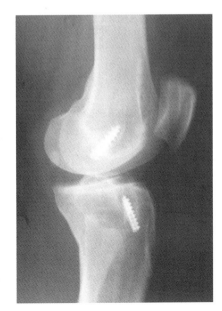

Figure 6.46 Anterior femoral and tibial tunnel placement. From Schenck RC Jr. Injuries of the knee. In: Bucholz RW, Heckman JD, eds. *Rockwood and Green's Fractures in Adults*. Vol 2. 5th ed. Philadelphia, PA: Lippincott Williams & Wilkins; 2001:1845-1938.

- Anatomy (Figure 6.47)
  - Blood supply—middle geniculate
  - Two bundles
    - Anterolateral—flexion
      - Single bundle and tension 90°
      - Larger
    - Posteromedial—extension
- Diagnosis
  - Most common injury mechanisms
    - Direct blow to anterior tibia—dashboard
    - Flexed knee with foot plantar flexed
    - Hyperextension bicruciate injury

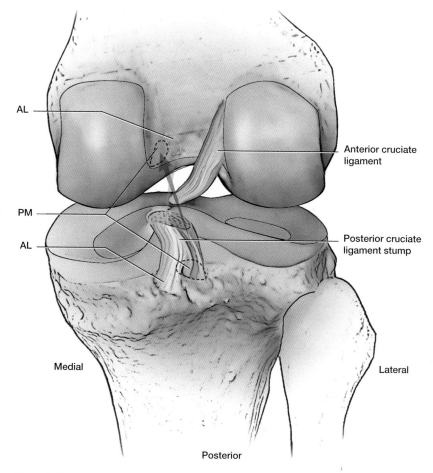

Figure 6.47 Posterior cruciate ligament anatomy. From Wang D, Cheung EC, Joshi NB, McAllister DR. Inlay posterior cruciate ligament reconstruction. In: Johnson DL, ed. *Master Techniques in Orthopaedic Surgery: Reconstructive Knee Surgery.* 4th ed. Philadelphia, PA: Wolters Kluwer; 2017:323-333.

- Clinical tests
  - Posterior drawer test—most sensitive
  - Quadriceps active test—anterior translation at 70° to 90° of flexion
  - Posterior sag test—100% specific
- Natural history
  - Short term
    - Most athletes return to same level l of activity without limitation.
    - Residual laxity (KT-1000) does not correlate with function.
    - Restoring quad strength is critical.
  - Long term
    - Variable prognosis
    - Medial and patellofemoral arthrosis
- Treatment
  - Nonoperative
    - Immobilize with daily ROM in extension for 1 month—decreases posterior sag
    - Quadriceps strengthening
  - Surgical
  - Indications
    - Young patients with grade 3 tears
    - Displaced posterior cruciate ligament (PCL) bony avulsions or "peel-off tears"
    - Two or more ligament injury tears, including the PCL
    - Failure on conservative measures
  - *Cruciate reconstruction is definitive management (Figure 6.48).*
  - Avulsion repair acutely
  - Single bundle
    - Re-creates the anterolateral bundle
    - Usually more appropriate in the multiligamentous setting
    - Transtibial
      - Risk to posterior neurovascular structures
      - Neurovascular bundle (popliteal artery) within 4 mm of posterior horn lateral meniscus
    - Inlay—reduces the killer curve
  - Double bundle—re-creates anterolateral and posteromedial bundles
    - Tensioned at 90 and re-creating the 1 cm anteromedial tibial step-off
- Postoperative rehabilitation
  - Knee extension to reduce stress on graft
  - Quadriceps strengthening
  - Early on—avoid active hamstring exercises

COLLATERAL LIGAMENTS
Medial Collateral Ligament

- Overview and diagnosis
  - Resists valgus and ER
  - Superficial—primary restraint
  - Valgus blow to weight-bearing flexed knee
  - Examination at 0° and 30° (Figure 6.49)
    - If stable in 0° extension—grade 1 or 2
    - If increased laxity—grade 3 with injury to posteromedial corner of knee
      - Consider ACL or PCL
      - Consider multiple ligament injury
  - MRI—not needed for primary medial collateral ligament (MCL)

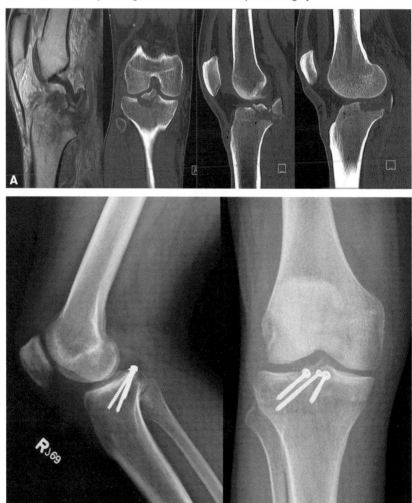

Figure 6.48 A, Posterior cruciate ligament (PCL) avulsion. B, Surgical repair.

- Treatment
  - Isolated MCL
    - Treat nonoperatively in hinged brace
    - Weight bearing as tolerated, early motion
    - Return to sports/activity as tolerated—typically 2 to 6 weeks
  - Combined MCL and ACL
    - Nonoperative MCL; surgical reconstruction of ACL when ROM restored
    - Some advocate early surgical repair of grade 3 MCL and cruciate reconstruction
  - Combined MCL and PCL
    - Most advocate primary repair of MCL, reconstruction of the PCL

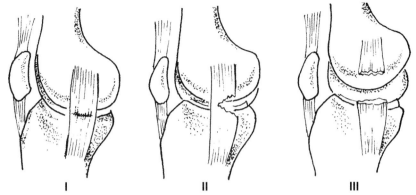

Figure 6.49 Medial collateral ligament (MCL) injuries. Grade 1: microscopic strain. Grade 2: partial tear. Grade 3: complete tear. From Wilckens JH, Urquhart M. Medial collateral ligament injury. In: Frassica FJ, Sponseller PD, Wilckens JH, eds. *The 5-Minute Orthopaedic Consult.* 2nd ed. Philadelphia, PA: Lippincott Williams & Wilkins; 2007:250-251.

Lateral Collateral Ligament (LCL) and PCL Injuries

- Anatomy of the posterolateral corner
  - LCL
  - Popliteus complex
    - Muscle-tendon
    - Popliteofibular ligament
  - Other structures that are included in the posterolateral knee—arcuate ligament, fabellar ligament, biceps, and iliotibial (IT) band
  - Varus stress at 0° and 30°
- Diagnosis of posterolateral corner injury—Dial test (Figure 6.50)
  - Increased ER at 30°
    - >15° of difference is significant.
    - Posterolateral instability—Key is asymmetrical ER.
  - Increase only at 30°: isolated PLC injury
  - Increase at both 30° and 90°: combined PLC and PCL injury
- Isolated LCL injury
  - Very uncommon
  - Carefully assess for associated cruciate injury
  - Nonoperative treatment for grades 1 and 2
  - Consider primary repair versus anatomic reconstruction in grade 3
- Combined lateral and cruciate injury
  - Reconstruction of both cruciate and lateral side
  - Timing is controversial.
    - Many advocate immediate primary repair of all posterolateral injuries.
    - With use of reconstruction, can delay surgery
- Chronic ligament deficiency and severe varus
  - Correct varus first
  - Take care of bony malalignment before ligament repair

MULTIPLE LIGAMENT INJURIES

- Knee dislocation
  - Direction of dislocation
    - Anterior—most common
    - Lateral—more common than medial
    - Posterolateral—irreducible

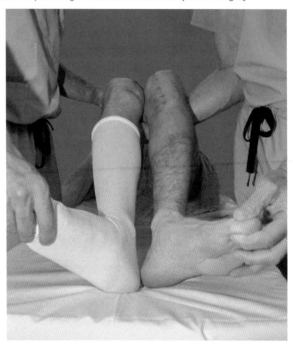

Figure 6.50 Dial test. From LaPrade RF, Moulton SG, Cram TR, Kennedy NI. PLC reconstruction with tibial/fibular-based tunnels: anatomic reconstruction. In: Johnson DL, ed. *Master Techniques in Orthopaedic Surgery: Reconstructive Knee Surgery.* 4th ed. Philadelphia, PA: Wolters Kluwer; 2017:391-405.

- Vascular injury
  - Incidence following anterior knee dislocation is 30% to 50%—transection or intimal tearing
    - High velocity—24%
    - Low velocity—4.8%
  - 25% incidence to popliteal artery—Popliteal artery is tethered between adductor hiatus proximally and soleus arch distally.
  - Amputation rate
    - 6% for revascularization <6 hours
    - 11% for revascularization <8 hours
    - 86% for revascularization >8 hours
- Neurologic injury
  - High velocity—26%
  - Low velocity—19%
  - 25% (16%-40%) incidence to peroneal nerve
  - Half result in permanent neurologic deficit
- Imaging
  - MRI—for surgical planning
  - Neurovascular examination
    - Closed reduction
    - Repeat examination
      - Pulses normal
        - Serial monitoring
        - Consider arteriography

- - Pulses abnormal
    - · Vascular consult
    - · Arteriography
  - Arteriography
    - Should be considered for all knee dislocation patients if questionable findings on physical examination
    - Identifies
      - Vascular tear
      - Thrombosis
      - Intimal tear
      - Vasospasm
    - Complication rate <2%
    - 5% false-positive rate
- Surgical treatment
  - Indications for immediate surgery
    - Open dislocation
    - Irreducible dislocation—posterolateral
    - Arterial injury
    - Compartment syndrome
  - Timing of definitive surgery
    - Immediate (within 2-3 weeks)
      - ACL + PCL + LCL
      - PCL + LCL
      - ACL + PCL + MCL—grade 3 injuries or distal tears
      - PCL + MCL—grade 3 injuries or distal tears
    - Delayed
      - ACL + PC—intact collaterals
      - ACL + PCL + MC—grade 1/2 where intact

MENISCAL INJURY AND REPAIR

- Diagnosis
  - Loss of motion—Extension loss indicates bucket-handle tear.
  - Joint line tenderness
  - Provocative tests for meniscal tears
    - McMurray
    - Apley
    - Thessaly
  - ACL injuries
    - Acute ACL injury—lateral meniscal tear associated
    - Chronic ACL injuries—medial meniscal tears
    - Repair—improved with ACL reconstruction
      - In the setting of ACL reconstruction, the healing rate for meniscal repair is 80%.
      - Isolated meniscal repair with no ACL tear, the healing rate is 70%.
- Nonoperative treatment
  - Management predicated on symptoms
  - Stable tears (Figure 6.51)
    - Short ≤1 cm long
    - ≤3-mm displacement with probing
  - Partial thickness—degenerative tears with OA
- Surgical treatment
  - Location of tear—**#1 factor in the success of meniscal repair is the blood supply.**
  - Vascular zones of meniscus (Table 6.1, Figure 6.52)
    - Highest success—red zone or most vascularized area
    - Lowest success—white zone

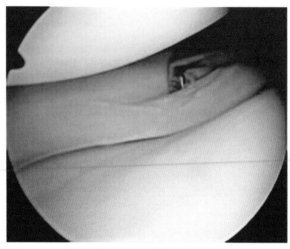

Figure 6.51 Stable meniscal tear. From Lopez-Vidriero E, Johnson DH. Meniscus resection. In: Johnson DH, ed. *Operative Arthroscopy*. 4th ed. Philadelphia, PA: Lippincott Williams & Wilkins; 2013:615-626.

- Partial meniscectomy
  - >80% satisfactory function at 5 years
  - 50% of patients have Fairbank radiographic findings at 5 years
  - Predictors of long-term success
    - <40 years of age
    - Normal alignment
    - Minimal arthritis
    - Single fragment
- Surgical repair
  - Inside out—gold standard (Figure 6.53)
    - Medial meniscus
      - Caution: saphenous nerve
    - Lateral meniscus
      - Caution: common peroneal nerve
  - Outside in—anterior tears
  - All inside—risk is damage to articular cartilage with improper insertion
  - Success rates
    - Stable knees—80%
    - Repair in conjunction with ACL—90%
    - Ligamentous unstable knees decrease success rate of repair from 70% to 95% down to 30% to 70%.

Table 6.1. Vascular Zones of the Meniscus

Zone	Location	Vascular Status
Red	Peripheral	Vascularized
Red-white	Middle third	Avascular
White	Central third	Avascular

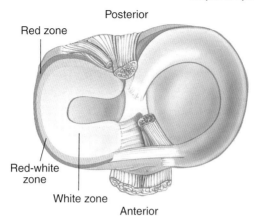

Figure 6.52 Meniscal vascular zones. From Azar FM, Bonnaig NS. Arthroscopic meniscectomy. In: Miller MD, ed. *Operative Techniques in Sports Medicine Surgery*. 2nd ed. Philadelphia, PA: Wolters Kluwer; 2016:367-377.

- **Fixation strengths—vertical suture (202N) > horizontal suture = most implants > meniscal arrow (96N)**
- Meniscal allograft
  - Noyes—"investigational"
    - 50% failure in 96 allografts with 10-year follow-up

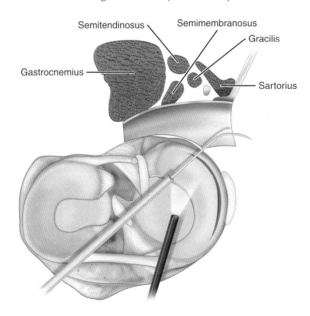

Figure 6.53 Inside-out medial meniscus repair. From Sgaglione NA, Myers K, Bitterman A. Meniscal repair. In: Miller MD, ed. *Operative Techniques in Sports Medicine Surgery*. 2nd ed. Philadelphia, PA: Wolters Kluwer; 2016:378-391.

  - Approximately 70% successful in "ideal patient"—fresh-frozen tissue, sizing crucial, and bone blocks performed better.
  - Indications
    - Young (<50 years) with pain
    - Status post total meniscectomy
    - Stable
    - Grade 3 or less chondral damage
  - Contraindications
    - Uncorrected extremity alignment
    - Instability
    - Significant chondral changes
  - Correct alignment before allograft
- Discoid meniscus (Figure 6.54)
  - Lateral more often than medial
  - 5% incidence
  - More common in Asians
  - Wrisberg variant lacks peripheral attachment.
  - Usually asymptomatic—surgery only if torn or snapping
  - Central tears treated with saucerization
  - Peripheral tears repaired when possible
- Meniscal cyst (Figure 6.55)
  - Strong association with degenerative tears
  - Horizontal cleavage tears of the lateral meniscus
  - Decrease in the size with knee flexion
  - Aspiration or scope and internal decompression
  - Open cystectomy for recurrence

ARTICULAR CARTILAGE INJURIES
Osteochondritis Dissecans

- Overview
  - Disease of the subchondral bone and the adjacent cartilage in young patients (Figure 6.56)
  - More common in adolescents and young children
    - Juveniles have open physes and better prognosis.

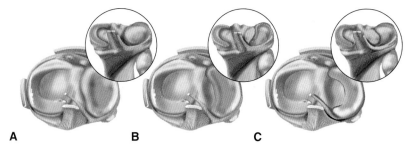

A   B   C

Figure 6.54 Classification of discoid meniscus: complete (A), incomplete (B), and Wrisberg variant (C). From Goodbody CM, Lee RJ, Ho-Fung VM, Ganley TL. Discoid meniscus: overview, epidemiology, classification, assessment. In: Cordasco FA, Green DW, eds. *Pediatric and Adolescent Knee Surgery*. Philadelphia, PA: Wolters Kluwer; 2015:231-235.

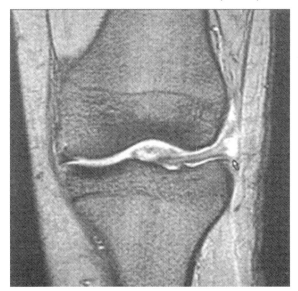

Figure 6.55 Meniscal cyst.

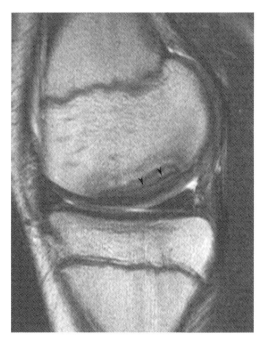

Figure 6.56 Osteochondritis dissecans. From Berquist TH. Knee. In: *MRI of the Musculo-skeletal System*. 6th ed. Philadelphia, PA: Wolters Kluwer; 2013:319-459.

- More common in males and bilateral in up to 25%
- 70% of cases in posterolateral aspect of MFC, 15% to 20% in central LFC, 5% to 10% in patella
- Etiology unknown—possible trauma or vascular
- Guhl staging
  - A—intact lesions
  - B—lesions with early separation
  - C—partially detached lesions
  - D—crater with loose bodies
- Nonoperative treatment
  - Limitation of activities as well as protected weight bearing with use of splints or crutches until patient free of symptoms
  - Continue conservative management for at least 3 months
  - Most juvenile osteochondritis dissecans cases and open physes can be successfully managed nonoperatively.
- Surgical treatment
  - If continued symptoms and recurrent effusions after at least 3 months of conservative management
    - Stable lesion—drilling (Figure 6.57)
      - Anterograde
      - Retrograde
    - Unstable lesion—internal fixation
      - Possible bone graft
      - Removal of loose fragment

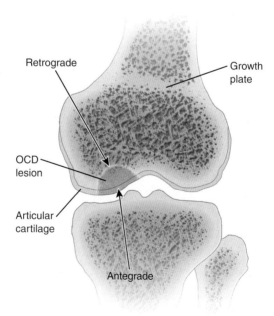

Figure 6.57 Retrograde and antegrade drilling of osteochondritis dissecans (OCD) lesions. From Burrus MT, Diduch DR. Osteochondritis dissecans and avascular necrosis. In: Miller MD, ed. *Operative Techniques in Sports Medicine Surgery*. 2nd ed. Philadelphia, PA: Wolters Kluwer; 2016:441-455.

Full-Thickness Grade 4 Defects

- Abrasion chondroplasty
  - Remove loose flaps and produce smooth margins to prevent propagation
  - Deteriorates with time
- Drilling/microfracture
  - Fibrocartilage formed.
  - Drilled into subchondral bone
  - Pluripotent cells escape from the marrow cavity.
  - Clot forms over defect and fibrocartilage forms.
  - Results better than abrasion, but type I collagen is not as durable as articular cartilage
  - Microfracture should be considered primary treatment option for full-thickness defects.
- OATS
  - Defects up to 2.5 cm^2
  - Plugs of varying diameters are harvested from low contact area (notch or supero-lateral aspect lateral femoral condyle).
- Allograft—medium to large lesions

Treatment Algorithm

- Correction of instability and malalignment critical to success of any procedure
- Lesions ≤1 cm
  - Observation
  - Abrasion chondroplasty
  - Microfracture
  - Osteochondral autograft transfer
- Lesions 1 to 2 cm
  - Abrasion chondroplasty
  - Microfracture
  - Osteochondral autograft transfer
- Larger than 2 cm
  - Lesions 2 to 3.5 cm
    - Fresh osteochondral allograft
    - Autologous chondrocyte implantation (ACI)
  - Lesions 3.5 to 10 cm—ACI
  - Multiple lesions (two or three)—ACI

EXTENSOR MECHANISM INJURIES AND PAIN

Patellofemoral Pain with Instability

- Medial patellofemoral ligament (MPFL)—main passive restraint to lateral translation (Figure 6.58)
- Medial dislocation—iatrogenic
- Nonsurgical management—first line
- Surgical indications
  - Osteochondral loose bodies
  - Recurrent instability—after PT
- Caton-Deschamps (CD) index—distance from the inferior patella articular margin to the tibial plateau/length of patella articular surface
  - Patella alta > 1.2
  - Baja < 0.8
- Recurrent (conservative management fails)
  - CT or MRI
    - Congruence—subluxation

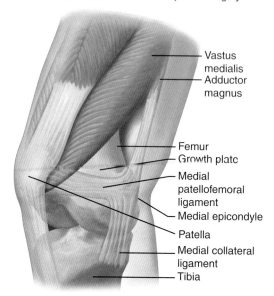

Figure 6.58 The MPFL tethers the medial patella to the medial condyle of the femur. From Wall EJ, Albright JC, Steward SR. Acute patellar and chronic patellar instability. In: Flynn JM, Sankar WN, eds. *Operative Techniques in Pediatric Orthopaedic Surgery*. 2nd ed. Philadelphia, PA: Wolters Kluwer; 2016:371-381.

- MPFL—reconstruction
  - No patella alta or dysplasia
    - Patella alta (CD ratio > 1.2)—add distalization of tibial tubercle (TT)
    - Patella tilt—add lateral release
- Lateral malposition
  - MPFL + medialization of TT with osteotomy
    - Fulkerson anteromedialization
    - Q-angle
      - Essentially the quadriceps vector—the resultant angle connecting a point near the anterior superior iliac spine (ASIS) to the midpoint of the patella
      - Males—15° is normal
      - Females—18° is normal
    - Tibial tubercle to trochlear groove (TT-TG) distance
      - Normal 12 mm, abnormal > 20 mm
      - CT or MRI
      - Lateralizing force that is applied to patella during quad contraction

Patellofemoral Pain without Instability

- Assess spine, hip, knee, and foot mechanics
- MRI—chondral injuries or ligamentous injuries
- CT—dynamic patella tracking and evaluating TT-TG distance
- Always start with nonsurgical treatment for 12 months.
- Surgical treatment—only after failure of at least 12 months of PT
  - Chondral flap—arthroscopy
  - Alta—distalization and arthroscopy

- Tight retinaculum—perform lateral release after failure of conservative measures, plus:
  - Lateral patellofemoral angle <11°
  - Positive lateral tilt without subluxation

Patellas and Quadriceps Tendons

- Ruptures
  - Patient age
    - <40 years—patellar tendon
    - >40 years—quadriceps tendon
  - Quadriceps ruptures 3 times more frequently
  - Indirect trauma—falling on partially flexed knee
  - Eccentric loading of the extensor mechanism and usually associated with predisposing factors—obesity, DM, thyroid conditions, rheumatoid arthritis, gout, systemic lupus erythematosus, and chronic renal failure
  - Palpable gap
  - Extensor disruption—unable to straight leg raise
  - Radiographs
    - Patella shifted inferiorly with quadriceps rupture
    - Patella shifted superiorly with patellar tendon rupture
  - Anatomic repair gives best results.
  - Generally results of quadriceps repairs better
- Tendinopathy
  - Active individuals, usually when increasing activities
  - Eccentric contractions, such as jumping sports
  - Usually occurs at attachment sites
  - Presentation and classification (Blazina)
    - 1—Pain after activity
    - 2—Pain during and after activity
    - 3—Limits function
  - X-rays—spurring at attachment sites
  - MRI—thickening of tendon
  - Treatment
    - Conservative
      - Activity modification, rest, and progress to flexibility and eccentric strengthening
      - Never corticosteroid injection
    - Surgery only if conservative management fails

HIP

Hip Arthroscopy

- Indications
  - Labral tear—symptomatic
  - Loose bodies
  - Synovial chondromatosis
  - Femoroacetabular impingement (FAI)
    - Cam—femoral head
    - Pincer—acetabulum
  - Chondral injuries
  - Instability
  - Snapping hip
  - Ligamentum teres injuries
  - Staging avascular necrosis
- Contraindications
  - Limitation capsular mobility

- Ankylosis
- Advanced OA
- Protrusio acetabuli
- Severe osteoporosis
- Grade 3 or 4 heterotopic ossification (HO)
- Portals
  - Anterolateral
    - First established
    - Superior anterior corner of greater trochanter
    - Least risk to neurovascular structures—superior gluteal nerve
  - Anterior
    - Starting point—line from the tip of greater trochanter intersecting with line from ASIS
    - 45° cephalad and 30° midline
    - Working portal
    - Risks—femoral artery, femoral nerve, lateral femoral cutaneous nerve, and lateral circumflex artery
  - Posterolateral
    - 2 to 3 cm posterior to tip of greater trochanter
    - Sciatic nerve at risk
- Complications
  - Complications rate—1% to 3%
    - Traction and compression injuries
      - Pudendal nerve, peroneal branch of sciatic, and lateral femoral cutaneous
      - Limit to less than 2 hours
      - Intermittent traction
    - Iatrogenic articular damage—underreported
    - Pressure necrosis
    - Instrument breakage

Femoroacetabular Impingement

- Categories (Figure 6.59)
  - Cam
    - Abnormalities that are femoral based, such as aspherical head, reduced head neck offset—a large, abnormally shaped femoral head jammed into acetabulum during normal motion, especially flexion
    - Most common in young, active males
  - Pincer
    - Acetabulum-based disorders such as acetabular retroversion—abnormal contact between acetabular rim and femoral neck
    - Middle-aged women engaged in athletic activity
- Clinical presentation
  - Young adult with slow onset of groin pain
  - Pain exacerbated by athletic activity, walking, or long period of sitting
  - Limitation of hip motion, especially IR and adduction with hip flexed
  - Impingement test almost always positive—flexion, adduction, IR (Figure 6.60)
  - Associated bony abnormalities (dysplasia and impingement disease)
- Imaging
  - Radiographs
    - Standing true AP, lateral—bony abnormalities
    - AP pelvis—assess acetabular anatomy and sphericity of femoral head (Figure 6.61)
    - Center edge angle—dysplasia
    - Cross table lateral in 15° IR
  - MR—chondral and labral lesions (Figure 6.62)

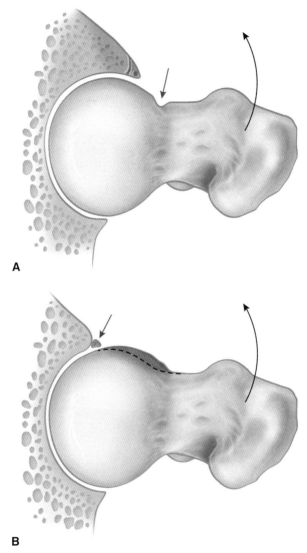

A

B

Figure 6.59 A, Pincer impingement is the result of contact between an abnormal acetabular rim and a normal femoral head-neck junction. B, Cam impingement is the result of contact between an abnormal femoral head-neck junction and the acetabulum. From Larson CM, Birmingham PM. Scope for femoroacetabular impingement. In: Miller MD, ed. *Operative Techniques in Sports Medicine Surgery*. 2nd ed. Philadelphia, PA: Wolters Kluwer; 2016:395-305.

- Treatment
  - Femoroacetabular osteoplasty
    - Open—surgical dislocation
    - Trochanteric flip to preserve femoral head blood supply by preserving deep branch medial femoral circumflex artery

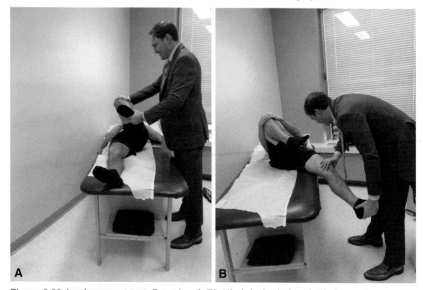

Figure 6.60 Impingement test. From Lynch TS. Hip injuries in baseball players. In: Ahmad CS, Romeo AA, eds. *Baseball Sports Medicine*. Philadelphia, PA: Wolters Kluwer; 2019:386-300.

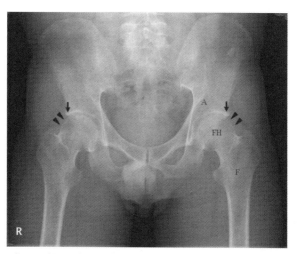

Figure 6.61 Radiographic evidence of both pincer-type impingement with acetabular overcoverage of the femoral heads (arrows) and cam-type impingement with asphericity of the femoral head-neck junctions (arrowheads). From Sandell LJ, Takebe K, Hashimoto S, Gill CS. Articular cartilage and labrum: composition, function, and disease. In: Clohisy JC, Beaulé, della calle CJ, et al, eds. *The Adult Hip: Hip Preservation Surgery*. Philadelphia, PA: Wolters Kluwer; 2015:31-41.

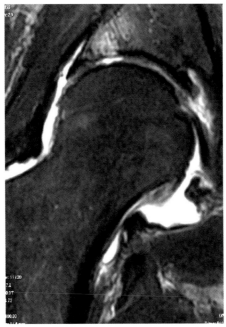

Figure 6.62 Magnetic resonance imaging (MRI) arthrogram showing femoroacetabular impingement with pincer and labral lesions. From Safran M, Kalisvaart M, Stanich MA. Hip arthroscopy: the basics. In: Miller MD, ed. *Operative Techniques in Sports Medicine Surgery*. 2nd ed. Philadelphia, PA: Wolters Kluwer; 2016:276-287.

- Arthroscopy
- Arthroscopy + limited open approach
- Complications
  - HO
  - Trochanteric nonunion—surgical dislocation
  - Sciatic nerve palsy
  - Femoral neck fracture—depth of femoral head neck junction osteochondroplasty should be limited to <30% diameter of femoral neck.

Sports Hernia

- Mechanism of injury—extension and abduction
- Most common in soccer and ice hockey players
- Abdominal ± groin injury
  - Abdominal—rectus, external oblique, transversalis tear
  - Groin—adductor longus tear
- Repair rectus and adductor release or lengthening

Bursitis

- At least 13 consistent bursae around hip region
  - Most common: trochanteric, iliopsoas, ischial, iliopectineal
  - Difficult to differentiate

- May coexist with tendinitis, tendinosis, friction syndromes
- Almost always nonoperative treatment

Snapping Hip Syndrome

- External—IT band tracks over greater trochanter
  - Most common
- Internal—iliopsoas tendon over femoral head
  - Audible snapping with extension of a flexed, abducted, and externally rotated hip
- Intra-articular—labral tears
  - Usually clicking rather than snapping
- Diagnosis
  - Generally clinical
  - X-rays may show loose bodies.
  - MRI arthrogram—diagnostic
  - Iliopsoas bursography
- Conservative treatment—first line
  - 6 to 12 months to resolve
  - Stretching
  - Rest and avoidance of symptoms
- Surgical treatment
  - Internal—iliopsoas fractional lengthening
  - External—Z-plasty of the IT band
  - Intra-articular—hip arthroscopy

SHOULDER

SHOULDER ANATOMY

- Proximal humerus
  - **Greater tuberosity**—insertion—**supraspinatus (SS)** (suprascapular nerve), **infraspinatus (IS)** (suprascapular nerve), **teres minor** (axillary nerve)
  - **Lesser tuberosity**—insertion—**subscapularis** (upper/lower subscapular nerve)
  - Rotator cuff (RTC)—provides stability and concavity compression of the glenohumeral joint
  - Bicipital groove—splits the lesser and greater tuberosity
  - **Biceps pulley**—prevents medial subluxation; composed of **coracohumeral ligament** and **superior glenohumeral ligament** (SGHL)
  - Humeral head is retroverted with respect to the shaft, an average of approximately 20° (range, 15°-45°).
  - Blood supply—anterolateral ascending branch of anterior circumflex artery
  - Rotator interval (Figure 7.1)
    - Borders—medial coracoid base, superior SS tendon (which is immediately posterior to bicipital groove), subscapularis inferiorly
    - **Contents—coracohumeral ligament, SGHL, long head of biceps** (intra-articular portion), capsule (Figure 7.2)
    - **Important points**
      - Inferior instability with arm in adduction
      - Posterior translation with arm flexed, adducted, and internal rotation

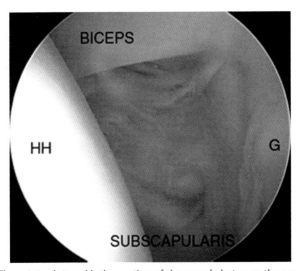

Figure 7.1 The rotator interval is the portion of the capsule between the supraspinatus and subscapularis. Arthroscopically, it is seen bordered by the biceps, subscapularis, humeral head (HH), and glenoid (G). From Delaney RA, Simovitch RW, Miller LR, Higgins LD. Arthroscopic capsular releases for loss of motion. In: Miller MD, ed. *Operative Techniques in Sports Medicine Surgery.* 2nd ed. Philadelphia, PA: Wolters Kluwer; 2016:124-133.

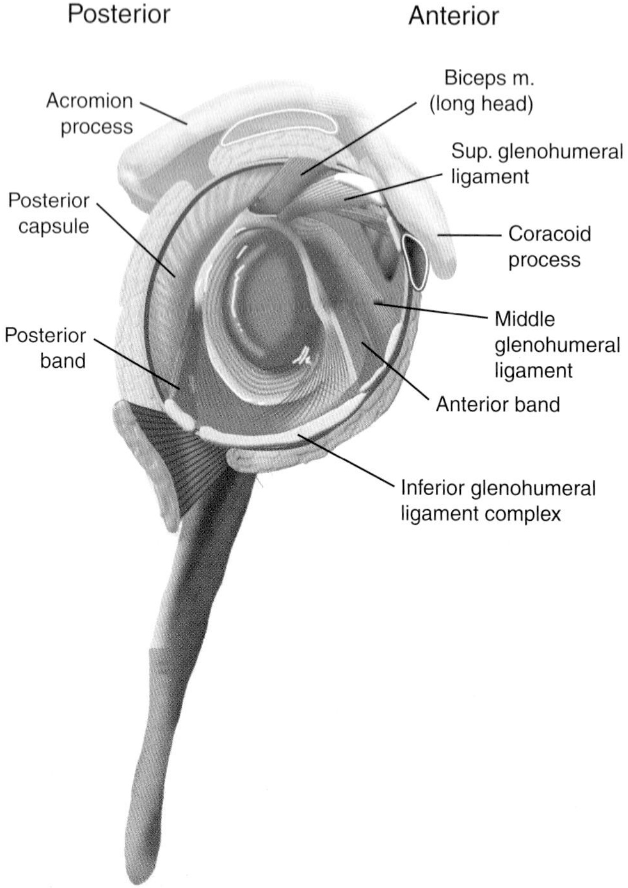

Posterior   Anterior

Figure 7.2 Shoulder anatomy of the glenohumeral ligaments and rotator interval. From Khair MM, Lehman JD, Gulotta LV. Gross and arthroscopic anatomy of the glenohumeral joint. In: Dodson CC, Dines DM, Dines JS, et al, eds. *Controversies in Shoulder Instability*. Philadelphia, PA: Lippincott Williams & Wilkins; 2014:3-10.

- With intact rotator interval, the sulcus sign decreases with external rotation (ER).
  - Adhesive capsulitis—contracture
- Glenohumeral ligaments (Figure 7.3)
  - Middle glenohumeral ligament (MGHL)—limits anterior instability in ER and abducted to 45°
  - Inferior glenohumeral ligament (IGHL)—limits anterior and posterior translation
    - Major stabilizer of arm when ER and abducted between 45° and 90°
- Dynamic restraints—important in multidirectional instability (MDI)
  - RTC muscles
    - Concavity—compression
    - Contract to center and stabilize humeral head on glenoid

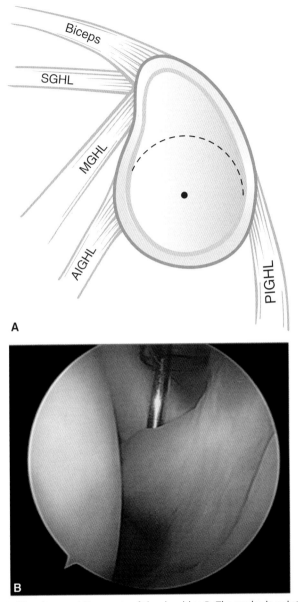

Figure 7.3 A, Glenohumeral ligaments of the shoulder. B, The probe is pointing to the middle glenohumeral ligament (MGHL). Subscapularis is also shown. C, The probe is pointing to the inferior glenohumeral ligament (IGHL). Humeral head and glenoid are also shown. AIGHL, anterior inferior glenohumeral ligament; PIGHL, posterior band of the inferior glenohumeral ligament; SGHL, superior glenohumeral ligament. A: From Burkhart SS, Lo IK, Brady PC. Understanding and recognizing pathology. In: *Burkhart's View of the Shoulder: A Cowboy's Guide to Advanced Shoulder Arthroscopy*. Philadelphia, PA: Lippincott Williams & Wilkins; 2006:53-109.

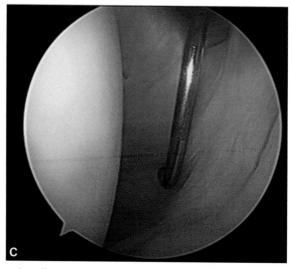

Figure 7.3 (*continued*)

- Scapula
  - Three borders: superior, medial, and lateral
  - **Acromion**—three ossifications centers—meta, meso, and pre
    - Failure of fusion of any results in **os acromiale; meso, most common**
  - Acromioclavicular joint—prevents horizontal translation of distal clavicle (superior and posterior most important)
    - Gliding joint, contains articular disk
  - **Coracoid**—"lighthouse" of the shoulder
    - Origin—short head of the biceps, coracobrachialis; insertion—pectoralis minor
      - Ligaments—coracoacromial (CA), coracoclavicular
  - **Stabilizers**
    - Trapezius
    - Serratus anterior
    - Levator scapulae
    - Rhomboid group
- Clavicle
  - First bone in the body to ossify, last to fuse
- Coracoclavicular ligaments
  - **Conoid** (posterior and **medial**), **trapezoid** (anterior and **lateral**)
    - Prevent vertical translation distal clavicle
- Glenoid
  - Shallow and relatively flat
  - Labrum provides stability and depth.
  - Version—average neutral to 5° retroversion
  - Central bare area
  - Ligaments
    - **SGHL**—restricts anterior translation with the arm in **adduction**
    - **MGHL**—restricts anterior translation with the arm at **45°**
    - Abduction and ER

- **IGHL**
  - Anterior band—restricts anterior-inferior translation with arm in **90° of abduction and ER**
  - Posterior band—restricts posterior-inferior translation with arm in internal rotation and adduction
- **Vessels**
  - Lateral border of the first rib subclavian artery becomes the axillary artery.
  - Axillary artery—three parts in relation to the pectoralis minor (Figure 7.4)
    - Medial to pectoralis minor—supreme thoracic
    - Deep to the pectoralis minor
      - Thoracoacromial
        · Acromial
        · Deltoid
        · Pectoral
        · Clavicular
      - Lateral thoracic
    - Inferior to pectoralis minor
      - Anterior humeral circumflex
      - Posterior humeral circumflex—quadrilateral space with axillary
        · Posterior inferior humeral head
      - Subscapular
        · Thoracodorsal
        · Circumflex scapular
- **Brachial plexus (Figure 7.5)**
  - Roots—C5 to T1
  - Trunks—upper, middle, and lower
  - Division—each trunk has an anterior and posterior division.
  - Cords—posterior, lateral, and medial
  - Branches—innervate upper extremity
  - Long thoracic—serratus anterior and medial winging
  - Spinal accessory—trapezius and lateral winging
  - Suprascapular—suprascapular notch (SS and IS) and spinoglenoid (IS)

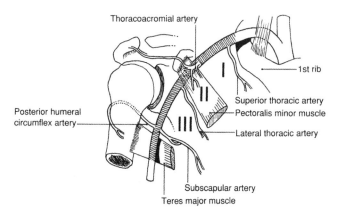

Figure 7.4 Axillary artery in relationship to adjacent structures. A: From Beavers FP, Simon KB. Axillobifemoral bypass. In: Scott-Conner CEH, ed. *Scott-Conner & Dawson Essential Operative Techniques and Anatomy*. 4th ed. Philadelphia, PA: Lippincott Williams & Wilkins; 2014:e36. B: Reprinted with permission from Williams A. *Massage Mastery*. Philadelphia, PA: Lippincott Williams & Wilkins; 2012.

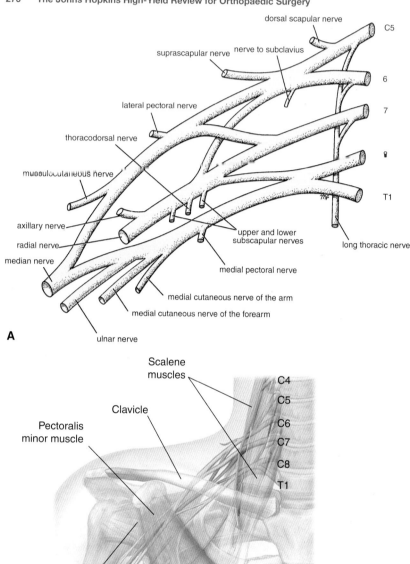

Figure 7.5 Brachial plexus. A: From Snell RS. *Clinical Anatomy*. 7th ed. Philadelphia, PA: Lippincott Williams & Wilkins; 2003. B: From Bell BR, Yan J-G, Matloub H. Primary treatment of neonatal brachial plexus palsy. In: Chung KC, ed. *Operative Techniques in Plastic Surgery*. Vol 4. Philadelphia, PA: Wolters Kluwer; 2020:2948.

- Commonly tested anatomic relationships
  - Pectoralis major—distance from the upper border to articular surface humeral head is approximately 5.6 cm.
  - **Musculocutaneous nerve** courses through the **coracobrachialis** on average **5 to 8 cm from tip of coracoid.**
  - **Axillary nerve**—anterior branch—**10 to 25 mm from inferior glenoid**
  - Posterior branch—5 cm (average) from lateral tip of acromion
  - Suprascapular nerve—1.5 cm from posterior glenoid rim
  - Radial nerve—most commonly crosses from posterior to anterior compartment at the deltoid insertion, more specifically approximately 14 cm from lateral epicondyle
  - **Quadrilateral space**
    - Medial border—triceps (long head)
    - Lateral border—humerus
    - Superior border—teres minor
    - Inferior border—teres major
    - **Contains axillary nerve, posterior circumflex vessels**
  - **Triangular space**
    - Inferior border—teres major
    - Medial border—long head of the triceps
    - Lateral border—humerus
    - **Contains radial nerve**
  - **Long thoracic nerve injury—serratus anterior palsy** → medial scapular winging
  - **Spinal accessory nerve injury—trapezius palsy** → lateral scapular winging
  - Winging based on direction of inferior border of scapula
- Surgical approaches
  - **Deltopectoral approach**—workhorse (Figure 7.6)
    - Most common for arthroplasty, trauma, and open instability
    - **Cephalic vein**
      - Marks the interval between the pectoralis major (medial and lateral pectoral nerves) and the deltoid (axillary nerve)
      - Move vein laterally to decrease bleeding
    - Deltoid (axillary)—pectoralis (medial and lateral pectoral nerves)
    - Deep
      - Identify coracoid and conjoint
      - Stay lateral
      - Musculocutaneous nerve can be injured with vigorous retraction conjoint tendon.
    - **Risks**
      - Axillary nerve
      - Musculocutaneous nerve—retraction
      - Anterior humeral circumflex
  - **Posterior approach**
    - Used to access scapula (open reduction internal fixation), posterior glenoid/labrum
      - Glenoid and posterior capsular shift
      - Scapular neck fractures
      - Glenoid fractures
      - Glenoid osteotomy
    - Interval—teres minor (**axillary nerve**) and IS (**suprascapular nerve**)
    - Risks
      - Quadrilateral space—axillary nerve and posterior humeral circumflex
      - Suprascapular nerve from retraction

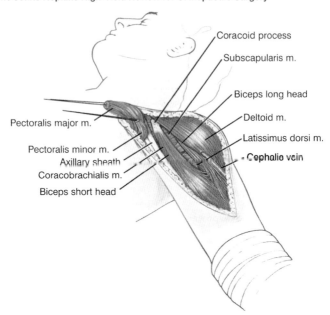

Coracoid process

Subscapularis m.

Biceps long head

Deltoid m.

Latissimus dorsi m.

Cephalic vein

Pectoralis major m.

Pectoralis minor m.

Axillary sheath

Coracobrachialis m.

Biceps short head

Figure 7.6 Deltopectoral approach. From Malawer MM, Wittig JC, Kellar-Graney K. Proximal humerus resection with endoprosthetic replacement: intra-articular and extra-articular resections. In: Wiesel SW, ed. *Operative Techniques in Orthopaedic Surgery*. Vol 2. 2nd ed. Philadelphia, PA: Wolters Kluwer; 2016:2208-2221.

- Lateral approach
  - Used for open RTC repair, tuberosity fractures, proximal humerus fractures (beware posterior branch axillary nerve approximately 7 cm)
  - No true internervous plane
  - Can use natural raphe between anterior and posterior deltoid (split) or take down deltoid from anterolateral acromion
  - Risk—axillary if deltoid split pass 5 cm

SHOULDER ARTHROSCOPY (Figure 7.7)

- Posterior portals
  - Initial diagnostic (1)
  - Posterior 7 o'clock (7) (posterior labrum and MDI)
- Anterior portals—2 (5 o'clock) and 6 (superior)
  - Diagnostic
  - Labrum procedures
    - Bankart (2)
    - Biceps tenotomy and superior labrum anterior to posterior (SLAP) (6)
  - Distal clavicle
- Lateral portals (3 and 4)
  - RTC, subacromial decompression, and distal clavicle
- SLAP repair portals
  - Neviaser (9)
  - Port of Wilmington (10)
  - Transcuff portal (11)

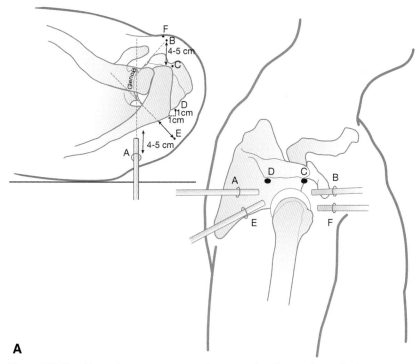

A

Figure 7.7 Shoulder arthroscopy ports. A, Common glenohumeral portals. (*A:* Posterior portal—starting. *B:* Anterosuperior—labrum. *C:* Anterolateral—subacromial. *D:* Posterolateral—labrum. *E:* Posteroinferior—labrum. *F:* Anteroinferior—Bankart.) B, Common subacromial portals. (*A:* Posterior—starting. *B:* Anterolateral—subacromial [rotator cuff]. *C:* Anteroinferior—Bankart. *D:* Neviaser—SLAP. *E:* Anterosuperior—labrum.) From Burkhart S, Lo IK, Brady PC, Denard PJ. *The Cowboy's Companion: A Trail Guide for the Arthroscopic Shoulder Surgeon.* Philadelphia, PA: Lippincott Williams & Wilkins; 2012.

SHOULDER ARTHRITIS

- Types
  - Osteoarthritis (OA)
  - Rheumatoid arthritis (RA)
  - Osteonecrosis
  - Instability arthropathy
  - RTC arthropathy—up to 50% in RA versus 10% in OA
  - Post-traumatic arthritis
  - Crystalline arthropathy
  - Hemophiliac arthropathy
- History
  - Pain—insidious onset, progressive; often occurs at night
  - **Loss of range of motion (ROM)—specifically ER**
  - Loss of function—simple tasks, activities of daily living
  - Crepitus
  - If avascular necrosis—evaluate risk factors (high-dose intravenous steroids), evaluate other joints (hip, knee)

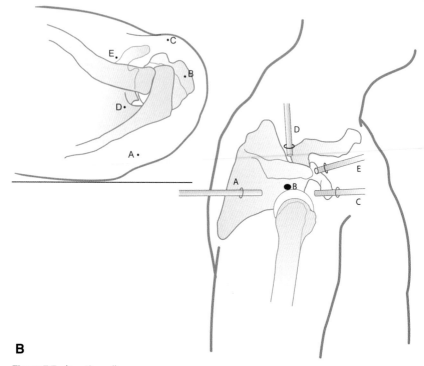

B

Figure 7.7. (*continued*)

- Physical examination
  - ROM (active and passive)—assess all planes, **commonly global loss**, endpoint pain
  - RTC strength—can be difficult to assess with severe motion loss/pain
- Imaging
  - **Radiographs**
    - Anteroposterior (Figure 7.8)—humeral head osteophytes (inferior), joint space narrowing, acromial–humeral interval (normal approximately 1 cm), cystic change (head and glenoid)
    - **Axillary—glenoid version and wear, posterior subluxation** (reference coracoid)
  - Computed tomography (CT) scan—best assessment of glenoid, including bone stock available
  - Magnetic resonance imaging (MRI)
    - Assess RTC if cannot determine on examination
    - If decreased acromiohumeral interval or previous RTC surgery
    - Stage avascular necrosis
- **Nonoperative management**
  - Activity modification
  - Ice/heat
  - Nonsteroidal anti-inflammatory drugs (NSAIDs)/acetaminophen
  - Corticosteroid injections
  - Physical therapy (maintain ROM)
  - Injections—cortisone/viscosupplementation
- Surgical management
  - Arthroscopic debridement—less predictable in moderate/severe, posterior subluxation

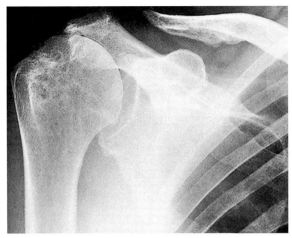

Figure 7.8 Rheumatoid arthritis from chronic rotator cuff tear showing upward migration of the humeral head secondary to rotator cuff tear, characteristic tapered erosion of the distal end of the clavicle, erosions of the humeral head, and a substantial degree of periarticular osteoporosis. From Greenspan A, Gershwin ME. Inflammatory arthritides. In: *Imaging in Rheumatology: A Clinical Approach*. Philadelphia, PA: Wolters Kluwer; 2018:201-268.

- Restorative—resurfacing, osteotomy
- Salvage—resection, arthrodesis (30°-45° of abduction, 10°-30° of flexion, 20°-45° of internal rotation)
- Interposition arthroplasty—alternative to total shoulder arthroplasty (TSA) in young patients, many substances tried, high failure rate (>50%)
- **Arthroplasty—TSA, reverse total shoulder arthroplasty (RTSA)**

SHOULDER ARTHROPLASTY

Hemiarthroplasty

- RTC deficient—moment arm
  - Must have CA ligament
- Fractures—three- and four- part fractures
- Risk of glenoid failure—active
- Important points on outcome and technique
  - RTC integrity determines postoperative function.
  - Fractures—tuberosities most important
  - Excellent for pain relief
  - Long term—progressive glenoid degenerative joint disease
- Technique
  - Correct version—The fin of the prosthesis should be slightly posterior to biceps groove.
  - Height—Pectoralis major tendon to top of prosthesis around 53 mm (Figure 7.9)

Total Arthroplasty

- Indications
  - RTC and deltoid intact
  - Sheer stress—glenoid
  - Soft tissues—crucial to success
  - OA—60% of TSAs

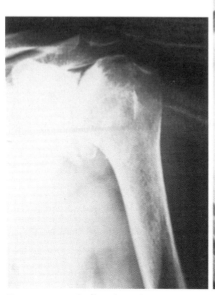
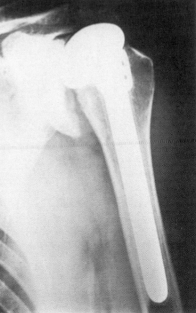

Figure 7.9 Hemiarthroplasty for osteoarthritis of the shoulder. From Throckmorton TW, Sperling JW, Cofield JH. Shoulder arthroplasty for osteoarthritis. In: Morrey BF, Sperling JW, eds. *Joint Replacement Arthroplasty: Basic Science, Elbow and Shoulder*. 4th ed. Philadelphia, PA: Lippincott Williams & Wilkins; 2011:303-311.

- 65 years of age
- Men more often than women
- Monoarticular
- Anterior capsule and subscapular contracture
- **RTC infrequently torn (only 5%-10%)**
- RA
- Post-traumatic arthritis
- Avascular necrosis
- Dislocation arthropathy
- In all patients
  - Pain that has failed to respond to nonoperative measures
  - Unacceptable functional decline
- Contraindications
  - Absolute—active infection
  - Relative—RTC deficiency, Charcot arthropathy, severe brachial plexopathy, intractable instability
  - **TSA with RTC deficiency** results in glenoid loosening (GH instability → **rocking horse**).
  - If small RTC intraoperatively, can repair (not contraindication)
- Imaging
  - Radiography—Evaluate glenoid bone stock with relation to the coracoid
  - CT scan—glenoid version and bone loss
- Retroverted glenoid—CT evaluation
  - No bone loss—eccentric anterior reaming
  - Bone loss—if there is more than 15° of retroversion, an allograft will be needed to reconstruct the glenoid.

- Approach
  - Deltopectoral most common
  - No difference in outcomes, subscapular peel versus subscapular osteotomy
- Glenoid
  - Normal glenoid is neutral or slightly anteverted.
  - OA—posterior glenoid wear, retroversion
  - RA—central/medial wear (loss of lateral offset)
  - Glenoid component
    - Peg
    - Polyethylene
    - Convex
    - Uncemented—lower rate of loosening
- Technique
  - Humeral head—placed to recreate normal humeral head version (20°-30° of retroversion)
  - Start point for humeral stem—5 mm posterior and medial to bicipital groove
  - Attempt to restore neutral version to glenoid (Figure 7.10)
  - Outcomes of **biconcave glenoid, inferior** to others
- Rehabilitation
  - Sling/abduction for 4 to 6 weeks (surgeon-dependent)
  - Must **protect subscapularis** (avoid extreme ER)
  - If subscapular repair fails—anterior/superior instability/escape
    - **Physical examination— positive belly-press/lift-off/bear-hug**
- Outcomes
  - **Pain—most predictable benefit** (>90% patient with good relief)

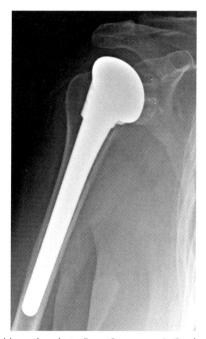

Figure 7.10 Total shoulder arthroplasty. From Greenspan A, Gershwin ME. Treatment of the arthritides and arthropathies. In: *Imaging in Rheumatology: A Clinical Approach.* Philadelphia, PA: Wolters Kluwer; 2018:114-140.

- In those with persistent pain, typically an explainable cause (intraoperative/ postoperative complication)
- Long-term improvement in pain, shoulder ROM, shoulder strength
- **Complications**
  - Overall—12% to 14%
  - **Glenoid loosening** most common—revise only if symptomatic
  - **Nerve injury**—axillary nerve most common
  - Infection
    - Acute versus chronic—same as all prosthetic joints
    - *Propionibacterium acnes*—Follow cultures for at least 2 weeks
  - Instability/soft-tissue imbalance
  - Periprosthetic fracture
  - Subscapularis failure—protect postoperatively
- Hemiarthroplasty versus TSA
  - **TSA with superior outcomes**—patient satisfaction, functional outcomes, ROM, decreased revision rates
  - Indications for hemiarthroplasty becoming more limited (with increased use of RTSA)
  - Outcomes after conversion TSA to hemiarthroplasty not as high (requires repeat subscapularis takedown)
  - Hemiarthroplasty can result in glenoid erosion and medial wear over time (monitor).

Reverse Total Arthroplasty

- **Mechanics**
  - Reverses ball and socket
  - **Center of rotation is medialized** (maximizes deltoid function/recruitment) (Figure 7.11).
  - Lowering humerus increases/re-tensions deltoid
- **Indications**
  - RTC arthropathy
  - Post-traumatic—nonunion/malunion
  - Revision—failed hemiarthroplasty/TSA, instability after TSA, failure of tuberosities to heal
  - Fracture—displaced proximal humerus fracture in elderly or otherwise not amenable to open reduction internal fixation
- Contraindications
  - Infection
  - Nonfunctioning deltoid/neuromuscular disease
  - Insufficient glenoid bone stock for baseplate
  - Young age/high activity level
  - Noncompliance/medical comorbidities precluding surgery
- **Complications**
  - **Overall rates high—19% to 68%**
  - Fracture—humerus, acromion, glenoid
  - **Infection**—higher rate than TSA, similar to TKA/THA; *Propionibacterium acnes*
  - Dislocation/instability—usually anterior—adduction/extension/internal rotation
    - Rate may increase if irreparable subscapularis.
  - Hematoma
  - Nerve injury—axillary nerve, brachial plexus
  - Loosening/failure
  - **Scapular notching**—decrease with inferior glenosphere tilt
  - Deltoid dysfunction
  - Complication rate doubles for revision surgery.
  - Learning curve—rates decreased with experience (number performed)

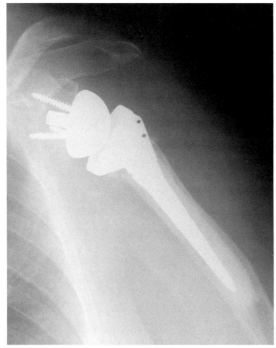

Figure 7.11 Reverse prosthesis with a convex cementless glenoid component fixed with screws and a cemented concave humeral component. Note the large distance between the acromion and proximal humerus, reflecting the distal translation of the center of rotation and consequent increased deltoid tensioning. From Sanchez-Sotelo J. Reverse total shoulder arthroplasty. In: Morrey BF, Sperling JW, eds. *Joint Replacement Arthroplasty: Basic Science, Elbow and Shoulder.* 4th ed. Philadelphia, PA: Lippincott Williams & Wilkins; 2011:275-283.

ELBOW

ELBOW ANATOMY

- Overview
  - **Bony anatomy**—ROM in two planes
    - Flexion and extension
    - Supination and pronation
  - **Bony stability**
  - Coronoid
  - Olecranon
  - *Radial head—a secondary stabilizer to valgus stress*
- **Axis of rotation**
  - *Center of trochlea to the center of the capitellum*
- Bony anatomy
  - *Radial head—secondary stabilizer to valgus stress*
    - **Important in ulnar collateral ligament (UCL) injuries**
  - **Terrible triad**
    - **Coronoid fracture/UCL injury/radial head fracture**
- Medial side anatomy
  - **UCL—has three bundles**

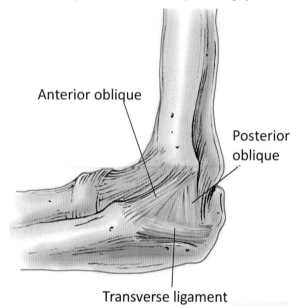

Figure 7.12 Anatomy of the medial elbow ligamentous complex. The ulnar collateral ligament complex comprises three ligaments: the anterior oblique, posterior oblique, and transverse ligaments. From Safran MS, Kalisvaart M. Arthroscopic treatment of chondral injuries and osteochondritis dissecans In: Hunt TR, ed. *Operative Techniques in Hand, Wrist, and Elbow Surgery*. 2nd ed. Philadelphia, PA: Wolters Kluwer; 2016:122-132.

- *Anterior bundle—most important in valgus stability*
  - **Anterior band**
  - **Posterior band**
  - **Reconstruction for pitchers or valgus instability**
- **Posterior bundle**
  - *ROM*
  - **Tight flexion**
  - **Contracted limits flexion**
- **Transverse ligament (Figure 7.12)**
- Lateral side anatomy
  - **Lateral ulnar collateral ligament (LUCL) complex**
    - *LUCL*—**lateral humeral epicondyle to supinator crest**
    - **Radial collateral ligament**
    - **Annular ligament (Figure 7.13)**
  - Functional ROM (Table 7.1)
    - Almost any question on elbow contracture or limited ROM will test on functional ROM.
    - Joint forces:
      - Radiohumeral—60%
      - Ulnohumeral—40%

LIGAMENT INJURIES OF THE ELBOW

UCL Injuries

- History—pain in late cocking phase or early acceleration phase of the throwing cycle
- Physical examination

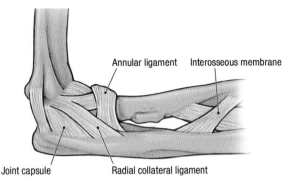

Figure 7.13 Annular ligament. From Detton AJ. The upper limb. In: *Grant's Dissector*. 16th ed. Baltimore, MD: Wolters Kluwer; 2017:23-72.

- Valgus stress test
- Milking maneuver
- Moving valgus test
- Stress radiographs
  - Greater than >3 mm difference from contralateral extremity
  - MRI arthrogram is a gold-standard test
    - T sign on MR arthrogram—contrast underneath tear (Figure 7.14)
- Treatment
  - Nonoperative—rehabilitation and physical therapy
    - Rest
    - Physical therapy to improve mechanics
    - Trunk-scapular kinesis, forearm pronation, flexor-pronator-flexor carpi ulnaris
  - Surgical indication
    - **High-level throwers**
    - **Fail conservative management—continues to have pain or unable to have a stable elbow**
    - Reconstruction techniques for examination purposes
      - Reconstruct anterior bundle
        - Usually use palmaris longus or gracilis tendon as graft choices
        - Jobe or docking technique
      - Jobe technique
        - Ulnar nerve transposition to minimize ulnar nerve symptoms postsurgery
      - Docking technique complications
        - Medial antebrachial cutaneous (MABC) nerve injury
        - Fracture
        - Stiffness and loss of motion common

Table 7.1 Functional Range of Motion

Motion	Normal	Functional
Extension	0°	30°
Flexion	145°	130°
Pronation	80°	50°
Supination	90°	50°

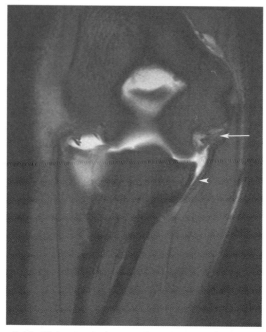

Figure 7.14 T1-weighted fat-saturated magnetic resonance arthrogram (MRA) demonstrating a tear of the proximal ulnar collateral ligament (UCL) (arrow). Note also a partial tear of the distal UCL, which is partially detached from its insertion in the sublime tubercle, the so-called T sign (arrowhead). From Greenspan A, Beltran J. Upper limb II: elbow. In: *Orthopedic Imaging: A Practical Approach*. 6th ed. Philadelphia, PA: Wolters Kluwer Health; 2015:164-267.

LUCL Injuries

- Mechanisms of injury
  - Elbow dislocation
  - Iatrogenic—any surgery for lateral epicondylitis
- Posterolateral rotary instability
  - Most common pattern of instability of the elbow
  - History and symptoms
    - Clicking or locking with pushing off or elbow extension (push-ups)
    - Elbow most unstable in supination and extension
    - Most stable flexion and pronation
  - Physical examination
    - Best test—lateral pivot shift
    - Supinate, valgus, and axial compression—bring elbow from extension to flexion, which reduces the radial head (Figure 7.15)
  - Treatment
    - Physical therapy to strengthen dynamic stabilizers (muscles around elbow)
    - Surgical indication
      - Failure of conservative management and continued instability
      - Reconstruction technique
        · Graft—gracilis or palmaris longus
        · Isometric point from lateral epicondyle to supinator crest

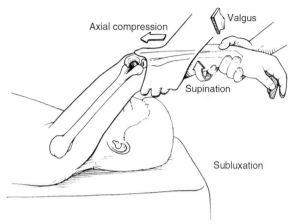

Figure 7.15 Lateral pivot shift test. From O'Driscoll SW, Bell DR, Morrey BF, Posterolateral rotatory instability of the elbow. *J Bone Joint Surg Am.* 1991;73(3):440-446.

OVERUSE TENDON INJURIES

- Lateral epicondylitis (tennis elbow)
  - Anatomy—main tendon involved is the extensor carpi radialis brevis (ECRB)
  - Histology—angiofibroblastic hyperplasia
  - History
    - Pain on the lateral side of the elbow
    - Patients complain of pain with typing, using a mouse, playing tennis (usually with the backhand), or golf (lead arm).
    - Can progress to decreased grip strength and difficulty shaking hands
  - Physical examination
    - Pain with resisted wrist extension
    - Tenderness lateral epicondyle
    - Do not get confused with radial tunnel—**pain distal to ECRB tendon and located over supinator/brachial wad**
    - Also can have both in 10% of the cases
  - Treatment
    - Nonoperative
      - 80% of patients with newly diagnosed lateral epicondylitis report symptomatic improvement after 1 year.
      - Physical therapy with emphasis on eccentric strengthening
    - Surgical—*for the examination*
      - There will be no recommendation for surgery.
      - The only question will be from complications from surgery and remember LUCL iatrogenic injury.
      - **Other question that might be asked:** Which is the better procedure, arthroscopy or open technique? Same results
      - Arthroscopy complication—nerves (radial)
      - Open complication—LUCL
- Medial epicondylitis (golfer elbow)
  - Histology—angiofibroblastic hyperplasia
  - History
    - Pain on the medial side of the elbow
    - Usually the dominant arm
  - Physical examination
    - Pain with resisted wrist flexion and forearm pronation

- Throwers—must rule out UCL injury
- Tenderness medial epicondyle—pronator teres insertion
- Treatment
  - Nonoperative
    - Physical therapy with emphasis on eccentric strengthening
  - Surgical
    - *Rarely* surgical
      - Must rule out physical therapy to even consider surgery
      - 12 months of failed conservative management
    - Open
      - Complication—MABC

TRAUMATIC TENDON INJURY
Distal Biceps

- Presentation
  - Usually an eccentric contraction—lengthening phase of the contraction "negative"
  - Lifting
  - Pain and ecchymosis
- Physical examination
  - Hook test—palpating the biceps tendon
- Treatment
  - Failure to repair the distal biceps tendon will result in:
    - 40% to 50% loss supination strength
    - 10% to 30% loss in flexion strength
    - 10% to 15% loss grip strength
  - Surgical complications
    - Single incision
      - Posterior interosseous nerve injury—usually placing a retractor radial
      - Lateral antebrachial cutaneous (LABC)
        - Commonly injured during the one-incision approach
        - Nerve needs to be retracted because it is commonly seen in the once incision approach.
    - Two-incision technique
      - Synostosis (Figure 7.16)
      - LABC

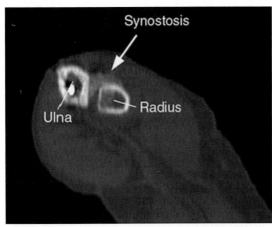

Figure 7.16 Axial computed tomography (CT) scan demonstrating radioulnar synostosis, a complication of distal biceps tendon repair. From Sutton KM, Dodds SD, Ahmad CS, Sethi PM. Surgical treatment of distal biceps rupture. *J Am Acad Orthop Surg.* 2010;18:139-148.

Distal Triceps

- History
  - *If see in vignette involving anabolic steroid use, think triceps.*
  - Systemic diseases
  - Corticosteroid injection
  - Meds—fluoroquinolones
- MRI—demonstrates avulsion olecranon
- Physical examination—weakness on elbow extension
- Treatment—surgical
  - Operative repair recommended—must maintain strength in extension
  - Reattachment—surgically with bone tunnels or suture anchors
  - Fracture fragments of less than 50% may be excised if unable to fix.

OSTEOCHONDRITIS DISSECANS (OCD) OF THE CAPITELLUM

- Physical examination
  - Excessive or repetitive compressive force—maximum at ball release
  - Lateral elbow pain—younger patients
  - *Important to evaluate ROM*
    - Locking or catching
    - Extension loss
    - Classification: stable versus unstable
- Treatment
  - *Nonsurgical*
    - Avoid activity
    - Rest
  - *Surgical indications*
    - Mechanical or unstable
    - Loose bodies
    - Intra-articular cartilage instability
- See Chapter 6, Sports Medicine, for Little Leaguer elbow (medial epicondyle apophysitis) and posterior Impingement

OSTEOARTHRITIS
Arthritis in Adults

- *RA*
- **Post-traumatic**
- **Osteoarthritis—male heavy laborers**
- Diagnosis
  - *Loss of motion*
  - Pain
  - Ulnar neuropathy
- Radiographs
  - Standard views
  - CT scan
- Treatment—nonoperative
  - ROM and function
    - **Improve ROM**
    - *Decrease pain*
  - NSAIDs
  - *Do not consider elbow arthroplasty until age 65.*

Arthritis in Younger Patients

- **Capsular contraction and osteophytes**
  - Goal of surgery—Release capsule and remove osteophytes
  - Ulnar neuropathy in up to 50% of patients—ulnar neurolysis
    - **Severe limited ROM**
  - *Open approach*
    - Collateral ligament sparing—medial or lateral approach
    - Outerbridge-Kashiwagi—olecranon fossa fenestration
  - *Arthroscopic approach*
    - Radial nerve highest at risk
    - If flexion less than 90°, release posterior band UCL and posterior capsule—ulnar neurolysis
  - *Ulnohumeral distraction arthroplasty*
    - Allograft or autograft
    - Higher demand patients
- **Total elbow arthroplasty (Figure 7.17)**
  - Indications
    - Patients aged >65 years with severe elbow arthritis
    - Complex distal humerus fracture in elderly with poor bone stock
    - **RA—best survival**
    - Chronic instability
  - Two types
    - Linked—constrained
      - Most common
    - Unlinked—collateral ligaments intact
  - Approach
    - Triceps splitting
    - Bryan-Morrey triceps reflecting approach
  - *Survival excellent at 10 to 15 years*
    - Best in RA
  - *Complications—high*
    - Aseptic loosening—constrained implant
    - Infection
    - Wound
    - Instability—unlinked implants
    - Triceps—During the Morrey approach, the triceps may have decreased force if not repaired correctly.

ELBOW DISLOCATION

- Mechanism—axial compression, valgus, forearm supination
- Treatment
  - *Early protected ROM*
  - *Loss of extension most common complication*
  - *Chronic instability—***posterolateral instability**—LUCL
  - Surgical repair (rarely)
    - Unstable arc of motion from 60° to full flexion
    - Significant fracture
  - *Surgical algorithm*
    - 50% coronoid present for stability
    - 50% olecranon present for stability
    - *Radial head secondary stabilizer to valgus*

- Bone first and then ligaments
- If instability persists: *Remember injury starts lateral to medial* (Figure 7.18)

LOSS OF MOTION

- *Functional ROM*
  - **Flexion/extension = 30° − 130°**
  - **Supination/pronation = 50°/50°**
- *Treatment*
  - Early ROM following injury is the key to prevention.
  - Surgical—If refractory and no improvement after 3 to 6 months

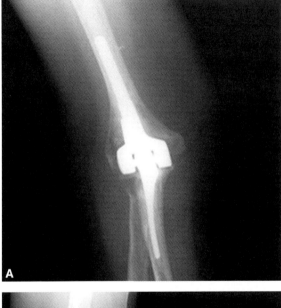

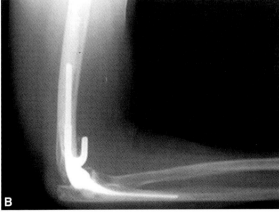

Figure 7.17 Total elbow arthroplasty. A, AP image of a total elbow arthroplasty. B, Lateral view of a total elbow arthroplasty.

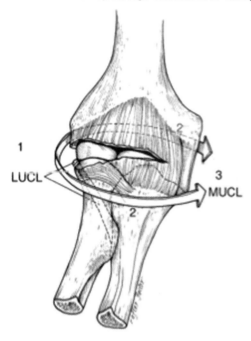

Figure 7.18 The ring of instability with elbow dislocations describes the progression of stresses from the lateral ulnar part of the lateral collateral ligament to the anterior capsule and, finally, ending with injury to the medial ulnar collateral ligament (MUCL). LUCL, lateral ulnar collateral ligament. From O'Driscoll SW, Morrey BF, Korinek S, An K-N. Elbow subluxation and dislocation: a spectrum of instability. *Clin Orthop.* 1992;280:186-197.

ELBOW ARTHROSCOPY (Figure 7.19)

- **Indications**
  - Lateral epicondylitis
  - UCL reconstruction—Diagnostic arthroscopy can be helpful for the diagnosis if MRI still questionable of instability.
  - Articular cartilage pathology
  - OCD
  - Debridement of osteophytes
  - Removal of loose bodies
  - Intra-articular fractures
  - Synovitis—arthroscopy helpful for synovectomy
- Contraindications
  - *Ulnar nerve transposition*
    - Identify ulnar nerve—especially in ulnar nerve subluxation
- *Risks*
  - Distend elbow joint
  - *Injury superficial cutaneous nerves*
    - *Proximal portals decrease risk*
    - *RA and contracture increase risk*
    - *Direct lateral—LABC*
    - *Anteromedial*
      - MABC
      - Median nerve
      - Brachial artery
    - *Anterolateral—radial nerve*
    - *Posterolateral and posterocentral portals only*
    - *No posteromedial portal—ulnar nerve*

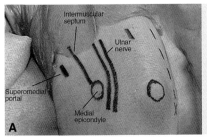
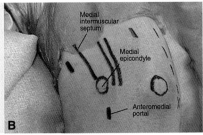
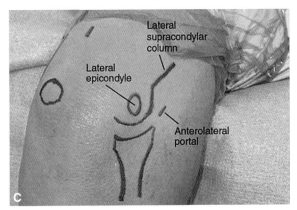
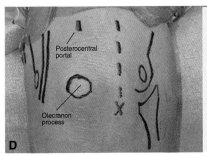
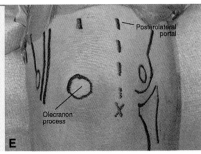

Figure 7.19 A, The proximal anteromedial portal (or superomedial portal) is just anterior to the intramuscular septum and 2 cm proximal to the medial epicondyle. Care must be taken to avoid the ulnar nerve. B, The anteromedial portal is approximately 2 cm anterior and 2 cm distal to the medial epicondyle. This portal augments the proximal anteromedial portal and is helpful for working in the medial recess of the elbow. Care must be taken to avoid the medial antebrachial cutaneous nerve. C, The anterolateral portal also is favored to decrease the risk of radial nerve injury. Compared with the proximal anterolateral portal, this placement is more proximal and somewhat anterior. Creating this portal under direct visualization, after establishment of a medial portal, helps avoid injury to lateral structures. D, The posterocentral portal, the safest portal, is placed in the midline 3 cm proximal to the tip of the olecranon process. E, The direct lateral portal (or soft-spot portal) is at the center of the triangle formed by the lateral epicondyle, olecranon process, and radial head. Care must be taken to avoid the posterior antebrachial cutaneous nerve. F, The posterolateral portal (or proximal posterolateral portal) is 2 to 3 cm proximal to the tip of the olecranon process at the lateral border of the triceps tendon. The medial and posterior antebrachial cutaneous nerves are most at risk. From Abboud JA, Ricchetti ET, Tjoumakaris F, Ramsey M. Elbow arthroscopy: basic setup and portal placement. *J Am Acad Orthop Surg.* 2006;14(5):312-318.

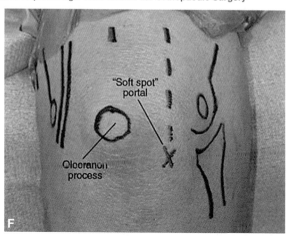

Figure 7.19 (*continued*)

8 Foot and Ankle
Nigel N. Hsu and Casey Jo Humbyrd

ANATOMY

- Ligaments
  - Lateral
    - Anterior talofibular ligament (ATFL)
    - Calcaneofibular ligament (CFL)
    - Posterior talofibular ligament
    - Syndesmosis
      - Anterior inferior tibiofibular ligament (AITFL)—35% of strength
      - Posterior inferior tibiofibular ligament (PITFL)—**40% of strength**
      - Interosseous ligament—21% of strength
  - Medial
    - Deltoid ligament complex
    - Calcaneonavicular ligament
- Windlass mechanism
  - Plantar fascia tightens as the metatarsophalangeal (MTP) joints extend and **lock the tarsal bones into a rigid column.**
- Gait mechanics
  - Stance phase
    - Heel strike
      - Hindfoot eversion **unlocks the transverse tarsal joints** for shock absorption.
      - Tibialis anterior—eccentric contraction
    - Foot flat
      - Gastrocnemius-soleus complex—eccentric contraction
    - Midstance
      - Hip extensors and quadriceps—concentric contraction
    - Heel off
      - Hip flexors—concentric contraction
  - Swing phase
    - Toe off
      - Hindfoot inversion **locks the transverse tarsal joints** for rigid lever arm.
      - Gastrocnemius-soleus complex—concentric contraction
    - Midswing
      - Tibialis anterior—concentric contraction
    - Terminal swing
      - Hamstring—decelerate

FOREFOOT

Hallux Valgus

- Definition
  - **Valgus deviation of the great toe** with **varus deviation of the first metatarsal (MT)**
- Patient history
  - More common in women
  - Pain over medial eminence
  - Difficulty with footwear
- Physical examination
  - Hallux—valgus and pronation
- Imaging (Figure 8.1)
  - Hallux valgus angle (HVA) <15°

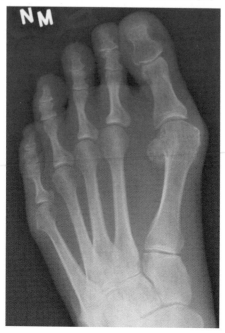

Figure 8.1 Hallux valgus. From Walker R, Hamilton P, Singh S. Scarf osteotomy. In: Easley ME, ed. *Operative Techniques in Foot and Ankle Surgery.* 2nd ed. Philadelphia, PA: Wolters Kluwer; 2017:41-50.

- Intermetatarsal angle (IMA) <9°
- Distal metatarsal articular angle (DMAA) <15°
- Hallux valgus interphalangeus angle (HVI) <10°
- Access congruency of the first MTP
- Treatment
  - Soft-tissue release (modified McBride procedure)
  - First MTP fusion—first MTP joint arthritis
  - Lapidus (first tarsometatarsal [TMT] joint fusion)—**instability of first TMT joint**
  - Distal chevron osteotomy—IMA <13° and HVA <40°
  - Proximal osteotomy—IMA ≥13° and HVA ≥40°
  - Biplanar osteotomy—**to correct a DMAA >15°**; may also need a proximal osteotomy
  - Akin osteotomy (proximal phalanx medial closing wedge osteotomy)—HVI >10°
- Hallux rigidus
  - Definition—first MTP arthritis and stiffness
  - History—pain and swelling of the first MTP
  - Physical examination
    - **Decreased dorsiflexion**
    - **Positive axial grind test**
  - Imaging (Figure 8.2)
    - Grade 0—normal radiograph, stiffness on examination
    - Grade 1—mild dorsal osteophyte, mild pain on examination
    - Grade 2—moderate dorsal osteophyte, <**50% joint space narrowing**, moderate pain on examination

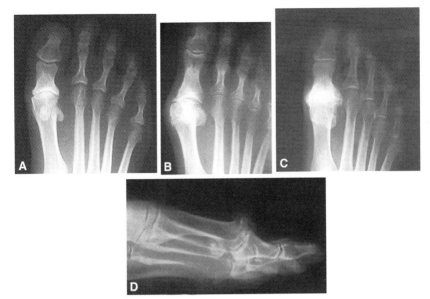

Figure 8.2 Hallux rigidus. A, Grade 1: hallux rigidus. B, Grade 2: hallux rigidus. C, Grade 3: hallux rigidus. D, Lateral view of hallux rigidus. From San Giovanni TP. Arthrosurface hemiCAP resurfacing. In: Easley ME, ed. *Operative Techniques in Foot and Ankle Surgery.* 2nd ed. Philadelphia, PA: Wolters Kluwer; 2017:154-175.

- Grade 3—severe dorsal osteophyte, >50% joint space narrowing, major stiffness, pain at extreme range of motion (ROM), **no pain at midrange**
- Grade 4—severe dorsal osteophyte, >50% joint space narrowing, major stiffness, pain at extreme ROM, **pain at midrange**
- Treatment
  - Nonoperative—Morton extension, that is, stiff foot plate with extension under great toe
  - Operative
    - Dorsal cheilectomy—grades 1 and 2
    - First MTP arthrodesis (fuse in 10°-15° of dorsiflexion)—grades 3 and 4

Lesser Toe Deformities

- Hammer toe
  - Definition
    - **Distal interphalangeal (DIP) joint extension**
    - **Proximal interphalangeal (PIP) joint flexion**
    - **MTP joint normal (slight extension)**
  - Treatment
    - Nonoperative—footwear modification to high toe box
    - Operative
      - Flexible deformity
        - Flexor tenotomy
        - Flexor-to-extensor tendon transfer
      - Fixed deformity
        - PIP arthroplasty
        - PIP arthrodesis

- Claw toe
  - Definition
    - **DIP flexion**
    - **PIP flexion**
    - **MTP hyperextension**
  - Treatment
    - Nonoperative—footwear modification to high toe box
    - Operative
      - Flexible deformity
        - Extensor digitorum brevis (EDB) tenotomy, extensor digitorum longus lengthening, flexor-to-extensor tendon transfer
      - Fixed deformity
        - PIP arthroplasty/arthrodesis, MTP joint capsulotomy, extensor lengthening
        - Shortening (Weil) osteotomy
- Mallet toe
  - Definition
    - **DIP flexion**
    - **PIP normal**
    - **MTP normal**
  - Treatment
    - Nonoperative—footwear modification to high toe box
    - Operative
      - Flexible deformity—flexor tenotomy
      - Fixed deformity—DIP arthroplasty/arthrodesis
- Crossover toe
  - Definition—**second toe lies dorsomedially relative to hallux**
  - Treatment
    - Nonoperative—toe taping/splint
    - Operative
      - Flexor-to-extensor tendon transfer, medial collateral ligament release
      - EDB transfer to the intermetatarsal ligament
      - Shortening (Weil) MT osteotomy
- MTP dislocation
  - Definition
    - Multiplanar instability
    - **Plantar plate disruption**
    - Walk on "marble in the ball of the foot"
  - Treatment
    - Nonoperative—taping, footwear modification, MT pads
    - Operative
      - Weil osteotomy
      - Plantar plate repair
      - Flexor-to-extensor tendon transfer
      - EDB transfer to the intermetatarsal ligament
- Bunionette
  - Definition
    - Bony prominence over lateral MT head
      - **Type I—Enlarged fifth MT head or lateral exostosis**
      - **Type II—Congenital bow of fifth MT**
      - **Type III—Increased 4 to 5 IMA**
  - Treatment
    - Nonoperative—footwear modification to wide-based shoes
    - Operative
      - Lateral condylectomy

  - Distal MT osteotomy
  - Oblique diaphyseal rotational osteotomy

Sesamoid Injuries

- Turf toe
  - Definition
    - Forced dorsiflexion—**avulsion of the plantar plate of the base of the phalanx and proximal migration of the sesamoids**
      - Grade 1—capsular strain
      - Grade 2—partial capsular tear
      - Grade 3—complete plantar plate tear
  - Treatment
    - Nonoperative—stiff insole, toe taping
    - Operative—plantar plate repair
- Sesamoid fracture
  - Boot immobilization
  - Transition to sesamoid relief pad
  - Surgery-excision versus open reduction and internal fixation (ORIF)
- Sesamoiditis
  - Rest, ice, compression, and elevation
  - Footwear modification

Fifth MT Base Fracture

- Zone 1—**avulsion fracture (pseudo-Jones fracture)**
  - Hindfoot inversion—peroneus brevis or plantar fascia
  - Protected weight bearing in shoe/boot
- Zone 2—**metaphyseal-diaphyseal junction, extend into fourth and fifth intermetatarsal articulation (Jones fracture)**
  - Forefoot adduction
  - Nonweight bearing
  - Intramedullary screw fixation in elite athletes
- Zone 3—**proximal diaphysis fracture**
  - Repetitive microtrauma
  - **Vascular watershed region**
  - Increased risk of nonunion
  - Nonweight bearing
  - Intramedullary screw fixation with sclerosis/nonunion or athletes

MIDFOOT

Lisfranc Injury

- Definition
  - TMT fracture/dislocation
  - Lisfranc ligament—**medial cuneiform to base of second MT; plantar ligament**
- History
  - Axial loading of a plantar-flexed foot
  - Sports injuries
  - Motor vehicle accident
- Physical examination
  - Severe pain and swelling
  - **Plantar ecchymosis**

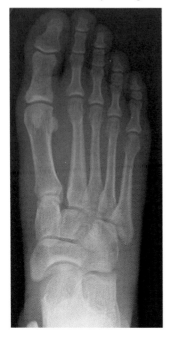

Figure 8.3 Lisfranc injury. Isolated disruption of second tarsometatarsal joint. From Early JS, Kitaoka HB, Campbell JT. Tarsometatarsal (Lisfranc) reduction and fixation. In: Kitaoka HB, ed. *Master Techniques in Orthopaedic Surgery: The Foot and Ankle*. 3rd ed. Philadelphia, PA: Lippincott Williams & Wilkins; 2013:229-248.

- Imaging (Figure 8.3)
  - Widened gap between first and second MTs
  - Fleck sign—first intermetatarsal space
  - **Weight-bearing view**
  - Abduction stress view
- Treatment
  - Nonoperative—cast immobilization for 8 weeks until no displacement on weight bearing or stress views
  - Operative
    - ORIF
    - Primary arthrodesis
      - **Purely ligamentous injury**
      - Intra-articular comminution

Midfoot Arthritis

- Definition—arthritis of the naviculocuneiform, intercuneiform, or MT cuneiform joint
- History—midfoot pain with push-off
- Physical examination
  - Arch collapse
  - Midfoot collapse
  - Tenderness to palpation in midfoot
- Imaging (Figure 8.4)
  - Meary angle
  - Longitudinal arch collapse
  - Loss of joint space

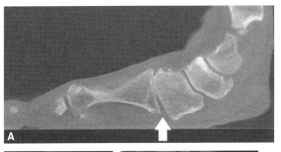

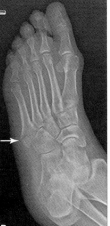
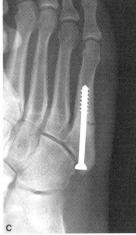

Figure 8.4 Jones Fracture (A) Midfoot. (B) Pseudo-Jones. (C) Oblique radiograph obtained at 8-month follow-up after open reduction and internal fixation (ORIF) (A) from Chou L B. *Orthopaedic Knowledge Update*. Wolters Kluwer, 2020. (B) From Sherman SC, Ross C, Nordquist E, Wang E, Cico S. *Atlas of Clinical Emergency Medicine*. Wolters Kluwer 2015. (C) Flatow E, Colvin AC, *Atlas of Essential Orthopaedic Procedures* 2ed. Wolters Kluwer 2019.

- Treatment
  - Nonoperative—orthotics
    - Arch support
    - Stiff shoe with rocker
    - Cushioned heel
  - Operative—**midfoot arthrodesis to correct midfoot collapse**

HINDFOOT

Fractures

- Talus fracture
  - Talar neck fracture, Hawkins classification (Figure 8.5)
    - Type I—**nondisplaced**
    - Type II—**subtalar dislocation**
    - Type III—**subtalar and tibiotalar dislocation**
    - Type IV—**subtalar, tibiotalar, and talonavicular (TN) dislocation**
  - Talar body fracture
  - Lateral process fracture
  - Talar head fracture
- History
  - Motor vehicle accident or fall from height
  - Forceful dorsiflexion
  - Snowboarding—**lateral process fracture**
- Physical examination—swelling, ecchymosis, and deformity

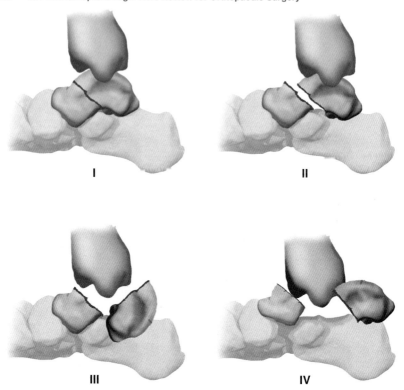

Figure 8.5 Hawkins classification of talar neck fractures. From Stewart DS II, McGarvey WC. Injuries of the foot. In: Brinker MR, ed. *Review of Orthopaedic Trauma*. 2nd ed. Philadelphia, PA: Lippincott Williams & Wilkins; 2013:187-209.

- Imaging
  - Canale view—talar neck
  - Computed tomography (CT) is the gold standard.
- Treatment
  - Nonoperative (nondisplaced fractures)—cast immobilization for 8 to 12 weeks
  - Operative—ORIF
- Calcaneus fracture
  - Intra-articular
    - Posterior facet fracture
    - **High energy**—motor vehicle accident, fall from height
    - Axial loading
    - Essex-Lopresti
      - Joint depression
      - Tongue-type (Figure 8.6)
    - Sanders classification
      - Type I—nondisplaced posterior facet
      - Type II—1 fracture line
      - Type III—2 fracture lines
      - Type IV—≥3 fracture lines

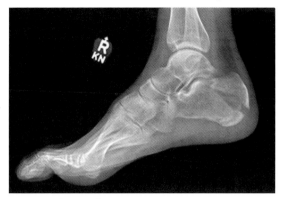

Figure 8.6 Tongue-type calcaneus fracture.

- Extra-articular—tuberosity avulsion fracture of the Achilles tendon
- Anterior process
  - Avulsion of the bifurcate ligament
  - Inversion and plantarflexion
- Physical examination
  - Heel—**shortened, widened, varus deformity**
- Imaging (Figure 8.7)
  - Harris view
  - Broden view—posterior facet
  - Bohler angle—20° to 40°
  - Gissane angle—130° to 145°
  - CT—gold standard

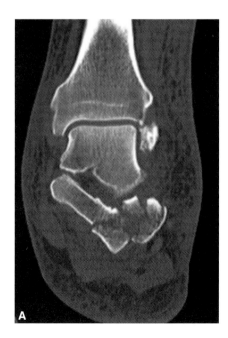

Figure 8.7 Calcaneus fracture. (A) Coronal CT scan and (B) Sagittal CT scan demonstrating comminuted, intra-articular calcaneus fracture.

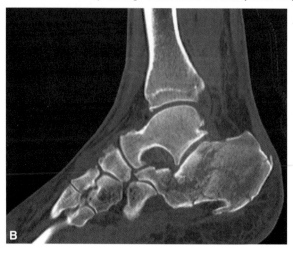

Figure 8.7 *(continued)*

- Treatment
  - Nonoperative (nondisplaced fractures)—cast immobilization
  - Operative (Sanders types II-IV)—ORIF
    - Extensile lateral approach—30% wound complication
    - Sinus tarsi approach
    - **Worse outcome with higher fracture types versus lower types**
    - **Subtalar arthritis is common.**

Post-traumatic Calcaneus

- Definition
  - Previous calcaneal fracture with loss of height
  - Anterior impingement—**anterior ankle pain**
  - Hindfoot pain
- Treatment—autograft or allograft bone-block arthrodesis
  - **Restore hindfoot height**
  - Less successful at correcting varus

NERVES

Tarsal Tunnel Syndrome

- Definition
  - **Compressive neuropathy of the tibial nerve in the tarsal tunnel**
  - Causes—engorged vessels, pigmented villonodular synovitis, ganglion cyst, tendinopathy, tenosynovitis, lipoma/tumor, perineural fibrosis, osteophytes, sustentaculum tali fracture, tarsal coalition, accessory muscle
- History
  - **Plantar foot burning pain**
  - Symptoms worse with prolonged standing, walking
- Physical examination
  - **Positive Tinel sign**
  - Intrinsic foot wasting
  - Compression test
  - Pes planus
- Imaging
  - Electromyography (EMG)
  - Magnetic resonance imaging (MRI)—mass-occupying lesion (Figure 8.8)

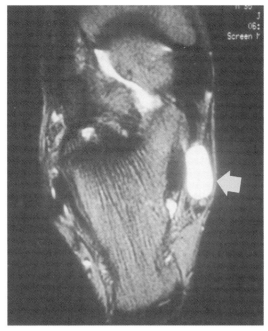

Figure 8.8 Tarsal tunnel syndrome caused by a ganglion cyst (arrow). From Helms CA, Vinson EA. Magnetic resonance imaging of the foot and ankle. In: Klein JS, Brant WE, Helms CA, Vinson EA, eds. *Brant and Helms' Fundamentals of Diagnostic Radiology*. 5th ed. Philadelphia, PA: Wolters Kluwer; 2019:1416-1427.

- Treatment
  - Nonoperative
    - **Nonsteroidal anti-inflammatory drugs (NSAIDs), vitamin B$_6$, tricyclic antidepressants**
    - Orthosis to correct hindfoot valgus
  - Operative—tarsal tunnel release

Morton Neuroma

- Definition—compressive neuropathy of the interdigital nerve **(most common between third and fourth MTs)**
- History
  - Burning pain with weight bearing in plantar web space radiating to the toes
  - Narrow toe box shoes
  - Relieved by removing shoes
- Physical examination
  - **Mulder click**
  - Differentials include metatarsalgia and MTP synovitis
- Imaging—conventional radiographs and MRI can rule out other abnormality.
- Treatment
  - Nonoperative
    - Footwear modification with wide toe box shoes
    - MT pads
    - Cortisone injections

- Operative—neuroma excision
  - Dorsal approach
  - Incise transverse intermetatarsal ligament
  - Stump retraction
  - **Most common complication is stump neuroma.**

TENDON DISORDERS
Peroneal Tendons

- Definition
  - Tendinitis, tenosynovitis, tendon subluxation
  - Peroneus brevis degenerative tears
- History
  - Chronic lateral ankle pain after ankle sprain
  - Eversion and dorsiflexion—**superior peroneal retinaculum injury**
  - Cavovarus foot
- Physical examination
  - Tenderness over peroneal tendon
  - Tendon subluxation
  - Pain with dorsiflexion and eversion
- Imaging
  - Conventional radiography: avulsion fracture of fifth MT base or os peroneum
  - Ultrasonography: subluxation/dislocation
  - MRI: peroneus quartus muscle or low peroneus brevis muscle belly
- Treatment
  - Nonoperative
    - Cast / boot immobilization in acute injuries
    - Physical therapy and bracing for chronic tendinosis
  - Operative
    - **Superior peroneal retinaculum repair and fibular groove deepening**
      - Peroneal tendon subluxation
    - Tenosynovectomy, debridement, and repair of degenerative tears
      - Peroneus brevis tears
    - **Lateralizing calcaneal osteotomy to correct hindfoot varus**

Posterior Tibial Tendon (PTT) Dysfunction (Table 8.1)

- Definition
  - Adult-acquired flatfoot deformity
  - Collapsed longitudinal arch—loss of support from secondary structures
    - Spring ligament complex
    - Plantar fascia
    - Plantar ligaments

Table 8.1 Deforming Forces and Deformity for Posterior Tibial Tendon (PTT) Deformity and Charcot-Marie Tooth (CMT) Disease

| | Position | | | Deforming Forces | | | |
Disorder	Forefoot	Midfoot	Hindfoot	Posterior Tibialis	Anterior Tibialis	Peroneus Brevis	Peroneus Longus
PTT deformity (see Figure 8.9)	Abducted	Planus	Valgus	Weak	Normal	Normal	Weak/Normal
CMT disease (see Figure 8.12)	Adducted	Cavus	Varus	Normal	Weak	Weak	Normal

- Talar head medial migration and uncoverage
- Hindfoot valgus
- Forefoot abduction
- Classification
  - Stage I
    - Tenosynovitis, no deformity
    - Normal single-limb heel rise
    - Normal radiograph
  - Stage IIA
    - Flatfoot deformity, flexible hindfoot
    - **Inability to perform single-limb heel rise**
    - Arch collapse on conventional radiographs
  - Stage IIB
    - Flatfoot deformity, flexible hindfoot, **forefoot abduction**, >40% TN uncoverage
    - Inability to perform single-limb heel rise
    - Arch collapse on conventional radiographs
  - Stage III
    - Flatfoot deformity, **rigid hindfoot valgus, rigid forefoot abduction**
    - Inability to perform single-limb heel rise
    - Arch collapse and subtalar arthritis on conventional radiographs
  - Stage IV
    - Flatfoot deformity, rigid hindfoot valgus, rigid forefoot abduction, **deltoid ligament compromise**
    - Inability to perform single-limb heel rise
    - Arch collapse, subtalar arthritis, talar tilt on conventional radiographs
- History
  - Medial ankle/foot pain
  - Progressive flatfoot deformity
- Physical examination
  - Flexible or fixed deformity
  - **Single-limb heel rise**
- Imaging (Figure 8.9)
  - **Negative Meary angle**
  - **TN uncoverage**
  - Forefoot abduction

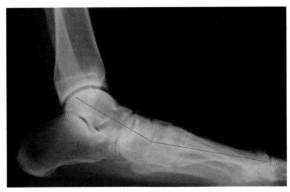

Figure 8.9 Posterior tibial tendon deformity. Any break from a straight line in the talo–first metatarsal angle demonstrates sag and abduction of the arch. From Guyton GP. Flexor digitorum longus transfer and medial displacement calcaneal osteotomy. In: Easley ME, ed. *Operative Techniques in Foot and Ankle Surgery*. 2nd ed. Philadelphia, PA: Wolters Kluwer; 2017:423-431.

- Treatment
  - Nonoperative
    - Ankle-foot orthosis, physical therapy
    - Orthotic with arch support, medial heel wedge
  - Operative
    - PTT debridement
    - Flatfoot reconstruction—stage II
      - Medial displacement calcaneal osteotomy and/or lateral column lengthening
      - Tendo-Achilles lengthening (TAL) or gastrocnemius recession
      - **Cotton osteotomy** (dorsal open wedge osteotomy of the cuneiform) for fixed supination
      - Flexor digitorum longus (FDL) or flexor hallucis longus (FHL) tendon transfer into navicular
    - Triple arthrodesis—stage III
    - Tibiotalocalcaneal arthrodesis—stage IV

Achilles Tendon Ruptures

- Definition—rupture can be insertional or midsubstance (Figure 8.10)
- History—reports a "pop" or "kicked in the back of the leg"
- Physical examination
  - **Thompson test**
  - Palpable gap
- Imaging
  - Radiography—lateral ankle shows disruption of Kager triangle
  - Ultrasonography—useful
  - MRI—gold standard
- Treatment
  - Nonoperative—**functional bracing**, equivalent to surgical at one year

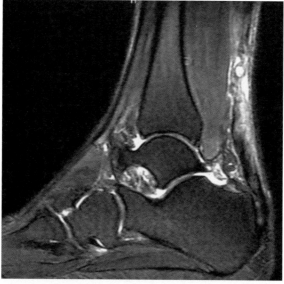

Figure 8.10 Midsubstance Achilles rupture. Radiographs demonstrating severe midfoot Charcot deformity with joint destruction and foot collapse.

- Operative
  - Open repair—wound complication
  - Percutaneous Achilles tendon repair—risk of sural nerve damage
  - Reconstruction, V-Y advancement, FHL transfer—chronic ruptures with large defect

Achilles Tendinopathy

- Definition—degenerative changes in the tendon because of **vascular supply** 2 to 6 cm proximal to insertion
- History—Achilles tendon pain and swelling
- Physical examination—tendon thickening and tenderness
- Imaging—MRI will show extent of tendon involvement.
- Treatment
  - Nonoperative—physical therapy with **eccentric exercise**, NSAIDs
  - Operative
    - Achilles tendon debridement
    - Achilles tendon reconstruction
    - FHL/FDL tendon transfer

ANKLE SPRAINS

High Ankle Sprains

- Definition—syndesmosis injury
- History—**external rotation**
- Physical examination
  - Syndesmosis tenderness
  - Squeeze test
- Imaging—**external rotation stress radiograph**
- Treatment
  - Nonoperative—boot immobilization
  - Operative
    - Syndesmosis screw fixation
    - Suture button fixation

Low Ankle Sprain

- Definition
  - ATFL and CFL injury
  - **ATFL—loose in dorsiflexion, tight in plantarflexion**
  - **CFL—tight in dorsiflexion, loose in plantarflexion**
- History—inversion injury
- Physical examination
  - Anterior drawer test
- Imaging—Ottawa Ankle Rules indication for radiographs
  - Inability to bear weight
  - Medial or lateral malleolus tenderness
  - Fifth MT base tenderness
  - Navicular tenderness
- Treatment
  - Nonoperative
    - Boot immobilization
    - Physical therapy
  - Operative
    - **Anatomic reconstruction (Brostrom-Gould)**—shortening and reinsertion of ATFL and CFL
    - Nonanatomic reconstruction (Chrisman-Snook)
    - Arthroscopy

SYNDROMES

Diabetes

- Diabetic neuropathy
  - Foot ulceration
  - **5.07/10 g Semmes-Weinstein monofilament**
  - Total contact cast
  - Debridement of exposed bones
  - TAL for equinus contracture with forefoot ulcers
- Peripheral vascular disease
  - **Transcutaneous oxygen pressure predictive of healing**
  - Gangrene
- Claw toe
  - Motor neuropathy affecting intrinsic muscles in the foot
  - Toe ulceration
- Charcot arthropathy (Figure 8.11)
  - Lack of protective sensation
  - Bone and joint destruction
  - **Erythema, warmth, and swelling improves from elevation**
  - Total contact cast
  - Arthrodesis after the acute inflammation subsides
  - TAL often required

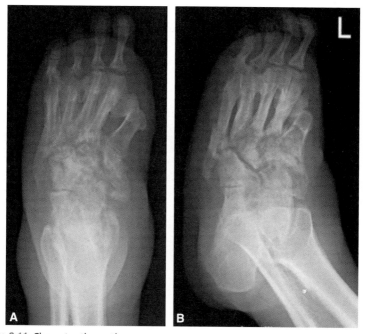

Figure 8.11 Charcot arthropathy.

- Infection
  - MRI to evaluate for abscess and osteomyelitis
  - Deep surgical culture and debridement
  - Targeted antibiotics

Charcot-Marie-Tooth Disease (see Table 8.1)

- Definition
  - Hereditary motor and sensory peripheral neuropathy
  - **Autosomal dominant, duplication of chromosome 17**
  - **Abnormal myelin sheath protein peripheral myelin protein 22**
- History
  - Onset in childhood or early adulthood
  - Weakness, gait abnormality
- Physical examination and imaging (Figure 8.12)
  - Forefoot cavus and hindfoot varus
  - **Unopposed peroneus longus to tibialis anterior**
  - Plantar-flexed first MT
  - Claw toe deformity from intrinsic wasting
  - Coleman block test—correct **flexible varus deformity**
- Treatment
  - Nonoperative
    - Bracing with lateral post
    - Rocker sole

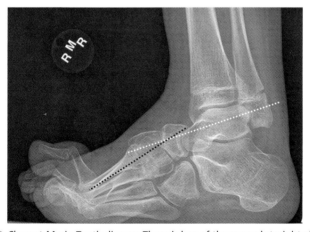

Figure 8.12 Charcot-Marie-Tooth disease. There is loss of the normal straight alignment of the first metatarsal (black line) with the talus axis (white line). The talar dome appears flattened, and the tibiotalar joint is rotated. From Ho-Fung A, Saptogino A, Cain T, et al. *Normal growth, normal development, and congenital disorders.* In: Lee EY, ed. *Pediatric Radiology: Practical Imaging Evaluation of Infants and Children.* Philadelphia, PA: Wolters Kluwer; 2018:1048-1084.

- Operative for flexible
  - First MT dorsiflexion osteotomy
  - Peroneus longus to brevis transfer
  - TAL
  - Lateral calcaneal osteotomy
- Operative for fixed deformity: Triple arthrodesis

CONGENITAL DEFORMITIES
Congenital Flat Feet

- Definition
  - Pes planovalgus
  - Familial—ligamentous laxity, flexible
- History—often not painful
- Physical examination
  - Forefoot abduction
  - Hindfoot valgus
  - Fallen arches
- Imaging—radiographs to rule out **tarsal coalition, congenital vertical talus, accessory navicular** (Figure 8.13)
- Treatment
  - Nonoperative
    - Observation in asymptomatic patients
    - Stretching **tight heel cord**
  - Operative
    - Medializing calcaneal osteotomy and/or lateral column lengthening (Evans)
    - Cotton osteotomy
    - Gastrocnemius recession or TAL
    - Arthroereisis screw (**controversial**)

Tarsal Coalitions

- Definition
  - Fusion of tarsal bones
  - Calcaneonavicular
  - Talocalcaneal

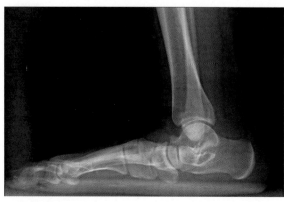

Figure 8.13 Pes planovalgus.

- History
  - Recurrent ankle sprains
  - Ankle pain with activities
- Physical examination
  - **Rigid flatfoot**
  - Limited subtalar motion
- Imaging
  - Radiographs
    - Calcaneonavicular coalition—**anteater nose sign**
    - Talocalcaneal coalition—**talar beaking; C sign** (Figure 8.14)
  - CT scan
  - MRI—fibrocartilaginous coalition
- Treatment
  - Nonoperative—immobilization with casting
  - Operative—surgical resection of coalition with interposition of fat graft

HEEL PAIN

- Plantar fasciitis
  - Inflammation of the plantar fascia at the calcaneus
  - Insidious onset of heel pain, often in the morning: "**first step pain**"
  - Tender to palpation at the **medial aspect of the calcaneal tuberosity**
  - Tight Achilles tendon
  - Stretching of plantar fascia and Achilles tendon
  - Night splints
  - Shockwave therapy
  - Surgical release

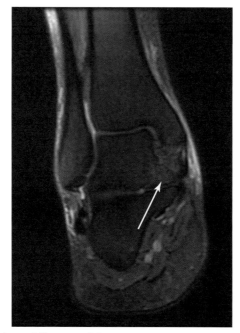

Figure 8.14 Talocalcaneal fibrous coalition.

- Baxter nerve
  - Lateral plantar nerve compression between fascia of abductor hallucis longus and quadratus plantae
  - **Common in runners**
  - EMG
  - Release of abductor hallucis fascia
- Calcaneus stress fracture
  - Bone scan or MRI helpful for diagnosis
  - Repetitive motion
  - Protected weight bearing and immobilization

ANKLE ARTHRITIS

- Ankle arthritis
  - Tibiotalar arthritis
  - **Most commonly post-traumatic**
  - Other causes include osteoarthritis, gout, rheumatoid arthritis, osteonecrosis, ankle instability, and PTT insufficiency
  - Pain and stiffness
  - Varus or valgus deformity
  - Weight-bearing radiographs show narrowing joint space, osteophytes, subchondral cysts, and deformity (Figure 8.15).

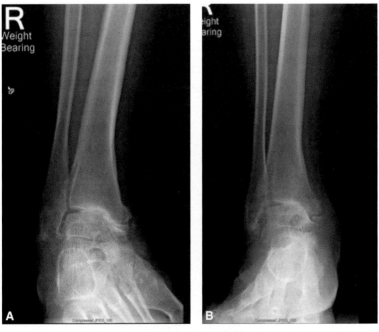

Figure 8.15 Ankle arthritis. AP, mortise and lateral radiographs demonstrating varus ankle arthritis with medial joint arthritis and wear, anterior spur, and sclerosis

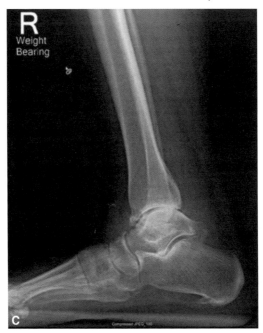

Figure 8.15 *(continued)*

- Ankle arthrodesis
  - Excellent pain relief
  - Young laborers
  - **Position of arthrodesis: neutral dorsiflexion, 5° valgus, 5° external rotation**
  - Subtalar arthritis develops
- Total ankle arthroplasty
  - Excellent pain relief
  - Complications with wound infection and revision

9 Spine

Jay S. Reidler, Eric Wei, A. Jay Khanna, Francis H. Shen, David J. Kirby, Varun Puvanesarajah, Matthew Hoyer, and Michael McColl

ANATOMY

Vertebral Column

- Overview
  - **33 vertebrae:** 7 cervical, 12 thoracic, 5 lumbar, 5 sacral (fused), and 4 coccygeal (fused)
  - Supports and protects spinal cord and nerve roots
  - Denis three-column theory (Figure 9.1)
    - **Anterior column**
      - **Anterior two-thirds of vertebral body and annulus**
      - Anterior longitudinal ligament (ALL)
      - Weight bearing in the erect position
    - **Middle column**
      - **Posterior one-third of vertebral body and annulus**
      - Posterior longitudinal ligament (PLL)
    - **Posterior column**
      - **Pedicles, facets, lamina, and spinous processes**
      - Posterior ligamentous complex (PLC)
        - Supraspinous ligament
        - Interspinous ligament
        - Ligamentum flavum
        - Facet capsules
      - Paravertebral musculature attachments
  - Typically, vertebral size increases caudally (more weight supported)
  - **Normal curvature**
    - Cervical lordosis
    - Thoracic kyphosis
    - Lumbar lordosis
    - Sacral kyphosis

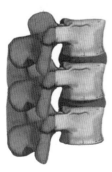 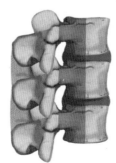 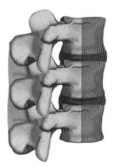

| Posterior column | Middle column | Anterior column |

Figure 9.1 Denis three-column theory. From Greenleaf R, Richman JD, Altman DT. General principles of vertebral bony, ligamentous, and penetrating injuries. In: Brinker MR, ed. *Review of Orthopaedic Trauma.* 2nd ed. Philadelphia, PA: Lippincott Williams & Wilkins; 2013:406-417.

- Cervical
  - **Atlanto-occipital joint**
    - Occipital condyles of the skull articulate with superior facets of the atlas.
    - Tectorial membrane—extension of PLL
    - **50% of head flexion/extension (~50°)**
  - C1 (atlas)
    - No vertebral body
    - No spinous process
    - Vertebral arteries travel through transverse foramen and then enter the foramen magnum (**to avoid injury, C1 dissection should not be >1.5 cm lateral from the midline in an adult**; Figure 9.2).
  - C2 (axis)
    - Odontoid process is the attachment site of the alar and cruciate ligaments.
      - **Transverse bands of cruciate ligament are the most critical for C1-C2 stability.**
    - Bifid spinous process
    - **50% of cervical rotation occurs at atlanto-axial joints (~50°).**
  - C3-C7 vertebrae
    - Bifid spinous process except for C7
    - Vertebral arteries **do not** travel in C7 transverse foramen.
    - **Subaxial spine** contributes to cervical motion: **lateral flexion (~60°), flexion/extension (~50°), and rotation (50°).**
- Thoracic
  - Costal facets articulate with the ribs, providing rigidity.
  - **Normal thoracic kyphosis is 20° to 50°.**
  - Largest transverse processes

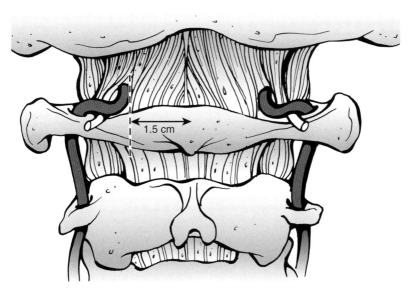

Figure 9.2 Anatomic relationship between C1 and the vertebral artery. From Schoenfeld AJ, Le HV, Bono CM. Cervical spine fractures and dislocations. In: Tornetta P III, Ricci WM, Ostrum RF, et al, eds. *Rockwood and Green's Fractures in Adults*. Vol 2. 9th ed. Philadelphia, PA: Wolters Kluwer; 2020:1817-1899.

- **T5—narrowest pedicle**
- Range of motion: flexion/extension (75°), lateral flexion (75°), and rotation (70°)
- Lumbar
  - **Normal lumbar lordosis is ~60° (range, 20°-80°).**
  - **Cauda equina begins at L1-L2.**
  - Range of motion: flexion/extension (85°), lateral flexion (30°), and rotation (10°)
- Sacrum
  - Five fused vertebrae
  - Four pairs of pelvic sacral foramina ventrally and dorsally
  - Sacral canal opens into sacral hiatus.
- Coccyx
  - Four fused vertebrae
  - "Tailbone"
  - Muscular attachments
    - Gluteus maximus muscle
    - External anal sphincter
    - Levator ani muscle (including coccygeus)
- **Facet joints**
  - Synovial joints that facilitate and limit spinal motion: flexion, extension, and rotation
  - Orientation varies with spinal level.
  - **Thin layer of hyaline cartilage between articulating surfaces**

Ligaments (Figure 9.3)

- **ALL**
  - Prevents hyperextension
  - Supports annulus fibrosus
  - Thick at center of vertebral body and thin at edges
- **PLL**
  - Prevents hyperflexion
  - Hourglass shape with wider and thinner sections over disks

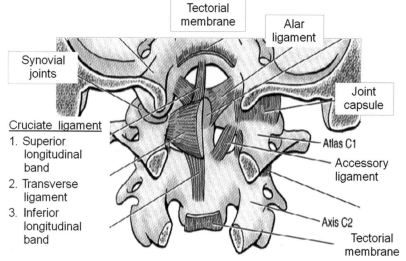

Figure 9.3 Ligaments in the upper cervical spine. From Meinhardt PA, Milam RA, Darden BV II. Cervical spine: plain radiography. In: Benzel EC, ed. *The Cervical Spine.* 5th ed. Philadelphia, PA: Lippincott Williams & Wilkins; 2012:278-290.

- **Ligamenta flava**
  - Connect laminae of adjacent vertebrae from axis to sacrum
  - **Hypertrophy may exacerbate nerve root compression.**
- **Denticulate ligaments**
  - Interconnect pia mater with dura mater
  - **Suspend and provide stability to the spinal cord**
  - Extend down to T12
- **Supraspinous ligament**
  - Continuation of ligamentum nuchae in cervical spine—C7 to sacrum
  - **Limits hyperflexion of the spine**
- Interspinous ligaments
  - Between adjacent spinous processes
  - Limits hyperflexion of the spine
- Intertransverse ligaments
  - Between transverse processes
  - Limits lateral flexion of the spine

Intervertebral Disks

- Overview
  - Twenty-three fibrocartilaginous disks starting at C2-C3 and ending at L5-S1
  - Constitutes 20% to 33% of vertebral column height—**aging causes disk dehydration and height decrease**
  - Cross-sectional areas of disks increase craniocaudally. L4-L5 disk space is largest.
- Vasculature
  - At birth, blood vessels that are present at endplates perforate intervertebral disk, extending into the annulus fibrosus.
  - **Normal adult intervertebral disk is avascular, with capillaries terminating at endplates; receives nutrients via passive diffusion.**
- Structure
  - **Annulus fibrosus—peripheral**
    - Outer layer—**type I collagen** fibers, obliquely oriented
    - Inner layer—fibrocartilage
    - **High tensile strength**
    - Superficial fibers of annulus fibrosus innervated by sinuvertebral nerves from dorsal root ganglia
  - **Nucleus pulposus—central**
    - Negatively charged proteoglycans
    - **Type II collagen**
    - Hydrophilic matrix
    - Approximately 88% water
    - No innervation
    - **High compressive strength**

Musculature

- **Extrinsic muscular** attachments—trapezius, rhomboids, serratus posterior, and latissimus dorsi
- **Intrinsic muscles**
  - Superficial
    - Splenius capitis and cervicis muscles
    - Lateral flexion of neck
  - Intermediate
    - Three erector spinae muscles—spinalis, longissimus, and iliocostalis muscles
    - Trunk extension and lateral flexion

- Deep
  - Semispinalis muscles—neck extension
  - Multifidus and rotatores muscles—stabilize and rotate vertebrae

Nervous System

- **Spinal cord (Figure 9.4)**
  - **Part of the central nervous system**
  - **Meninges** cover spinal cord
    - **Pia** mater (innermost layer)
    - **Arachnoid** mater—subarachnoid space (between pia and arachnoid mater)

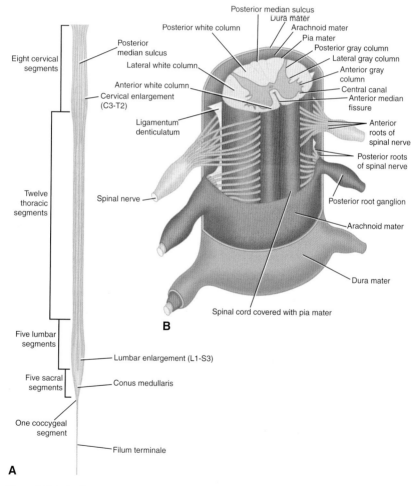

Figure 9.4 Spinal cord anatomy. A, Spinal segments demonstrating cervical and lumbar enlargements. B, Layers surrounding the spinal cord include the dura mater, arachnoid mater, and pia mater. From Splittgerber R. Spinal cord and ascending, descending, and intersegmental tracts. In: *Snell's Clinical Neuroanatomy*. 8th ed. Philadelphia, PA: Wolters Kluwer; 2019:131-184.

- Filled with cerebrospinal fluid (CSF)
- Mechanical protection
- Immune cells
  - **Dura** mater (outermost layer)
- **Terminates with conus medullaris at L1-L2, then transitions into cauda equina**
  - Filum terminale
  - Nerve roots
- Spinothalamic tracts carry sensory information.
  - **Lateral—pain and temperature**
  - **Ventral—light touch**
  - **Dorsal—deep touch, vibratory, and proprioception**
- Corticospinal tracts carry motor information.
  - Medial—upper extremities
  - Lateral—lower extremities
- Nerve roots
  - Thirty-one pairs of spinal nerves, exit through neural foramina
  - **Cervical roots 1 to 7** exit canal **above** the pedicle of the corresponding vertebrae and **cervical root 8** exits **below** C7 pedicle.
  - **All other spine roots** exit canal **below** the pedicles of the corresponding vertebrae.
  - Common deficits by nerve root are shown in Table 9.1.
- **Sympathetic chain**
  - **Twenty-two ganglia**—3 cervical, 11 thoracic, 4 lumbar, and 4 sacral
  - **Three cervical ganglia**—stellate, middle, and superior
    - **Injury of middle cervical ganglion leads to Horner syndrome.**

Blood Vessels

- Arterial
  - **Vertebral arteries**
    - Ascend through transverse foramen of C6-C1

Table 9.1 Common Deficits by Nerve Root

Nerve Root	Motor	Sensory	Reflex
C5	Shoulder abduction, elbow flexion (biceps)	Lateral arm	Biceps
C6	Elbow flexion (brachioradialis), wrist extension	Thumb, radial forearm	Brachioradialis
C7	Elbow extension, wrist flexion, finger extension	Middle finger	Triceps
C8	Finger flexion	Small finger, ulnar forearm	
T1	Finger abduction	Medial forearm/arm	
L1		Groin, iliac crest	Cremasteric
L2	Hip flexion, hip adduction	Anteromedial thigh	
L3	Hip flexion, hip adduction, knee extension	Anteromedial thigh	
L4	Knee extension, ankle dorsiflexion	Lateral thigh, anterior knee, medial leg	Patellar
L5	Ankle dorsiflexion, foot inversion, toe dorsiflexion, hip extension/abduction	Anterolateral leg, dorsal foot	
S1	Foot plantar flexion, foot eversion	Posterior leg, lateral foot	Achilles
S2	Toe plantar flexion	Plantar foot	
S3, S4	Bowel and bladder function	Perianal	

- Branches supply the posterior spinal arteries and the anterior spinal artery.
  - **Unite to form basilar artery**
- Three vertical arteries
  - **Anterior spinal artery**—runs down ventral median fissure
  - **Two posterior spinal arteries**—run down dorsal fissures
- Segmental arteries
  - Enter via intervertebral foramina along with nerve roots
  - **Artery of Adamkiewicz**
    - Largest segmental medullary artery
    - **Commonly left-sided and present between T8 and L1**
    - **Damage may cause paralysis**
- Venous
  - Parallels arterial supply pathways
  - There are also internal and external venous plexuses.

CERVICAL SPINE TRAUMA

Presentation and Initial Evaluation

- **Assume trauma patients have a cervical spine injury until confirmed otherwise**
  - Immobilize in rigid cervical collar, use spinal board for transport, and log roll for posterior examination
  - **Children**: Use **specialized board with occipital recess and body pad** to maintain spinal alignment.
- History
  - Often involves **high-energy** trauma such as motor vehicle accidents, falls from heights, and high-impact sports
  - Occurs more commonly in those >65 years of age and in men
  - Assess **mechanism of injury** and forces involved
    - Distraction, compression, hyperflexion, hyperextension, lateral flexion, rotational, or translation forces
    - **Distractive forces can cause ligamentous injuries** that are not apparent on initial imaging.
  - Incidence
    - C2 is the most commonly fractured vertebra (24%), followed by C6 and C7.
    - Subaxial spine (C3-C7) accounts for 65% of cervical fractures and 75% of cervical dislocations/subluxations.
- Physical examination
  - Examine for midline bony tenderness.
  - Complete neurologic examination, **including cranial nerves**, which can be involved in high cervical spine injuries
  - **Hoffman sign:** Flick finger nail and observe for reflexive thumb contraction, which may suggest cervical myelopathy or cord injury.
  - **Romberg sign:** Standing patient is asked to close eyes and stand still; swaying or imbalance suggests injury to cerebellum or dorsal column of the spinal cord that mediates proprioception.
  - In subacute setting, if there is no longer suspicion for fracture or dislocation:
    - **Lhermitte sign:** Maximally flex the neck and trunk. Radiating pain down the arms or spine suggests cervical spinal stenosis.
    - **Spurling sign:** Patient's head is extended and rotated to the side of suspected neural impingement and axially compressed. Radiating pain suggests cervical foraminal stenosis.
- Imaging
  - Cervical spine clearance without radiographic imaging
    - **National Emergency X-Radiography Utilization Study (NEXUS) low-risk criteria**
      - Patient must be awake and alert

- ◦ Patient cannot be intoxicated
- ◦ No neurologic deficits
- ◦ No painful, distracting injuries
- ◦ No posterior midline cervical spine tenderness
- • **Canadian C-spine rule** (CCR)
  - ▪ **Absence** of all high-risk factors that necessitate radiography
    - · Age ≥65 years
    - · Dangerous mechanism
    - · Paresthesias in extremities
  - ▪ **Presence** of any low-risk factors that suggest range-of-motion testing would be safe
    - · Simple rear-end motor vehicle collision
    - · Sitting position in the emergency department
    - · Ambulatory at any time
    - · Delayed (not immediate) onset of neck pain
    - · Absence of midline cervical spine tenderness
  - ▪ If criteria 1 and 2 are satisfied, test range of motion; if patient can rotate neck actively 45° to the left and right, cervical spine can be cleared without radiography.
  - • CCR has higher sensitivity and specificity for cervical spine injury and decreases radiography rates when compared with NEXUS criteria.
- • If the cervical spine cannot be cleared clinically, radiographs (anteroposterior [AP], lateral, odontoid views, and swimmer's view if needed to visualize cervicothoracic junction) and/or computed tomography (CT) should be obtained.
  - ◦ Inspect the following on the lateral cervical spine radiograph: **anterior vertebral line**, **posterior vertebral line**, **spinolaminar line**, and **spinous process line** (Figure 9.5).
  - ◦ **Prevertebral soft tissues** are normally ≤**6 mm at C2** and ≤**18 mm at C6.**
  - ◦ Order **magnetic resonance imaging (MRI)** if there is concern for **neurologic or major soft-tissue** (eg, ligamentous) injury as MRI provides the best visualization of spinal cord injury, disk herniation, and PLC disruption.
  - ◦ Order **magnetic resonance angiography or CT angiography** if there is concern for **vertebral artery injury.**
- ● Treatment principles
  - • Select operative versus nonoperative treatment according to specific patient-related factors: previous functional level, medical comorbidities, associated injuries, and the patient's personal wishes.
  - • **Surgical treatment usually aims to:**
    - ◦ **Reduce** spinal cord or nerve root **compression**
    - ◦ **Provide mechanical stability**, thereby preventing pain, deformity, and further neurologic injury

Occipital Condyle Fractures

- ● Often caused by axial loading of the skull on C1 lateral masses or by lateral hyperflexion injuries
- ● **Anderson and Montesano classification**
  - • **Type I: compression/impaction-type** fracture causing occipital condyle comminution
  - • **Type II: shear-type** fracture extending into the skull resulting from direct blow to the skull
  - • **Type III:** condylar-alar ligament **avulsion fracture** resulting from forced rotation and lateral bending
  - • Type I and type II injuries are usually stable and treated with cervical orthosis if there is no fragment displacement into the foramen magnum (alar ligaments and tectorial membrane usually preserved).

- **Type III injuries are more likely to be unstable**, requiring halo immobilization or occipitocervical arthrodesis.
  - Anterior pin placement when applying a halo should be **superolateral to the eyebrow to avoid supraorbital nerve injury.**

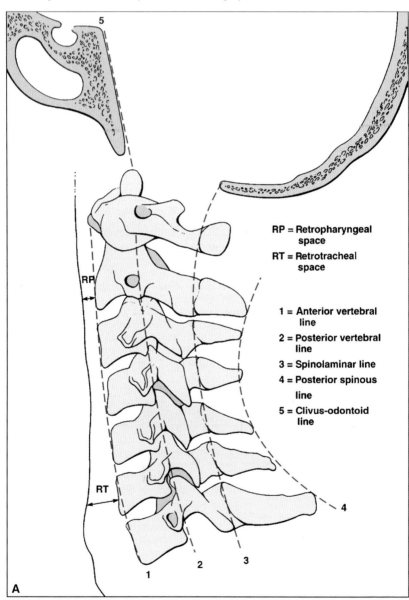

RP = Retropharyngeal
       space

RT = Retrotracheal
       space

1 = Anterior vertebral
      line

2 = Posterior vertebral
      line

3 = Spinolaminar line

4 = Posterior spinous
      line

5 = Clivus-odontoid
      line

Figure 9.5 Lateral cervical spine lines. A, When viewing lateral cervical spine radiographs, it is important to ensure there are no disruptions in the anterior vertebral, posterior vertebral, spinolaminar, posterior spinous, and clivus-odontoid lines. B, Lateral cervical spine radiograph demonstrating intact lines. From Greenspan A, Beltran J. Spine. In: *Orthopedic Imaging: A Practical Approach*. 6th ed. Philadelphia, PA: Wolters Kluwer Health; 2015:442-510.

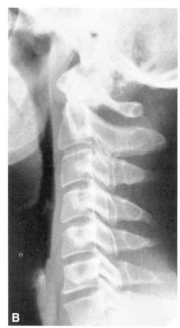

Figure 9.5 (*continued*)

Atlanto-Occipital Dissociation

- Usually highly unstable and involves **alar ligament and tectorial membrane disruption**
- **Traynelis classification**
  - Type I: **anterior** dislocation (occiput translated anteriorly relative to cervical spine)
  - Type II: **longitudinal** dislocation (occipital condyles distracted off of atlas)
  - Type III: **posterior** dislocation (occiput translated posteriorly relative to cervical spine)
- **Powers ratio** calculated on CT
  - Powers ratio = (**basion** to **posterior arch of C1** distance)/(**anterior arch of C1** to **opisthion** distance) (Figure 9.6)
  - Powers ratio >1 is suggestive of anterior dislocation.
- **Basion-dens interval** calculated on CT
  - Value of 9 to 12 mm also suggestive of atlanto-occipital dissociation
- Atlanto-occipital dissociations usually require posterior **occipitocervical arthrodesis** for maintenance of long-term stability.

C1-C2 Subluxation (Atlanto-axial Instability)

- **Atlanto-dens interval (ADI)**
  - In healthy adults—usually <3 mm for men and <2.5 mm for women
  - In children <15 years of age—usually <5 mm
- Chronic instability can usually be seen on **flexion-extension views**, although such views would usually be contraindicated after an acute trauma when instability is suspected.
- C1-C2 subluxation caused by forced flexion of the neck leads to:
  - **Rupture of the transverse ligament** (best seen on MRI) or
  - **Avulsion fracture of C1 lateral mass** via pull by the transverse ligament (fragment best seen on CT)

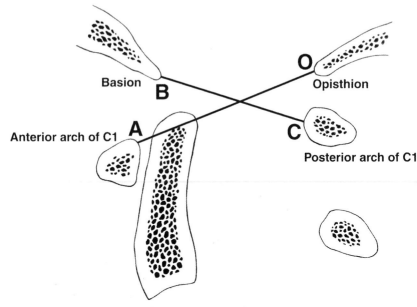

Figure 9.6 Powers ratio. Basion to posterior arch of C1 distance divided by anterior arch of C1 to opisthion distance. From Patel AA, Spiker WR, Ghanayem AJ. Functional anatomy of joints, ligaments, and disks. In: Benzel EC, ed. *The Cervical Spine.* 5th ed. Philadelphia, PA: Lippincott Williams & Wilkins; 2012:43-52.

- Treatment
  - Transverse ligament rupture—often requires C1-C2 arthrodesis because of instability and poor ligamentous healing potential
  - Avulsion fracture—often treated with halo immobilization because of potential for osseous healing of C1 lateral mass avulsion fracture
- Atlanto-axial rotatory subluxation
  - Caused by combined rotatory and flexion or extension forces; can occur spontaneously without any clear trauma
  - **Fielding classification** assesses:
    - Pivot point (odontoid or facet)
    - Transverse ligament competence
    - ADI
  - In about half of cases, the odontoid serves as the pivot point, the transverse ligament remains intact, and the ADI is <3 mm. Treat with gradual cervical halter traction with patient supine.
  - Rarely necessitates C1-C2 arthrodesis

C1 (Atlas) Fractures
- Caused by high-energy axial loads
- Fracture patterns
  - Anterior arch fractures
  - Posterior arch fractures
  - Transverse process fractures
  - Lateral mass fractures (often comminuted)
  - Burst fractures (ie, Jefferson fractures): combined anterior and posterior arch fractures

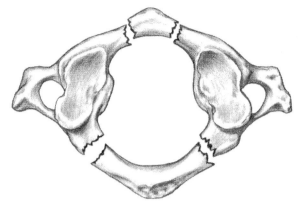

Figure 9.7 Jefferson fracture. From Morgan RA. Acute management of spine trauma. In: Swiontkowski MF, ed. *Manual of Orthopaedics*. 7th ed. Philadelphia, PA: Lippincott Williams & Wilkins; 2013:232-261.

- If isolated, C1 fractures are usually **not** associated with spinal cord injury because of the **large space available** for the cord at this level.
- Most fractures can be treated in cervical orthosis or halo immobilization if the transverse ligament remains intact.
- **Burst fractures (ie, Jefferson fractures; Figure 9.7)**
  - Usually involve lateral mass displacement away from the spinal canal
  - On odontoid radiographic view, if C1 right and left lateral mass overhang distance (compared with C2) is **greater than 7 to 8 mm, then the transverse ligament is considered ruptured** and the fracture is deemed unstable; this **necessitates C1-C2 arthrodesis** (or occipitocervical arthrodesis if inadequate C1 bony purchase).

C2 (Axis) Fractures

- Categories
  - Odontoid process fractures (~50% of C2 fractures)
  - Lateral mass fractures
  - Pars fractures (also known as "Hangman's fracture")
- **Odontoid process fractures (Figure 9.8)**
  - Result from hyperextension or hyperflexion injuries
  - Classified in relation to watershed area at the base of the dens, from which the odontoid process receives its vascular supply

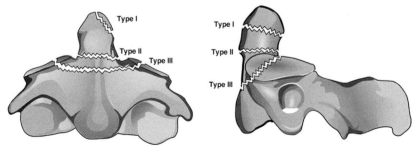

Figure 9.8 Odontoid process fractures. From Morgan RA. Acute management of spine trauma. In: Swiontkowski MF, ed. *Manual of Orthopaedics*. 7th ed. Philadelphia, PA: Lippincott Williams & Wilkins; 2013:232-261.

- · **Type I: apical avulsion** fracture (involves alar ligament)
- · **Type IIA: base** fracture at the junction of the odontoid process and C2 body—minimally displaced
- · **Type IIB: base** fracture—displaced with **anterosuperior to posteroinferior** oblique fracture line
- · **Type IIC: base** fracture—displaced with **anteroinferior to posterosuperior** oblique fracture line
- · **Type III: body** fracture in the C2 cancellous bone, possibly extending into lateral facets
- If isolated injuries, **type I and III fractures are usually stable and have good healing potential** with cervical collar (Type I) or halo immobilization (Type III).
- Type II fractures have a high nonunion rate and can often benefit from surgical fixation. **Nonunion risk factors:**
  - · Increased patient age
  - · Displacement >5 mm
  - · Posterior displacement
  - · Angulation >10°
  - · Smoking
- Type II fractures can be treated by **lag screw fixation** (**Type IIB pattern** is most likely to benefit from this technique) **or C1-C2 arthrodesis.**
- ● C2 lateral mass fractures
  - Caused by combined lateral bending and axial compression forces
  - Usually treated in cervical orthosis. Chronic pain may be an indication for later arthrodesis.
- ● **C2 pars fractures (Hangman fracture; Figure 9.9)**
  - This represents a traumatic spondylolisthesis of the axis caused by hyperextension and axial loading; involves fractures of bilateral pars interarticularis of C2.

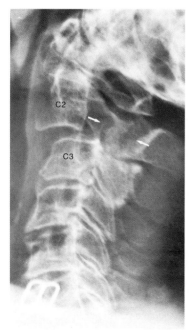

C2

C3

Figure 9.9 C2 pars (Hangman's) fracture. Lateral cervical spine radiograph showing fractures through the C2 pars interarticularis (arrows) with resulting C2–C3 subluxation following a hyperextension injury. From Greenspan A, Beltran J. Spine. In: *Orthopedic Imaging: A Practical Approach*. 6th ed. Philadelphia, PA: Wolters Kluwer Health; 2015:442-510.

- **Levine and Edwards classification** categorizes these fractures according to the degree of displacement, angulation, translation, and C2-C3 disk disruption.
  - Type I: nondisplaced, <3 mm translation, no angulation, C2-C3 disk intact
  - Type II: displaced, substantial C2-C3 angulation and >3 mm translation, C2-C3 disk disrupted
  - Type IIA: displaced, severe C2-C3 angulation but no translation, severe C2-C3 ligamentous complex disruption, hinging on the ALL
  - Type III: pars fracture with associated unilateral or bilateral C2-C3 facet dislocation
- Treatment
  - Type I: usually treated with cervical orthosis
  - Type II: if <5-mm displacement, can be reduced with axial traction and extension and then immobilized in halo; **if >5-mm displacement, usually requires surgical stabilization**
  - Type IIA: **should not be placed in traction** because of risk for ligamentous disruption; reduce with hyperextension alone and then halo immobilization
  - Type III: usually requires reduction followed by open reduction and internal fixation of C2, or arthrodesis of C2-C3 or C1-C3

C3-C7 (Subaxial) Injuries

- **Allen-Ferguson classification** system categorizes subaxial fractures and dislocations by injury mechanism (Figure 9.10).
  - Compressive flexion
  - Vertical compression
  - Distractive flexion
  - Compressive extension
  - Distractive extension
  - Lateral flexion
- **Subaxial injury classification** system builds on the Allen-Ferguson classification system, grading injuries by morphology, discoligamentous complex damage, and extent of neurologic compromise (Table 9.2).
  - Higher scores are more likely to require surgical treatment.
- Compressive flexion injuries
  - Cervical spine is axially loaded and flexed—indicates compression fractures without neurologic deficits; **can often be treated nonoperatively.**
  - In severe cases, can develop **triangular "teardrop" fracture** anteriorly, PLC disruption, and retrolisthesis, causing spinal canal compromise, which requires surgical treatment with anterior decompression and plating with or without posterior fixation.
- Vertical compression injuries
  - Pure axial loading can cause **burst fractures with retropulsion of bony fragments into the canal.**
  - Can be treated with anterior decompression and plating with or without posterior fixation
- Distractive flexion injuries
  - Most common mechanism causing **facet dislocations**
  - Subaxial facet dislocations (Figure 9.11)
    - Most commonly occur at C5-C6 and C6-C7 levels
    - Unilateral facet dislocations—usually involves <50% translation
    - Bilateral facet dislocations—usually involves >50% translation
      - Often associated with nerve root or spinal cord injuries; 30% of patients have complete spinal cord injuries
      - Use of MRI is controversial; most authors recommend **MRI before reduction** to rule out herniated disk, which occurs in ~7% of cases.

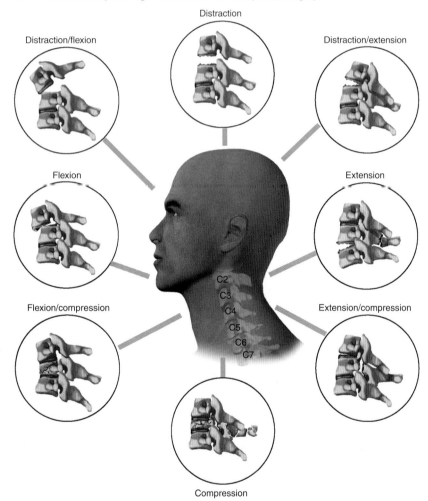

Figure 9.10 Allen-Ferguson system for categorizing subaxial fractures and dislocations by injury mechanism. From Greenleaf R, Richman JD, Altman DT. General principles of vertebral bony, ligamentous, and penetrating injuries. In: Brinker MR, ed. *Review of Orthopaedic Trauma.* 2nd ed. Philadelphia, PA: Lippincott Williams & Wilkins; 2013:406-417.

- If **herniated disk present**, proceed with **open** decompression and arthrodesis via anterior approach.
- If **no herniated disk present** and the patient is alert and cooperative, attempt **closed** reduction with traction.
- Extension injuries
  - Compressive extension injuries can cause unilateral or bilateral vertebral arch fractures; in most severe cases, there can be anterior ligamentous disruption with anterolisthesis.
  - Distractive extension injuries cause anterior ligamentous disruption and, in most severe cases, injury of the PLC with posterior displacement of the rostral vertebral body into the canal.

Table 9.2 Subaxial Cervical Spine Injury Classification System Scale

Characteristic	Points
Morphology	
No abnormality	0
Compression	1
Burst	+1 = 2
Distraction[a]	3
Rotation/translation[b]	4
Discoligamentous complex	
Intact	0
Indeterminate[c]	1
Disrupted[d]	2
Neurologic status	
Intact	0
Root injury	1
Complete cord injury	2
Incomplete cord injury	3
Continuous cord compression in setting of neurologic deficit (neuro modifier)	+1

[a] For example, facet perch, hyperextension.
[b] For example, facet dislocation, unstable teardrop, or advanced-stage flexion-compression injury.
[c] For example, isolated interspinous widening, magnetic resonance imaging signal change only.
[d] For example, widening of disk space, facet perch, or dislocation.
From Vaccaro AR, Hulbert RJ, Patel AA, et al; Spine Trauma Study Group. The subaxial cervical spine injury classification system. A novel approach to recognize the importance of morphology, neurology, and integrity of the disco-ligamentous complex. Spine (Phila Pa 1976). 2007;32:2365-2374.

Mechanism of Locking

Ruptured ligamentum flavum

Ruptured posterior longitudinal ligament

Detached anterior longitudinal ligament

Ruptured interspinous ligament

Ruptured supraspinous ligament

Perched facets

A

Figure 9.11 Facet dislocations. A, Bilateral facet dislocations result from combined hyperflexion and distraction forces. There is associated extensive damage to the posterior ligamentous complex. B, The facets become locked following anterior dislocation of the cephalad vertebral body. The inferior facets of the cephalad vertebra are anterior to the superior facets of the caudal vertebra. C, Lateral cervical spine radiograph showing C5–C6 bilateral locked facets. From Greenspan A, Beltran J. Spine. In: Orthopedic Imaging: A Practical Approach. 6th ed. Philadelphia, PA: Wolters Kluwer Health; 2015:442-510.

Locked Facets

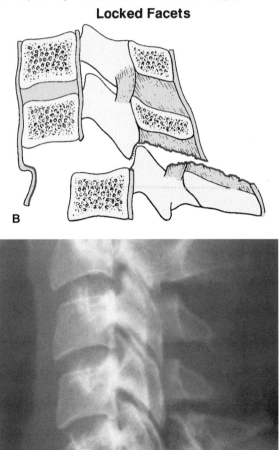

Figure 9.11 *(continued)*

- Treatment depends on stability and neurologic compromise, with most severe cases requiring surgical intervention.
- Lateral flexion injuries
  - Involve direct trauma to the side of the head, leading to distraction forces on the side of impact and compression contralaterally
  - Can result in ligamentous disruption and lateral mass fractures
  - Treatment depends on stability and neurologic compromise.

- Cervical spinous process avulsion fracture
  - Known as "**clay-shoveler fracture**"
  - Most common at C7
  - Results from musculoligamentous avulsive forces during sudden flexion/extension activities (eg, shoveling hard dirt)
  - Usually treated nonoperatively; can be excised if patient develops painful nonunion

THORACOLUMBAR SPINE TRAUMA

Etiology

- **Major causes** of thoracolumbar trauma: motor vehicle accidents (38%), falls, violence (gunshot wounds), and sporting accidents
- **Bimodal distribution** in young adults and the elderly
- Location of thoracolumbar spine trauma
  - **T11-L2 thoracolumbar junction/transitional zone** (50%)
    - Fulcrum for movement
    - L1 is the most commonly injured vertebra
  - **Thoracic spinal cord is more susceptible to injury with trauma.**
    - Decreased caliber of spinal canal relative to spinal cord compared with the lumbar spine
    - Tenuous blood supply because mid-thoracic spine is a watershed zone

Classification

- **Denis classification**
  - Assessment of spinal stability after traumatic injury
  - Classification characterizes the spine and associated soft tissue with the **three-column concept**:
    - **Anterior column**—anterior half of vertebral body, anterior half of vertebral disk space, and ALL
    - **Middle column**—posterior half of vertebral body, posterior half of vertebral disk space, and PLL
    - **Posterior column**—spine posterior to the PLL
  - **Unstable fracture—Two or more adjacent columns within same level are injured.**
- **AOSpine Thoracolumbar Spine Injury Classification**
  - Classifies fractures according to mechanism (type), morphology (subtype), and neurologic status
  - Incidence of neurologic injury increases with increasing AO classification, from 22% with Type A to 51% with Type C.
    - Type A: compression
    - Type B: distraction
    - Type C: translation
- **Thoracolumbar Injury Classification and Severity (TLICS) Scale** (Figure 9.12)
  - Injury severity classification determining need for surgical intervention in thoracolumbar injury
  - Thoracolumbar injury scored by injury morphology, PLC integrity, and neurologic status:
    - **Morphology**—compression (1), burst (2), translation (3), distraction (4)
    - **Neurologic status**—intact (0), nerve root (2), complete cord injury (2), incomplete cord injury (3), cauda equina (3)
    - **PLC integrity**—intact (0), injury suspected (2), injured (3)
  - Scoring
    - Score ≤3: nonoperative treatment
    - Score = 4: nonoperative or operative
    - Score ≥5: operative treatment

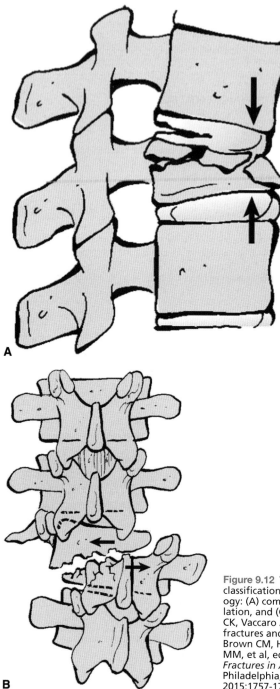

Figure 9.12 Thoracolumbar injury classification and severity scale morphology: (A) compression, (B) rotation/translation, and (C) distraction. From Kepler CK, Vaccaro AR. Thoracolumbar spine fractures and dislocations. In: Court-Brown CM, Heckman JD, McQueen MM, et al, eds. *Rockwood and Green's Fractures in Adults.* Vol 2. 8th ed. Philadelphia, PA: Wolters Kluwer Health; 2015:1757-1794.

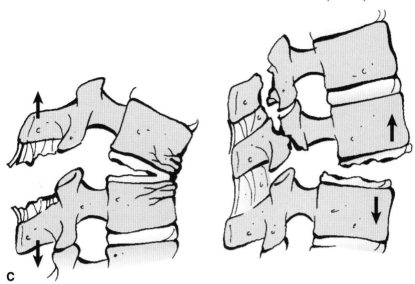

C

Figure 9.12 (*continued*)

Evaluation

- Initial management
  - Patient presentation
    - In a healthy patient, damage to vertebral columns is often caused by high-energy trauma.
    - Vigilance for associated injuries on the part of the evaluating physician is essential.
    - Patients with polytrauma, especially those involved in motor vehicle accidents, falls from height (>15 ft), high-impact sporting accidents, and gunshot wounds should be evaluated for spinal trauma.
  - Stabilization
    - 25% of spinal cord injuries are sustained during handling/transport from the scene and in the first stages of care.
    - Immediate **total spine immobilization** with hard collar, spine board, and use of the log-roll technique as soon as spinal trauma is suspected.
  - Assessment
    - Primary survey (ABCDE, advanced trauma life support)
    - Secondary survey
      - History should assess the following: mechanism of injury, preinjury functional status, neurologic change (sensorimotor), pain, urinary/bowel incontinence, previous spinal injuries/surgeries, predisposing conditions (eg, ankylosing spondylitis, diffuse idiopathic skeletal hyperostosis [DISH])
      - Physical examination
        - Mental status
        - Neurologic—American Spinal Injury Association examination every 4 to 6 hours to assess for changes (assess sensory, motor, reflexes, rectal examination—perianal sensation, volitional control, bulbocavernosus reflex)
        - Spine (tenderness, step-offs, interpedicular widening)
        - Pelvis
          - Sensory defect
          - Stable pelvis

- Associated injuries
  - One-third of thoracolumbar transition fractures have associated injuries.
  - 20% of associated injuries are missed.
  - **Common associated injuries**
    - Head injury (26%)
    - Chest injury
    - Long-bone fractures
  - **Intra-abdominal injuries** are commonly associated with **flexion-distraction injuries.**
    - Half of children with spinal trauma sustain intra-abdominal injuries.
  - **Burst fractures secondary to fall** are associated with **calcaneus** and **tibial plateau** fractures.
  - **Epidural hematomas** are common in **extension-type** injuries.
    - Extension-type injuries with worsening neurologic status should be evaluated with MRI.
- Imaging
  - CT
    - CT scan should be considered for evaluation of the thoracolumbar spine when spinal trauma is suspected.
    - High sensitivity and specificity for identifying osseous lesions
    - Indications: focal neurologic signs, signs of spine fracture, or trauma
    - CT of chest, abdomen, and pelvis also aids in identifying visceral organ damage.
  - Radiographs (full-length AP and lateral)
    - Acceptable method for evaluating osseous injury in spinal trauma
    - Upright radiographs are indicated for alignment evaluation after patients have been mobilized.
  - MRI
    - Indicated if soft-tissue injury is suspected (ie, ligamentous injury or spinal cord injury)

Mechanism and Treatment

- General considerations
  - Nonoperative treatment
    - Functional (no bracing)
      - Patients are mobilized and instructed to perform usual daily activity, limiting activity according to pain.
      - Only acceptable in stable fractures
    - Thoracolumbosacral orthosis (TLSO)
      - Can be used if the fracture is at T7 or lower
      - Brace must be worn whenever the patient is upright to 30° above horizontal
      - Worn for ≥12 weeks
      - Upright radiographs are required after initial mobilization to ensure acceptable spinal alignment
    - Reduction and cast stabilization
      - Patients are positioned to reduce the fracture and a restricting cast is placed.
      - Typically worn ≥12 weeks
      - Rarely used due to discomfort from cast and risk of developing pressure sores
      - Upright radiographs are required after initial mobilization to ensure spinal alignment.
  - Operative treatment
    - **Indications for surgery**
      - Fracture dislocation
      - Progressive neurologic defect
      - Incomplete neurologic defect
      - Cord compression with signs of neurologic deficits
      - Kyphosis >30°

- TLICS >4
- Mechanical instability
- Inability to tolerate closed treatment
- Timing
  - Consider treatment with urgent/emergent decompression in cases of progressive neurologic deficits and neurologic deficits with signs of cord compression, pending trauma clearance
  - In other cases, consider postponing surgery to optimize the patient's health
- Technique
  - **Posterior approach**
    - Most common method for internal stabilization
    - Decompression can be achieved indirectly via distraction and ligamentotaxis or directly via laminectomy and/or facetectomy.
    - Stabilization constructs available by this approach:
      - Monosegmental—Single-level fixation is possible in patients with intact pedicles and inferior endplate.
      - Short bisegmental—Two-level posterior fixation is the most common method.
      - Long bisegmental—Highly unstable fractures and patients unable to bear weight (McCormack load-sharing classification) require posterior long-segmental fixation.
    - Costotransversectomy
      - Removal of transverse process and part of rib allows for improved access to anterior column through the posterior approach.
  - **Anterior approach**
    - Allows for direct decompression of retropulsed fragments impinging on the spinal cord
    - Severely comminuted fractures
    - Kyphotic deformity
  - Combined approach
    - Rarely used
    - Burst fractures with major canal compromise and kyphosis >40°
- Outcomes
  - Kyphotic deformity tends to persist with nonoperative treatment.
    - Studies have not correlated kyphosis with pain or functional outcomes, although long-term outcomes are unclear.
    - Nonoperative treatment, 75% to 80%: minimal pain and return to work with no restrictions
  - Operative treatment allows for immediate stabilization and earlier mobilization.
- **Flexion-compression fractures**
  - Pathophysiology
    - As the spine flexes anteriorly, each vertebral body within the arc of flexion experiences compressive forces from the adjacent spinal elements (intervertebral disks and bodies).
    - Compressive forces increase at the anterior spine as torque increases with an increasing moment arm.
    - Fracture at the point of highest stress
      - Often **anterior wedge-compression fracture**
      - Lateral flexion can result in a lateral compression fracture
      - Vertebral height loss and kyphotic deformity
  - Treatment
    - Nonoperative
      - TLSO bracing with gradual return to activity
        - Pain is severe for these patients and often requires substantial medical treatment in the first month.
        - Obtain upright AP and lateral radiographs of the spinal level involved with initial mobilization to ensure proper alignment.

- Operative
  - If posterior ligamentous injury or neurologic deficit, use short two-level posterior stabilization
  - **Kyphoplasty use is limited to low-energy trauma fractures (osteoporotic/pathologic) because high-energy trauma can have fracture lines that would allow bone cement to enter the spinal canal.**
- **Flexion-distraction fractures**
  - Pathophysiology
    - Rapid flexion of the torso, as in a car accident with two-point seatbelt, creates a center of rotation.
    - Spinal components anterior to the center of rotation will sustain **compressive force,** whereas those posterior will sustain **distracting force.**
    - Ranges from distraction of all three columns to distraction of the posterior column with compression of the anterior column
    - Also known as "**chance**" or "seatbelt" fracture
    - **Bony chance** fractures can often be treated with **bracing** because of fracture healing potential; **ligamentous chance** fractures usually require **surgery** because of poor healing potential.
  - Treatment
    - Nonoperative
      - Neurologically intact, mechanically stable, and TLICS <4
      - Hyperextension cast or TLSO brace for 12 weeks
    - Operative
      - Complete or partial neurologic deficit with cord compression or TLICS >4
      - Short posterior constructs are sufficient because of the minimal comminution associated with the injury.
      - Ligamentum flavum should be decompressed or excised to avoid canal enfolding.
- **Axial compression fractures**
  - Pathophysiology
    - Mechanism: Vertical load on the neutral spine results in a comminuted fracture of the vertebral body.
    - Expulsion of comminuted fragments posteriorly into the spinal canal and interpedicular widening often seen
    - This is characterized as a **burst fracture.**
    - **McCormack classification** is a useful tool for determining the load-sharing capability of comminuted vertebral body fractures (Figure 9.13).
      - ≥7 points indicate severe comminution and likely failure of posterior segment stabilization.
  - Treatment
    - Nonoperative
      - No neurologic deficit and intact PLC
      - Hyperextension casting or bracing for 12 weeks
    - Operative
      - Neurologic deficit, disrupted PLC, or TLICS >4
      - Partial neurologic deficits secondary to fragment retropulsion can be decompressed from an anterior approach.
      - Complete neurologic deficits or disrupted PLC without neurologic deficit can be treated with posterior two-level fixation.
        - McCormack classification can be used to determine if posterior stabilization will suffice or if anterior stabilization is required.
- **Extension fractures**
  - Pathophysiology
    - "**Lumberjack fracture**"—caused by hyperextension and shear forces to the posterior spine resulting in tension at the anterior column, as with a rolling log

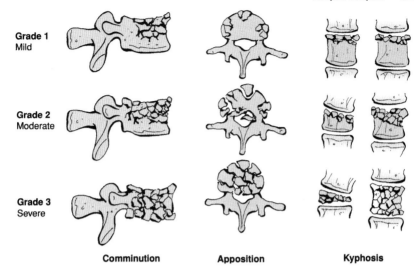

Grade 1
Mild

Grade 2
Moderate

Grade 3
Severe

Comminution   **Apposition**   **Kyphosis**

Figure 9.13 The load-sharing classification of spine fractures. From Gendelberg D, Bransford RJ, Bellabarba C. Thoracolumbar spine fractures and dislocations. In: Tornetta P III, Ricci WM, Ostrum RF, et al, eds. *Rockwood and Green's Fractures in Adults*. Vol 2. 9th ed. Philadelphia, PA: Wolters Kluwer; 2019:1900-1963.

- · Highly unstable—Fracture occurs in weight-bearing portion of the spine and is susceptible to translation.
- · Treatment: Immediate immobilization and surgical stabilization are required.
- · Associated with ankylosing spondylitis and DISH
- • Treatment
  - · Operative—long posterior construct with segmental stabilization
- ● **Translation fractures**
  - • Pathophysiology
    - · All three columns fail due to shear or rotational forces.
    - · Translation in the axial plane and discontinuity of the spinal canal
    - · Can result in a transverse fracture through the caudal vertebral body secondary to shear force from rotation of cephalad vertebra
    - · **This injury most often results in complete spinal cord injury (80%).**
  - • Treatment
    - · Operative—long posterior arthrodesis construct with segmental stabilization

Osteoporotic Fractures

- ● Pathophysiology
  - • **Compression fractures of the spine are the most common osteoporotic fractures.**
  - • Osteoporotic bones, and the defining decrease in bone mineral density, are weaker and more susceptible to fracture.
- ● Presentation
  - • Sudden localized back pain
  - • Minimal or no history of trauma
  - • **Previous vertebral compression fracture is greatest risk factor.**
- ● Treatment
  - • Nonoperative
    - · No neurologic deficit or instability

- Observation and medical treatment
  - Nonsteroidal anti-inflammatory drugs **(NSAIDs)** and narcotic analgesics—effective for pain in the acute phase
  - Extension **bracing**
  - **Antiosteoporotic medications**
    - Bisphosphonates have been shown to reduce the risk of future fracture.
    - Vitamin D mediates a dose-dependent fracture risk reduction.
    - Calcium
  - **Kyphoplasty**
    - Indicated for pain lasting longer than 1 month
    - **Considered safer than vertebroplasty because bone cement can be injected under lower pressure**
- Operative
  - Neurologic impairment, instability, or TLICS >4
  - Posterior approach
    - Multilevel segment stabilization (two to three segments above and below) is often required because the bone is fragile.
    - Decompression can be achieved through distraction and ligamentotaxis.
  - Anterior approach—appropriate if cord compression necessitates anterior decompression

SPINAL CORD INJURY

Background
- Epidemiology
  - There are 12 500 new spinal cord injuries per year in the United States.
  - Approximately 250 000 individuals in the United States have spinal cord injuries.
- Pathophysiology
  - **Direct injury** to neural tissue from trauma
  - **Indirect injury** to neural tissue secondary to damaged adjacent tissues that causes diminished perfusion, release of free radicals, and lipid peroxidation
    - **Methylprednisolone can help to limit each of these processes, but is controversial.**
  - Commonly associated with:
    - Spinal fractures
    - Head injuries
    - Damage to vertebral vasculature
- **American Spinal Injury Association Classification**
  - Level of neurologic injury is defined as **lowest spinal segment with motor function grade ≥3 and intact sensation** (provided the next rostral level is 5/5 and sensation intact).
    - **A: complete injury**—no preserved motor or sensory function in S4-S5
    - **B: incomplete injury**—below the level of injury, **some sensory** function is preserved; however, **no motor function is preserved**
    - **C: incomplete injury**—below the level of injury, **some sensory** and motor function is preserved; however, **more than half of muscle functions have a muscle grade <3**
    - **D: incomplete injury**—below the level of injury, **some sensory** and motor function is preserved, and **at least half of muscle functions have a muscle grade ≥3**
    - **E: normal**—sensory and motor functions are normal

Immediate Stabilization and Examination
- Stabilization—Injured patients should be immobilized before transport.
  - Cervical collar should be used.
  - Log-roll techniques should be used for examination of patient and placement on firm spine backboard.

- Advanced trauma life support protocol
  - **Primary survey (ABCDE)**
    - **A**irway maintenance
    - **B**reathing—In cases of spinal cord injury above C5, intubation may be required.
    - **C**irculation—Neurogenic shock may cause hemodynamic changes (see next).
    - **D**isability and neurologic assessment
    - **E**xposure of patient
  - Imaging
    - Radiographs or CT scans of the cervical spine are usually obtained first in trauma settings to assess for fractures/dislocations.
    - MRI is indicated when there is evidence of acute neurologic injury to assess for spinal cord injury, disk herniation, or other spinal canal compromise; can also obtain MRI to assess for ligamentous disruption that can cause spinal instability.

Neurogenic and Spinal Shock

- **Neurogenic shock**
  - Pathophysiology—**Acute spinal cord injury causes disruption in sympathetic nervous system activity.**
    - Decreased sympathetic tone and vascular resistance causes **hypotension.**
    - Unopposed vagal activity results in **bradycardia.**
      - Distinguishes neurogenic shock from hypovolemic/hemorrhagic shock, which usually causes hypotension and tachycardia
      - Note that in trauma patients with spinal cord injury, neurogenic and hypovolemic shock can occur concurrently.
  - Treatment
    - Initially, pulmonary artery catheterization is used to monitor fluid volume.
    - Vasopressors may be required to treat hypotension.
- **Spinal shock**
  - Pathophysiology
    - Spinal cord injury causes **temporary (usually 24-72 hours) loss of function and reflex.**
      - Hypotension
      - Bradycardia
      - Flaccid, areflexic/hyporeflexic paralysis
      - **Deficient bulbocavernosus reflex**
        - **Reflex return indicates that spinal shock has ended.**
        - **Full evaluation of neurologic deficit/level of injury cannot be performed until spinal shock has ended.**
        - Injuries to conus or cauda equina may permanently disrupt this reflex.
  - Phases
    - Phase 1: hyporeflexia/areflexia (~24-48 hours)
    - Phase 2: reflex return (bulbocavernosus reflex is usually one of the first to recover, 24-48 hours after Phase 1)
    - Phase 3: hyperreflexia (1-4 weeks after Phase 2)
    - Phase 4: spasticity (1-12 months or more after Phase 3)

Spinal Cord Injury Treatment

- **High-dose methylprednisolone**
  - **Use is controversial.**
  - Thought to improve perfusion, decrease lipid peroxidation, and decrease free radical release
  - National Acute Spinal Cord Injury Studies II and III recommend use in patients with nonpenetrating injuries to the spinal cord, but not the nerve roots; **only recommended if started within 8 hours of injury**

- 30 mg/kg methylprednisolone bolus given over 15 minutes
- 5.4 mg/kg/h maintenance infusion
  - Administer infusion for **24 hours if begun within 3 hours** of injury
  - Administer infusion for **48 hours if begun within 3 to 8 hours** of injury
- **Contraindications**
  - **>8 hours after injury**
  - **Penetrating spinal injury (eg, gunshot wounds)**
  - **Patient <13 years of age**
  - **Pregnancy**
  - **Infection**
  - **Injuries to peripheral nerves (brachial plexus, spinal roots)**
- Outcomes
  - Improvement of spinal cord function unclear
  - At level of spinal cord injury, may cause improvement in root function
- Acute closed reduction
  - Reduction using axial traction may be indicated for certain cervical injuries such as facet dislocation (see Cervical Spine Trauma section).
  - Abort procedure if neurologic deficit worsens with traction.
- Definitive treatment
  - Nonoperative—bracing
    - For patients with terminal metastatic cancer (<6-month life expectancy) and most gunshot wounds
  - Operative—decompression and stabilization
    - For patients with complete spinal cord injuries, incomplete spinal cord injuries whose neurologic recovery worsens or plateaus, or metastatic cancer with >6-month life expectancy
      - Prognosis—may recover nerve root function at level of spinal cord injury
    - May also be indicated in patients with gunshot wounds with cauda equina syndrome, a bullet retained in the thecal sac, or a bullet retained in the spinal canal with progressive neurologic deterioration
- **Complications of spinal cord injury**
  - **Autonomic dysreflexia**
    - Symptoms—**headache, agitation, anxiety, hypertension, and blurred vision**
    - Caused by **sympathetic overactivation** (eg, from fecal impaction/bladder distension)
  - Deep venous thromboembolism—prophylaxis with sequential compression device and/or anticoagulation may be indicated
  - Major depressive disorder—approximately 11% of spinal cord injury patients
  - Pressure ulcers
  - Urosepsis
  - Sinus bradycardia
  - Orthostatic hypotension
- Rehabilitation
  - Patients can learn to restore limited motor function
  - Tendon transfers may help to recover certain functions
  - Patient function by level of spinal cord injury
    - **C1-C3**
      - **Ventilator dependent**
        - Vital capacity <20% of normal
        - Cough absent or weak
        - Limited speech
      - **Electric wheelchair controlled by head/chin**
    - **C3-C4**
      - **Ventilator dependent**, with **potential to become independent**
      - **Electric wheelchair controlled by head/chin**

- C5
  - Ventilator independent
  - Distal upper extremity motor deficits—difficulty eating
  - May use **hand-controlled electric wheelchair**
- C6
  - Can feed/groom/dress oneself independently
  - **Manual wheelchair**, **sliding board transfers**
- C7
  - Improved upper extremity motor strength and function—can cut food with knife
  - **Manual wheelchair, independent transfers**
- C8-T1
  - Increased dexterity and strength in distal upper extremities
  - **Independent transfers**
- T2-T6
  - **Upper extremities have normal motor function.**
  - Patients are reliant on wheelchair.
- T7-T12
  - **Seated activities may be done without support because of improved abdominal muscle control.**
- L1-L5
  - Functions throughout lower extremities and bowel/bladder are variable.
  - **Variable need for bracing**
- S1-S5
  - Walking with little to no bracing or assistance
  - **Bowel/bladder and sexual functions variable**

Specific Clinical Syndromes

- Incomplete injury (Figure 9.14)
  - **Central cord syndrome**
    - Pathophysiology
      - Most common syndrome of incomplete spinal cord injury
      - Central gray matter of spinal cord is compressed (eg, anterior compression by osteophytes and posterior compression by an infolded ligamentum flavum).
        - Causes motor function deficit **(upper extremities worse than lower)**; sensory deficits are variable
  - Presentation
    - Hand weakness and diminished hand dexterity
    - Burning sensation in upper extremity
    - **Distal upper extremity muscles have more pronounced motor deficits than proximal muscles.**
  - Treatment
    - Operative versus nonoperative treatment remains controversial.
    - Prognosis is usually good, although full functional recovery is unpredictable and less likely in upper extremity than lower; **can have residual clumsiness in hands.**
  - **Anterior cord syndrome**
    - Pathophysiology—injury caused by:
      - Direct compression of anterior spinal cord—often from osteophyte growth
      - **Occlusion of the anterior spinal artery**
    - Presentation—**loss of pain and temperature sensation** and motor function below the level of spinal cord injury
      - Dorsal column sensation (vibration, deep pressure, and proprioception) usually preserved
      - Deficits usually worse in lower extremities than in upper extremities.
    - **Worst prognosis**—chances of motor recovery between 10% and 20%

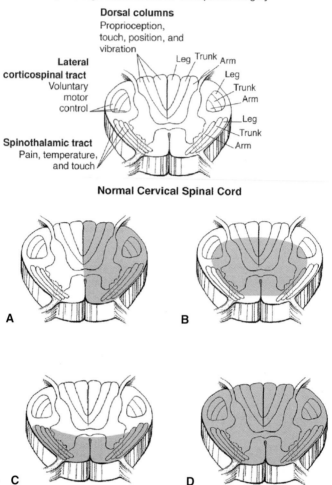

Figure 9.14 Spinal cord injury syndromes. A, Brown-Séquard syndrome. B, Central cord syndrome. C, Anterior cord syndrome. D, Complete spinal cord injury. From Woodward GA. Neck trauma. In: Fleisher GR, Ludwig S, eds. *Textbook of Pediatric Emergency Medicine*. 6th ed. Philadelphia, PA: Lippincott Williams & Wilkins; 2010:1376-1421.

- **Posterior cord syndrome**
  - Pathophysiology—rare injury **isolated to the posterior spinal column**
  - Presentation—**loss of vibration, deep pressure, proprioception sensation**, with preservation of pain and temperature sensation and motor function
- **Brown-Séquard syndrome**
  - Pathophysiology—**caused by injury to one side of the of spinal cord**, often penetrating trauma
  - Presentation
    - **Ipsilateral** to injury: **motor deficits**, sensory deficits **(proprioception, vibration)**
    - **Contralateral** to injury: sensory deficits **(pain, temperature)**

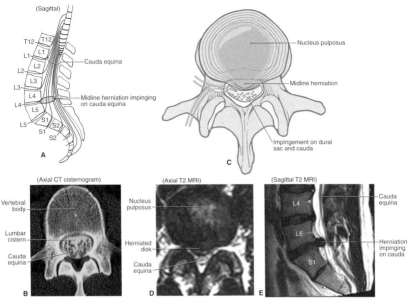

Figure 9.15 Cauda equina syndrome. A, Large central disc herniations can cause compression of the cauda equina. B, CT cisternogram showing the cauda equina in the lumbar cistern. C, Illustration of axial spinal demonstrating a midline disc herniation impinging on the cauda equina. D, E, Axial and sagittal T2 MRI showing a midline disc herniation impinging on the cauda equina. From Haines DE. Clinical syndromes of the CNS. Part I. Herniation syndromes of the brain and spinal discs. In: *Neuroanatomy Atlas in Clinical Context Structures, Sections, Systems, and Syndromes.* 10th ed. Baltimore, MD: Wolters Kluwer Health; 2019:297-308.

- **Good prognosis** for recovery of motor function, with 90% of patients returning to ambulation
- **Cauda equina syndrome (Figure 9.15)**
  - Pathophysiology
    - **Compression of lumbosacral terminal nerve roots** (cauda equina) caused by:
      - Herniated disk (most common)
      - Spinal stenosis
      - Trauma
      - Epidural hematoma
      - Tumor
    - Not a spinal cord injury, but rather injury to the nerve roots distal to the conus medullaris
  - Presentation
    - Symptoms
      - **Bilateral buttock/leg pain, as well as motor or sensory deficits**
      - **Bladder/bowel deficits (90%)**
        - Especially urinary retention
      - **Saddle anesthesia (75%)**
      - Erectile dysfunction
    - Physical examination
      - Leg weakness, sensory loss
      - Diminished lower extremity reflexes
      - Diminished perianal sensation
      - Diminished rectal tone

- Imaging
  - MRI can assess for cauda equina compression.
  - CT myelography—suitable alternative in patients who cannot undergo MRI
- Treatment
  - **Emergent surgical decompression**
  - Better outcomes if done **within 48 hours**
- Spinal cord injury without radiologic abnormality
  - Pathophysiology—occurs **more often in pediatric cervical spine injuries** because of skeletal flexibility
  - Presentation
    - Neurologic deficits/transient paresthesias
    - In severe cases, complete injury may be present.
    - No radiographic abnormality noted on radiographs or CT scans
    - MRI usually shows evidence of injury to the spinal cord, spinal ligaments, or vertebral bodies; evidence absent in 30% to 35% of patients.
  - Treatment
    - **Spine and blood pressure require monitoring and support.**
    - **External immobilization versus surgical treatment if there is evidence of spinal instability**

CERVICAL SPINE DEGENERATIVE CONDITIONS

Cervical Degenerative Disk Disease

- **Cervical degenerative disk disease** (or cervical spondylosis) can lead to discogenic neck pain, radiculopathy, and/or myelopathy. It can involve:
  - Disk degeneration (bulging, shrinking, desiccation)
  - Joint degeneration (bone spurs and arthrosis)
  - Ligamentum flavum thickening
  - Kyphosis resulting in a load transfer to facet and uncovertebral joints
- Commonly arises in patients 40 to 60 years of age and disproportionately affects men
- **Most common at C5-C6**
- Risk factors: smoking, frequent heavy lifting, and frequent long-distance driving
- **Discogenic neck pain**
  - Pain resulting from disk degeneration in the absence of other abnormalities
  - Typically normal examination with some decreased range of motion or pain in cervical motion
  - MRI shows degeneration in disk.
  - Treat with **anti-inflammatory medications and activity modification**
- **Cervical radiculopathy**
  - Compression of ≥ 1 nerve roots because of disk herniation, osteophytes of the uncovertebral or facet joints, and/or ligamentum flavum thickening
    - In the cervical spine, the **exiting nerve root** at a given level is usually affected; **at C5-C6, the C6 nerve root is affected** (Figure 9.16).
    - Involves biologic inflammatory mediators, including **substance P, bradykinin, and interleukins**
  - Symptoms include radiating pain (eg, **neck and scapular pain**), numbness, weakness, paresthesia, and loss of corresponding upper extremity reflexes
    - **Spurling test:** positive when radicular symptoms present as the neck is rotated and bent laterally
    - **Shoulder abduction sign:** positive when radicular symptoms resolve with shoulder abduction
    - Characteristics of each common radiculopathy:
      - **C5**—weakness in deltoid and biceps with diminished biceps reflex
      - **C6**—weakness in brachioradialis and wrist extensors with diminished brachioradialis reflex, thumb paresthesia

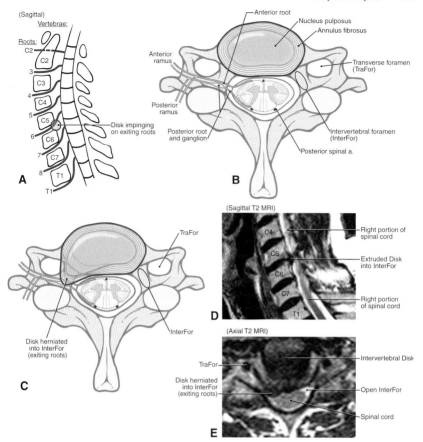

Figure 9.16 Cervical radiculopathy. A, A disc herniation at the C5–C6 disc level usually affects the C6 nerve root. B, Illustrations of the axial cervical spine anatomy and exiting C6 nerve root. C, A disc herniation impinges on the exiting nerve root. D, E, Sagittal and axial T2 MRI showing a disc herniation at the C5–C6 disc level impinging affecting the C6 nerve root. From Haines DE. Clinical syndromes of the CNS. Part I. Herniation syndromes of the brain and spinal discs. In: *Neuroanatomy Atlas in Clinical Context Structures, Sections, Systems, and Syndromes*. 10th ed. Baltimore, MD: Wolters Kluwer Health; 2019:297-308.

- **C7**—weakness in triceps and wrist flexors with diminished triceps reflex, middle finger paresthesias
- **C8**—weakness in distal phalanx flexors in fingers, small finger paresthesias
- Radiographs usually show osteophyte formation and disk space narrowing; lateral, flexion, and extension views recommended to assess alignment and stability.
- MRI may show disk degeneration and herniation with nerve root compression.
  - **High false-positive rate in patients >40 years** of age because many people of this age will have some degenerative changes.
- Nonoperative treatment
  - NSAIDs, corticosteroid injections, oral steroids, physical therapy, and immobilization in extreme cases
  - Improvement in ~75% of patients treated nonoperatively

- Operative treatment
  - Indications for surgery include progressive symptoms and/or failure of nonoperative treatments to alleviate symptoms.
  - Interventions
    - Anterior cervical discectomy and fusion **(ACDF)**
      - "Gold standard" treatment
      - **Smith-Robinson anterior approach**
      - Herniated disk and osteophytes are removed followed by a bone graft arthrodesis.
    - Anterior cervical **corpectomy** and arthrodesis
      - Smith-Robinson anterior approach
      - **Used when the vertebral body must be removed to address otherwise inaccessible abnormality behind the vertebra** that is causing compression
    - **Cervical disk arthroplasty**
      - Proposed as motion-preserving technology with potential to decrease adjacent segment disease
      - Early clinical trials suggest lower reoperation rate and quicker return to work compared with ACDF; however, long-term clinical trials are needed.
    - Posterior keyhole **laminoforaminotomy**
      - Used when the neural compression is caused by facet hypertrophy or lateral soft-disk herniation
      - Reduces risk of iatrogenic injury associated with an anterior approach
      - **More than 50% of the facet joints should be preserved to maintain spinal stability.**
  - Complications in operations
    - Pseudarthrosis in 5% to 10% of single-level arthrodesis patients and 30% in multilevel arthrodesis patients
    - **Recurrent laryngeal nerve or hypoglossal nerve injury** in 1% of patients
      - **Preoperative laryngoscopic examination** is indicated in patients undergoing a second ACDF approached through the contralateral side.
- Cervical myelopathy (Figure 9.17)

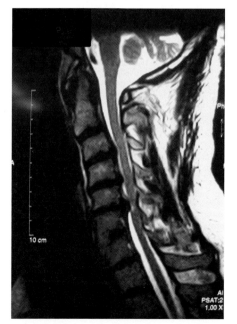

Figure 9.17 Cervical myelopathy. Sagittal T2-weighted magnetic resonance imaging shows multilevel cervical stenosis with cord signal change at most severe level, C5 to C6. From Nassr A, Ponnappan RK, Kang JD. Anterior decompression, instrumentation, fusion techniques: corpectomy, strut grafting. In: Bridwell KH, DeWald RL, eds. *The Textbook of Spinal Surgery*. Vol 1. 3rd ed. Philadelphia, PA: Lippincott Williams & Wilkins; 2011:236-252.

- Symptoms include **loss of hand dexterity, an ataxic gait, and occasionally urinary retention and/or frequency**
  - Physical examination
    - Weakness in extremities—lower extremity weakness suggests advanced disease
    - Pain sensation and proprioception dysfunction
    - **Hyperreflexia**
    - **Clonus**
    - **Wartenberg escape sign:** involuntary abduction of the fifth digit
    - **Grip and release test:** positive test if patient is unable to open and close fist 20 times in 10 seconds
    - **Hoffman sign:** Snapping middle finger at distal phalanx causes flexion of thumb and other fingers.
    - **Babinski test:** Stimulation of the sole of the foot causes an extension of the great toe.
    - **Lhermitte sign:** Extreme cervical flexion causes a shock sensation along spine and extremities.
- Often results from cervical stenosis; can be caused by age-related degeneration, trauma, or congenital differences.
  - **Absolute cervical stenosis** is defined by a canal diameter of <**10 mm**; **relative cervical stenosis** is defined by a **10- to 13-mm diameter**.
  - Lateral radiographs are the most useful image for determining canal diameter and Torg-Pavlov ratio (canal/vertebral body width).
    - **Torg-Pavlov ratio <0.8 suggests cervical stenosis.**
  - **Lumbar stenosis occurs in tandem in 20% of cases.**
- MRI can be used to determine the degree of compression and cord signal change.
- Most patients show a **slowly progressive disease with periods of stability followed by periods of deterioration.**
- A small percentage (<5%) of patients experience a sharp progressive decline over a few days to weeks.
- Imaging—MRI to assess degree of spinal cord compression and cord signal change
  - Compression ratio (smallest sagittal diameter/largest sagittal diameter) of <0.4 and signal changes on a T1 scan are associated with a poor prognosis.
  - Effacement of CSF space suggests functional stenosis.
- Treatment
  - Nonoperative, including NSAIDs, gabapentin, immobilization, and physical therapy
    - Patients with mild disease and no functional impairments
    - Poor surgical candidates
  - Surgical intervention—usually indicated because myelopathy is often progressive
    - **Anterior cervical decompression and arthrodesis**
      - Anterior approach **indicated in patients with kyphotic or lordotic cervical sagittal alignment**
      - Less blood loss, postoperative pain, and risk of infection than posterior approach
    - **Posterior laminectomy and arthrodesis**
      - For treating multilevel cord compression with kyphosis <10°
      - **If there is >10° fixed kyphosis, posterior approach alone contraindicated because of anterior bowstringing**
      - Laminectomy alone is rarely indicated because of potential for postlaminectomy kyphosis.
    - **Posterior cervical laminoplasty**
      - For treating multilevel cord compression with **kyphosis <13°**
      - **Contraindications include severe axial neck pain (should be fused) and kyphosis >13°**
      - **Motion-preserving treatment** (compared with ACDF/posterior arthrodesis), but higher blood loss than ACDF

- **Combined anterior and posterior approach** used in multilevel anterior cervical corpectomies, postlaminectomy kyphosis revisions, and multilevel stenosis correction in a rigid kyphotic spine
- **Cervical disk arthroplasty**
- Complications include:
  - Pseudarthrosis in 12% of single-level arthrodesis patients and 30% of multilevel arthrodesis patients
  - **Postoperative C5 palsy** in ~5% of patients
    - Can occur immediately after operation or have delayed onset many weeks later
    - Most patients recover, although it can take many months
  - Recurrent laryngeal nerve injury

Rheumatoid Cervical Spondylitis

- Present in 90% of patients with rheumatoid arthritis (RA) but often undiagnosed
- Declining prevalence because of increasing use of disease-modifying antirheumatic drugs
- Characterized by **instability in the occipitoatlantoaxial joints**
  - Includes three features: **atlanto-axial subluxation, basilar invagination, and subaxial subluxation**; they typically present in that order
- Symptoms include **axial neck pain and stiffness with occipital headaches** (caused by compression of C2 nerve).
  - Physical examination shows hyperreflexia, ataxic gait, and extremity weakness.
- Radiographic studies, including flexion and extension, needed to assess for instability and the posterior atlanto-dens interval (PADI).
  - **PADI <14 mm** is indication for surgery because of inadequate space available for the cord.
  - MRI is useful for assessing cord compression and the cervicomedullary angle.
- Atlanto-axial subluxation
  - In 50% to 80% of patients with RA
  - C1 subluxation on C2
    - Usually anterior subluxation, but other directions are possible
  - Caused by **pannus formation** between dens and C1 that destroys transverse ligament or dens
  - Treatment
    - Nonoperative if subluxation is stable (<3.5 mm of motion on flexion/extension radiographs)
    - **Surgical interventions**—indications include **PADI < 14 mm or ADI > 10 mm**
      - **C1 lateral mass—C2 pedicle/pars arthrodesis (Harms construct)**
        - Strongest and most common fixation
      - **C1-C2 transarticular screw fixation (Magerl)**
      - Odontoidectomy
      - **Occiput-C2 arthrodesis** for concurrent **basilar invagination**
- Basilar invagination (atlanto-axial invagination)
  - Dens penetrates the foramen magnum
  - 40% of patients with RA
  - **McGregor, Chamberlain, and McRae lines** can be used to diagnose through radiography
  - **Cervicomedullary angle <135°** on MRI is a surgical indication to prevent neurologic impairment.
  - Surgical interventions
    - Occipitocervical arthrodesis (occiput to C2)
    - Transoral or retropharyngeal odontoid resection
- Subaxial subluxation
  - 20% of patients with RA
  - Frequently presents with upper spine instability

- Caused by pannus formation in facet joints and uncovertebral joints leading to instability
- Radiograph showing a **subaxial subluxation of >4 mm suggests a cord compression** requiring surgical intervention.
- Surgical interventions
  - Posterior arthrodesis for concurrent atlanto-axial subluxation or basilar invagination; C1-C2 and occiput may be included
  - Complications include pseudarthrosis (10%-20% of cases) and degeneration in neighboring vertebrae.
  - Anterior spinal arthrodesis—to restore sagittal alignment

Ossification of the PLL (OPLL; Figure 9.18)

- Myelopathy resulting from **ectopic endochondral ossification in PLL**
- Common in Asian (especially Japanese) men
- Typically C4-C6
- **Correlated with low calcium levels or calcium absorption problems, obesity, diabetes, and physical stress on the cervical spine**
- Often **accompanies spondyloarthropathies and DISH**
- Symptoms can include those associated with myelopathy or radiculopathy, but often asymptomatic.
- Imaging should show ossification along the posterior side of the vertebral bodies within the spinal canal.
  - **CT is recommended** to better define ossification and classify as continuous (over several vertebrae), mixed, or localized.
- Treatment
  - Asymptomatic cases do not require treatment.
  - Surgical intervention for symptomatic cases

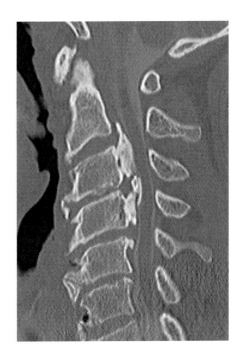

Figure 9.18 Ossification of the posterior longitudinal ligament. From Okawa A, Takahashi M, Sakai K, Shinomiya K. Surgery for ossification of the posterior longitudinal ligament: ventral approach. In: Benzel EC, ed. *The Cervical Spine*. 5th ed. Philadelphia, PA: Lippincott Williams & Wilkins; 2012:1031-1043.

- **Anterior approach is rarely** used, although it is more direct because dural ossification associated with **OPLL greatly increases the chance of dural tears.**
  - Indication for anterior approach is a kyphotic spine in which a posterior approach is unfeasible.
  - **Dural tears can be avoided using a float technique** in which the OPLL is left in place after corpectomy.
- **Posterior approach** is a more common and safer procedure but **requires a lordotic spine.**

THORACOLUMBAR SPINE DEGENERATIVE CONDITIONS

Thoracic Disk Herniation (Figure 9.19)

- Pathophysiology
  - Relatively uncommon
  - Typically middle/lower thoracic levels
    - T11-T12 is most common
  - Classification
    - **Protrusion:** bulging nucleus with intact anulus
    - **Extrusion:** disk through anulus, but restrained by the PLL
    - **Sequestration:** free disk material in canal
- Presentation
  - Symptoms
    - Chest/back pain
    - Radicular symptoms
      - **Band-like chest/abdominal pain or numbness**
      - Bowel/bladder deficits
      - Sensory deficits
      - Myelopathy
    - Arm pain with upper level herniations

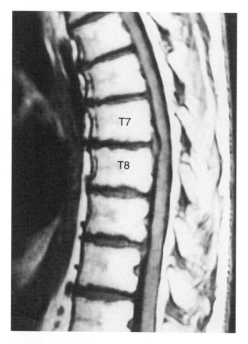

Figure 9.19 Thoracic disk herniation T7-T8 causing acute onset interscapular pain. From Yochum TR, Kettner NW, Barry MS, et al. Diagnostic imaging of the musculoskeletal system. In: *Yochum and Rowe's Essentials of Skeletal Radiology.* Vol 1. 3rd ed. Baltimore, MD: Lippincott Williams & Wilkins; 2005:485-678.

- Physical examination
  - Changes in dermatomal sensation
  - Myelopathy: upper motor neuron signs, including hyperreflexia, positive Babinski sign, and weakness
- Imaging
  - Radiographs: disk narrowing, osteophyte formation
  - MRI: best for showing disk herniation, high false-positive rate
- Treatment
  - Nonoperative—immobilization, analgesics, and injections
  - Operative—usually for patients with myelopathy and progressive neurologic symptoms
    - Discectomy approach
      - **Central herniated nucleus pulposus**
        - **Anterior transthoracic** approach—When performing thoracotomy or rib excision, **dissect along the superior aspect of ribs** to avoid neurovascular injury.
        - With or without arthrodesis or hemicorporectomy
      - **Lateral herniated nucleus pulposus**
        - **Posterior transpedicular or lateral extracavitary approach**
        - Usually requires arthrodesis

Lumbar Disk Herniation

- Pathophysiology
  - Tears in outer annulus causing herniation of nucleus pulposus
    - **Posterolateral**
      - Most common, because of weakness in PLL
      - Affects lower level **(traversing) nerve root**
    - **Foraminal/far lateral**—affects upper level **(exiting) nerve root**
    - **Central**
      - Typically associated with back pain only
      - May cause cauda equina syndrome
    - **Axillary**
      - May affect **exiting and traversing nerve roots**
  - Most common at L4/L5 and L5/S1 levels
  - More common in men (3:1)
- Presentation
  - Symptoms
    - Back pain—axial, lower back
      - Discogenic or mechanical
    - Leg pain—usually worsened with sitting
    - Cauda equina syndrome—less common
  - Physical examination
    - Motor—usually normal, may have focal deficits
    - Sensory—pain, numbness, or dysesthesia in legs
    - Reflexes—may have **weak reflexes**
    - Provocative tests
      - Supine/sitting **straight leg test**
        - Indicator for affected L4-S1 nerve root
        - With knee straight, 30° to 70° hip flexion reproduces symptoms in leg
        - **Lasègue sign:** hip flexion with knee flexion does not reproduce symptoms, but with knee extended does reproduce symptoms
      - **Contralateral straight leg test**
        - With knee straight, 30° to 70° hip flexion in asymptomatic leg causes symptoms in symptomatic leg.
        - More specific (especially for axillary herniation), less sensitive

- **Femoral tension sign**
  - Indicator for affected L2-L4 nerve root
  - With patient prone, combination of hip extension and knee flexion reproduces symptoms in thigh
- Imaging
  - Radiography
    - Better when taken upright rather than supine for assessment of instability; flexion-extension should be obtained
    - Decreased disk height
    - Disk degeneration
  - MRI
    - Should be obtained if pain lasts longer than 1 month or trauma/infection/cancer/cauda equina syndrome/motor deficit present
    - **Gadolinium indicated if need to distinguish recurrent disk herniation from fibrosis**
- Treatment
  - Nonoperative—90% of patients do not require surgery.
    - NSAIDs, muscle relaxants, oral steroids, and physical therapy
    - Corticosteroid injections
      - Epidural
      - Long-term improvement seen in approximately half of patients
  - Operative
    - Discectomy—best outcomes for patients with progressive weakness, correlated MRI findings, and tension signs
      - Approach
        - Can be done via open, microscope-assisted, endoscopic approaches
        - Usually performed with laminectomy, which allows access to central herniations**Foraminal herniations may require a paramedian (Wiltse) approach.**
      - Complications
        - Recurrent herniated nucleus pulposus
        - Dural tear
        - Discitis
        - Vascular catastrophe—**Damage to aorta or inferior vena cava can occur if anterior annulus is broken through.**
    - Arthrodesis—**performed if there is also evidence of mechanical instability**

Discogenic Back Pain

- Pain caused by disk degeneration, no nerve root impingement or other abnormality
- Presentation
  - Symptoms
    - Pain in lower back
    - Pain with axial loading, sitting, bending
    - No radicular symptoms
  - Physical examination
    - Pain in back is greater than pain in leg; aggravated by motion
    - Negative for nerve tension signs
  - Imaging
    - Radiograph—may show spondylosis, narrowed disk space
    - MRI—evidence of disk degeneration
      - T2: disk space shows diminished signal intensity
      - No herniation, annular tear, or stenosis
    - **Discography—controversial**

- Injecting contrast into disk space to increase pressure: positive when pain produced at abnormal levels (as seen on MRI) but not other levels (control levels)
- May cause annular tears and accelerate disk degeneration

- Treatment
  - Generally nonoperative treatment; surgery to be avoided
    - NSAIDs, physical therapy
    - Recovery
      - Within 1 week for >50% of patients
      - Within 1 to 3 months for 90% of patients
  - Operative
    - Discectomy with interbody arthrodesis: approaches include posterior midline, posterior transforaminal, anterior retroperitoneal, and direct lateral
    - Total disk arthroplasty—controversial and rarely indicated
      - Concerns about long-term results, safety, and cost
      - Considered by some for single-level degenerative disk without facet arthropathy

Lumbar Spinal Stenosis

- Pathophysiology
  - Nerve compression/ischemia caused by narrowing of spinal canal or neural foramina
    - Can be caused by compression from bone (osteophytes, spondylolisthesis) or soft tissue (herniated disks, cysts)
    - Can be congenital (short pedicles, medially located facets) or acquired (degeneration, trauma, inflammation)
  - Variations (Figure 9.20)
    - **Central stenosis**
      - Narrowing of central canal such that the cross-sectional area <100 mm^2 or the **AP diameter <10 mm**

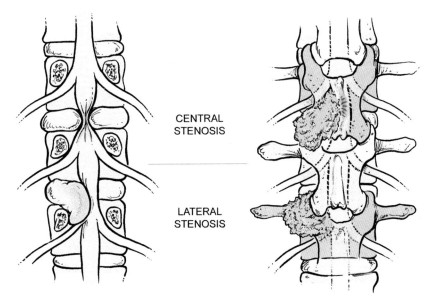

CENTRAL STENOSIS

LATERAL STENOSIS

Figure 9.20 Central stenosis versus lateral stenosis caused by disk pathology (left) and facet overgrowth (right). From Koval KJ, Zuckerman JD. *Atlas of Orthopaedic Surgery: A Multimedia Reference.* Philadelphia, PA: Lippincott Williams & Wilkins; 2004.

- Typically involves ligamentum flavum hypertrophy and/or bulging disk
- Causes **traversing nerve root compression**
- **Lateral/subarticular recess stenosis**
  - Caused by facet joint arthropathy and osteophyte formation (typically at the superior articular facet)
  - Causes **traversing nerve root compression**
- **Foraminal stenosis**
  - More common in lumbar region because of increased nerve root diameter and decreased foraminal diameter
  - Often caused by intraforaminal disk protrusion
  - Causes **exiting nerve root compression**

- Presentation
  - Symptoms
    - Back and radiating lower extremity pain or numbness
      - **Worse with back extension—standing/walking**
      - **Relieved with flexion activities—sitting**
    - Bladder/bowel dysfunction—less common
  - Physical examination
    - Limited back extension
    - Tension signs (straight leg raise) often negative, but can be positive in foraminal stenosis
    - **Kemp test**
      - Worsened radicular pain unilaterally with back extension—suggestive of foraminal stenosis
    - **Differentiating neurogenic and vascular claudication** (Table 9.3)
  - Imaging
    - Radiographs may show disk space narrowing, osteophyte formation, degenerative scoliosis, or spondylolisthesis.
    - MRI may show hypertrophy of facets or ligamentum flavum, lateral foramen/recess compression.
    - CT myelogram may show osteophytes (in better detail than MRI), trefoil canal, and central/lateral compression.
- Treatment
  - Nonoperative
    - NSAIDs, physical therapy, rest, and weight loss
    - **Epidural/transforaminal steroid injections may be effective over the short term.**
  - Operative—decompression performed in patients with progressive neurologic symptoms
    - Approach
      - Usually involves laminectomy and/or medial facetectomy
      - **Usually no arthrodesis unless there is evidence of instability (including that caused by laminectomy/facetectomy), degenerative spondylolisthesis/scoliosis**

Table 9.3 Differentiating Neurogenic and Vascular Claudication in Lumbar Spinal Stenosis

Parameter	Neurogenic Claudication	Vascular Claudication
Distal pulses/perfusion	Normal	Abnormal
Sitting	Symptoms relieved	Symptoms relieved
Standing	Symptoms induced	Symptoms relieved
Walking	Symptoms induced	Symptoms induced
Stairs	Ascending easier	Descending easier
Bicycling	Symptoms relieved	Symptoms induced

- Outcome
  - Increased function, decreased pain
  - Disease may recur above or below the level of decompression.

Degenerative Spondylolysis

- Pathophysiology
  - **Anatomic defect in the pars interarticularis**, accompanied by adjacent sclerosis
  - Develops during childhood and adolescence
  - Typically caused by **repetitive hyperextension** (eg, in football linemen, gymnasts, and weight lifters)
- Presentation
  - Symptoms
    - Often asymptomatic
    - Hamstring tightness
    - Knee contracture
    - Radicular pain
    - Bowel/bladder dysfunction
  - Physical examination
    - Reduced lordosis
    - Limited flexion/extension of lumbar region
    - Positive tension signs
    - Popliteal angle may show hamstring tightness
  - Imaging
    - Lateral radiograph
      - Pars interarticularis defects
      - Oblique angle may show pars interarticularis elongation ("Scottie dog" sign), as well as sclerosis.
    - Bone scans, CT, and single-photon emission CT may aid in anatomic and diagnostic assessment when radiographs are negative.
- Treatment
  - Nonoperative—usually preferred when not accompanied by spondylolisthesis
    - **Asymptomatic patients—observation, no activity restriction**
    - **Symptomatic patients—activity restriction, physical therapy**
    - **Acute symptomatic pars interarticularis stress fracture—TLSO**
  - Operative
    - **Pars interarticularis repair**
      - For patients with multiple L1-L4 isthmic defects
      - Approach
        - Posterior midline approach
        - Techniques include tension wiring, screw fixation, as well as screw and sublaminar hook
    - **Posterolateral decompression and arthrodesis**, particularly if there is also spondylolisthesis (see below)

Spondylolisthesis

- Pathophysiology
  - **One vertebra slipping forward on another**
  - **Wiltse-Newman classification** defines types of spondylolisthesis (Table 9.4).
  - **Meyerding classification** defines severity of disease according to amount of slip (Figure 9.21).
    - Grade I: 0% to 25%
    - Grade II: 26% to 50%
    - Grade III: 51% to 75%
    - Grade IV: 76% to 100%
    - Grade V: >100% (spondyloptosis)

Table 9.4 Wiltse-Newman Classification of Spondylolisthesis

Type	Pathology
I: Dysplastic	Congenital S1 superior facet dysplasia
II: Isthmic	Elongation or fracture of pars
III: Degenerative	Subluxation caused by facet instability
IV: Traumatic	Acute fracture of posterior arch, other than pars
V: Neoplastic/pathologic	Bony structure incompetence
VI: Postsurgical	Excessive resection of facets or arches

- **Degenerative spondylolisthesis** commonly occurs at **L4-L5.**
  - Sagittal instability of vertebrae caused by
    - Degeneration of intervertebral disk or facet joint
    - Ligamentous laxity
  - More common in women because of hormonal changes
  - More common in patients with sacralized/transitional L5 vertebrae or sagittally oriented facet joints
- **Adult isthmic spondylolisthesis** most common at **L5-S1**
  - Spondylolisthesis **caused by a pars interarticularis defect**
    - Relatively uncommon; 95% of patients with spondylolysis do not develop spondylolisthesis

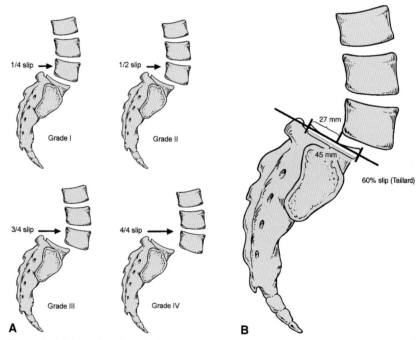

Figure 9.21 Meyerding classification system of spondylolisthesis. From Kuchera ML. Postural considerations in osteopathic diagnosis and treatment. In: Seffinger MA, ed. *Foundations of Osteopathic Medicine: Philosophy, Science, Clinical Applications, and Research.* Baltimore, MD: Wolters Kluwer; 2018:696-746.

- **Foraminal stenosis can occur because of fibrocartilaginous repair tissue of pars compressing exiting nerve root**
  - Associated with **increased pelvic incidence**
    - 70° to 80°, compared with normal pelvic incidence of 50° to 55°
    - This increases sacral slope and requires greater lordosis to preserve balance.
- Presentation
  - Symptoms
    - Back pain—relieved by flexion or sitting
    - Leg/buttock heaviness and cramps while walking or standing—relieved by sitting
    - Radicular symptoms
      - Central and lateral recess stenosis compresses traversing nerve root
      - Foraminal stenosis affects exiting nerve root.
    - Bladder/bowel deficits, cauda equina syndrome are rare
  - Physical examination
    - Difficulty walking an extended distance
    - Hamstring tightness
    - Radicular symptoms
  - Imaging
    - Radiograph
      - Lateral view shows vertebral slip.
      - **Flexion/extension studies may show instability**—defined as adjacent vertebra angle of **10°** or displaced by **4 mm** relative to adjacent segment.
    - MRI may show nerve compression.
    - CT can best assess bone abnormality.
- Treatment
  - Nonoperative—NSAIDs, physical therapy, injections
  - Operative—for patients with progressive symptoms in whom nonoperative treatment has failed
    - L5-S1 posterolateral decompression (laminectomy and foraminotomy) and arthrodesis—for patients with L5 spondylolysis and grade I-II spondylolisthesis
    - L4-S1 posterolateral decompression (laminectomy and foraminotomy) and arthrodesis—for patients with grade III to V isthmic spondylolisthesis
      - Approach
        - Posterior midline approach
        - With or without reduction
          - May correct sagittal alignment and kyphosis
          - **High risk of complications, including injury to the L5 nerve root** or other serious neurologic damage
      - Complications include pseudarthrosis, adjacent segment disease, dural tear, neuropathy, and infection

Synovial Facet Cysts

- Pathophysiology
  - Most common in lumbar spine—especially L4-L5
  - **Facet instability leads to synovium extrusion** from joint capsule and increased hyaluronic acid production
- Presentation
  - Symptoms
    - Back pain
    - Radicular symptoms if nerve root compressed
    - Neurogenic claudication

- Physical examination—nerve deficits associated with level of the cyst
- Imaging
  - Radiographs often normal
  - MRI may show the cyst
- Treatment
  - Nonoperative—NSAIDs, immobilization, and injections
  - Operative
    - **Laminectomy and decompression without arthrodesis** typically attempted first—can have recurrent back pain and cysts
    - Facetectomy and arthrodesis
      - **For patients with symptom recurrence after laminectomy**
      - Lower rate of recurrent back pain and cysts

SPINAL INFECTIONS

Background

- Epidemiology
  - Incidence 2% to 7% of all musculoskeletal infections
  - Mortality <5% in developed countries
  - Early diagnosis increases success of nonoperative treatment.
  - **Bimodal age distribution**: <20 years and 50 to 70 years
- Causes
  - Pyogenic: *Staphylococcus aureus* and *Streptococcus* are most common causative organisms
  - Tuberculosis (TB), fungal, parasitic less common
- Clinical presentation
  - **Nonspecific neck and back pain, worsening at night**
  - **Weight loss and poor appetite**
  - **Fever and night sweats**
  - Diagnosis requires high index of suspicion
- **Predisposing factors**
  - Diabetes; malnutrition; substance abuse (including intravenous drug abuse); human immunodeficiency virus infection; malignancy; long-term steroid use; chronic renal failure; liver cirrhosis; septicemia; RA; spinal fractures and paraplegia; infective endocarditis; sickle-cell disease; chronic alcoholism; spinal surgery; skin, dental, or other systemic infection
- Potential complications
  - Sepsis, neurologic deficits, spinal column bony destruction, kyphosis/Gibbus deformity, and psoas abscess (psoas major)

Diagnosis

- Laboratory tests
  - Erythrocyte sedimentation rate **(ESR)**
    - Ninety percent sensitivity for pyogenic spondylitis, low specificity
    - Average ESR 43 to 87 in pyogenic spondylitis
  - **C-reactive protein** blood test
    - Elevated in >90% of patients with spinal infection, low specificity but better predictor than ESR
  - **White blood cell count**
    - Moderate elevation with spinal infection
    - Low sensitivity—elevated in only two-thirds of patients
  - **Blood cultures**
    - Useful for identifying causative organism and targeting antibiotic treatment
    - Only two-thirds of blood cultures positive
  - **Urinary culture**—useful if urogenital tract suspected to be primary site of infection

- Imaging
  - Conventional radiographs
    - Earliest sign is **erosion at vertebral endplates**
    - Narrowed intervertebral disk space
    - Coronal or sagittal malalignment caused by bony destruction
  - CT scans
    - Sensitive to bony destruction and abnormalities
    - Abscess formation
  - **MRI with gadolinium**
    - Gold standard for imaging spinal infections
    - Sensitivity of 96%, specificity of 92%
    - Increased fluid signal
    - Helps differentiate between spinal infection and tumor
  - Radionuclide studies may be useful for those who cannot undergo MRI: three-phase technetium-99m bone scans, gallium-67 citrate scans, indium 111-labeled leukocyte scintigraphy
- Biopsy
  - CT-guided percutaneous biopsy—withhold antibiotics before biopsy
  - Endoscopic biopsy
    - Visualization
    - Debridement of infected tissues
  - Open biopsy
  - Specimens can be sent for gram stain and cultures (aerobic, anaerobic, fungal, mycobacteria)

Treatment

- Nonoperative
  - Long-term antibiotic treatment
  - **Monitor clearance of infection using ESR and C-reactive protein.**
  - Continue antibiotic treatment for 4 weeks after normalization of ESR and end of symptoms.
  - Immobilization with collar or orthosis
- Operative
  - **Absolute indications**
    - **Spinal cord or cauda equina compression**
    - **Progressive neurologic deterioration**
  - Relative indications
    - **Lack of clinical improvement** with 2 to 3 weeks of antibiotic treatment
    - **No known diagnosis** (absence of positive blood cultures and unable to obtain percutaneous biopsy)
    - **Progressive spinal deformity** with biomechanical instability
  - Key principles
    - Obtain cultures, surgical debridement, followed by antibiotic treatment
    - Neurologic decompression to address progressive neurologic deficit
    - Spinal stabilization
    - Perioperative neurophysiologic monitoring

Four Major Types of Spinal Infection

- **Pyogenic vertebral osteomyelitis:** infection in vertebral column (Figure 9.22)
  - Epidemiology
    - Most common form of spinal infection
    - Mean patient age of 50 to 60 years
    - Most common in lumbar spine

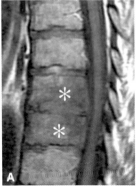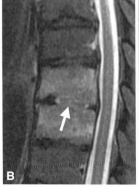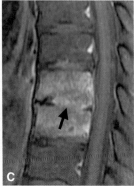

Figure 9.22 Pyogenic osteomyelitis with discitis. A, Sagittal T1 MRI shows two adjacent vertebral bodies (asterisks) with decreased signal intensity and an abnormal disc in between. B, Sagittal T2 MRI shows abnormal increase in signal intensity in the vertebral marrow as well as disc space (white arrow). C, Sagittal postcontrast T1 MRI shows disc enhancement (black arrow). These findings confirm the diagnosis of osteomyelitis/discitis. From Gaensler EHL, Purcell DD, Watanabe AT. Spine imaging. In: Klein JS, Brant WE, Helms CA, Vinson EN, eds. *Brandt and Helms' Essentials of Diagnostic Radiology*. 5th ed. Philadelphia, PA: Lippincott Williams & Wilkins; 2019:225-261.

- Causes
  - Hematogenous spread from distant site is most common mechanism
  - Direct spine trauma and open fractures
  - Iatrogenic (ie, spinal surgery)
  - Local spread of infection
- Causative organisms
  - *Staphylococcus aureus* most common
  - Others: *S. epidermidis*, group A *Streptococcus*, gram-negative infection, *Pseudomonas*, and *Salmonella*
- Diagnosis and treatment as described above.
- **Discitis:** disk space infection
  - Epidemiology
    - Primarily children, mean age of 7 years
    - Lumbar spine most common
  - Pathophysiology
    - Disk space infection from hematogenous spread
    - At birth, blood vessels present at endplates perforate cartilaginous intervertebral disk, extending into annulus fibrosus
    - **Normal adult intervertebral disk is avascular** (ie, small vessels disappear).
  - Causative organism
    - *Staphylococcus aureus*—most common causative organism in children
    - Gram-negative organisms are common causative organism in elderly patients.
    - *Salmonella* may be causative in patients with sickle-cell disease.
  - Imaging
    - Radiograph—**delayed findings; changes cannot usually be seen until 1 to 3 weeks**
      - Vertebral endplate blurring/bony destruction
      - Loss of normal lumbar lordosis
      - Narrowing of disk space
    - MRI with gadolinium—diagnostic test of choice
    - Bone scan
  - Treatment is usually with intravenous antibiotics for 4 to 6 weeks or longer
  - Complications
    - Narrowing of disk space

- Fusion of adjacent vertebra
- Back pain
- **Epidural abscess:** infection in spinal canal between dura mater and surrounding adipose tissue
  - Epidemiology
    - Most common in adults aged >60 years
    - Posterior thoracic and lumbar regions
  - Pathophysiology
    - Bacterial infection leading to the collection of pus in epidural space
    - **Most commonly originates from distant focus** such as skin infection or dental abscess
    - **Can be caused by local spread from vertebral osteomyelitis or osteodiscitis** and is more likely to cause systemic symptoms
  - Imaging
    - Radiographs usually normal
    - MRI with gadolinium
      - Differentiation between pus and CSF
      - Gadolinium enhances pus on T1-weighted images, indicated by ring-enhancing lesion
    - CT with myelogram—90% sensitive for epidural abscess
  - Nonoperative treatment such as intravenous antibiotics and bracing may be attempted for small abscess without neural compression or neurologic deficits; however, this remains controversial.
  - **Operative treatment indicated for neurologic deficits, compression of neural elements on imaging, failure of antibiotic treatment, spinal instability**
    - Decompressive laminectomy with irrigation and debridement when abscess can be accessed posteriorly
    - Anterior abscesses may require anterior approach and strut grafting
- **Spinal tuberculosis**
  - Epidemiology
    - Fifteen percent of patients with TB have extrapulmonary manifestation.
    - Thoracic spine is most common site of extrapulmonary TB.
  - Pathophysiology
    - Granulomatous spinal infection—*Mycobacterium tuberculosis*
    - Respiratory system is local source
    - **Spreads beneath ALL**
    - Can have multiple contiguous levels or skip lesions
    - Vertebral body destruction leads to **Gibbus deformity.**
    - Paraspinous abscesses, typically anterior
    - Preservation of disk distinguishes from pyogenic infection
  - Presentation
    - Often occurs in immunocompromised patients
    - Severe kyphosis in chronic infection
  - Imaging
    - **Chest radiograph is key diagnostic step** in diagnostic work-up when any suspicion of TB—abnormal in two-thirds of patients.
    - Spine radiographs
      - Preservation of disk distinguishes from pyogenic infection during early infection.
      - Severe kyphosis and disk destruction in late infection
    - CT can define bony destruction.
    - MRI with gadolinium can detect abscesses, soft tissue, and neural element involvement.
  - Treatment
    - **Nonoperative if no neurologic deficits or instability—orthosis and antitubercular treatment for 9 to 12 months (rifampin, isoniazid, pyrazinamide, ethambutol)**
    - **Operative** for progressive neurologic deficit, limited antibiotic efficacy, spinal instability, and correction of severe kyphosis

ACKNOWLEDGMENTS

We would like to thank each of the authors for their contributions to this section:

Part 1 – Spine Anatomy: Jay S. Reidler, Eric Wei, A. Jay Khanna, and Francis H. Shen

Part 2 – Cervical Spine Trauma: Jay S. Reidler and A. Jay Khanna

Part 3 – Thoracolumbar Spine Trauma: David J. Kirby, Varun Puvanesarajah, Jay S. Reidler, and Francis H. Shen

Part 4 – Spinal Cord Injury: Matthew Hoyer, Jay S. Reidler, and A. Jay Khanna

Part 5 – Cervical Spine Degenerative Conditions: Michael McColl, Jay S. Reidler, and A. Jay Khanna

Part 6 – Thoracolumbar Spine Degenerative Conditions: Matthew Hoyer, Jay S. Reidler, and Francis H. Shen

Part 7 – Spinal Infections: Eric Wei, Jay S. Reidler, and Francis H. Shen

10 Oncology and Pathology

Adam S. Levin

EVALUATION AND STAGING

- **Staging**
  - Musculoskeletal Tumor Society **(MSTS, Enneking)** staging—anatomic, surgical staging system
    - Benign tumors
      - **Latent**—**narrow zone of transition** on radiographs
      - **Active**—may grow but **without clear cortical destruction**
      - **Aggressive**—expansile **destructive**
    - Malignant tumors
      - **Low grade (stage I)**
        - IA—intracompartmental
        - IB—extracompartmental
      - **High grade (stage II)**
        - IIA—intracompartmental
        - IIB—extracompartmental
      - **Metastatic (stage III)**
  - American Joint Committee in Cancer **(AJCC)** staging—prognostic staging system for sarcomas
    - Soft tissue sarcomas
      - Low grade (stage I)
      - High grade (stage II), and either large (>**5 cm**) or deep to fascia
      - High grade (stage III), large (>**5 cm**), and deep to fascia
      - Metastatic (stage IV)
    - Bone sarcomas
      - Low grade (stage I)
        - IA: ≤8 cm
        - IB: >8 cm
      - High grade (stage II)
        - IIA: ≤8 cm
        - IIB: >8 cm
      - **Skip metastases (stage III)**—another discontinuous lesion in the same bone
      - Distant metastasis (stage IV)
- **Imaging**
  - **Radiography**
    - Good detail on aggressiveness of bone tumors
    - Localization gives keys to likely diagnosis.
    - Calcifications of soft tissue lesions can give clue to diagnosis.
  - **Computed tomography (CT)**
    - Improved osseous detail for cortical erosion or scalloping at the primary lesion
    - **Chest CT** part of standard staging workup for malignant bone or soft tissue tumors
  - **Magnetic resonance imaging (MRI, Figure 10.1)**
    - Excellent soft tissue detail for tumor extent
    - **Gadolinium** enhancement can determine cystic versus solid masses, degree of vascularity.
    - MRI of the entire compartment or bone to assess for skip metastases
  - **Positron emission tomography (PET)**
    - Fluorodeoxyglucose assesses metabolic activity of lesions
    - Good for detecting lymph node metastases, occult masses, or hematologic malignancy

- **Bone scan**
  - **Technetium-99-methylene diphosphonate**
  - Labels site of increased bone turnover
  - **30% of myeloma** lesions will be **cold** on bone scan—improved yield with metastatic skeletal survey.
- **Biopsy principles**
  - How to perform a biopsy (optimally, by treating surgeon)
    - Incise **along the limb salvage incision**

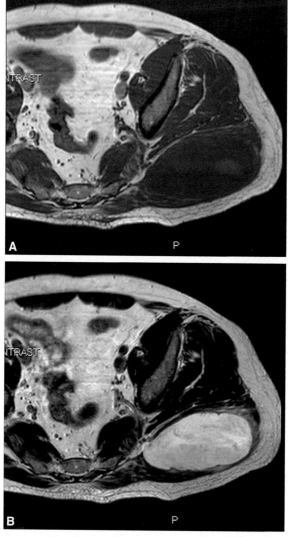

Figure 10.1 A large mass that is deep to the fascia may be concerning for soft tissue sarcoma. Soft tissue sarcoma MRI appearance will often be isointense to muscle on T1-weighted images (A), hyperintense on T2-weighted images (B), and often with heterogeneous enhancement (C).

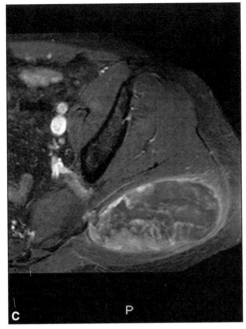

Figure 10.1 (*continued*)

- Approach with minimal soft tissue flaps/dissection
- Avoid contamination of critical structures—neurovascular, joints
- Minimize stress risers, protect the limb after biopsy
- Practice **meticulous hemostasis**—avoid postoperative hematoma
- Deflate tourniquet before closure
- If leaving a drain, in-line with the incision and close to the end
- Histopathology principles
  - Careful handling of specimen
  - Lymphoma very delicate, nondiagnostic biopsy common
  - **Fresh, sterile collection** to allow for immunohistochemical stains, flow cytometry
  - Certain tissue types are difficult to assess on frozen section.
    - Lipomatous masses
    - Calcified bone
    - Langerhans cell histiocytosis (LCH)
    - Cartilage
- Adjuvant treatments
  - Chemotherapy
    - Cytotoxic medications target rapidly growing cells.
      - Antiangiogenic agents—vascular endothelial growth factor inhibitors, tyrosine kinase inhibitors
      - Intercalating agents—doxorubicin
      - Alkylating agents—vincristine, ifosfamide
      - Topoisomerase inhibitors—etoposide
      - Antifolate—methotrexate
      - Nucleoside analogs—gemcitabine

- Targeted chemotherapy options developed for specific pathways
  - Mechanistic target of rapamycin inhibitors—rapamycin, everolimus
- **Radiation**
  - **Deoxyribonucleic acid (DNA) damage** induces apoptosis of rapidly dividing cells.
- **Local adjuvants**
  - Advances cell death locally at the site of tumor excision
  - **Often used in benign aggressive tumors** (giant cell tumor)
  - Commonly used local adjuvants
    - Cryosurgery
    - Argon beam coagulation
    - Low-intensity pulsed ultrasound
    - Radiofrequency ablation
    - Radiation therapy
    - Polymethyl methacrylate
    - Phenol
- Molecular biology of musculoskeletal tumors
  - **Common translocations**
    - t(9;22)—*EWS, CHN1*—extraskeletal myxoid chondrosarcoma
    - **t(11;22)**—*EWS, FLI1*—**Ewing family of tumors** (also t[21;22])
    - t(12;22)—*EWS, ATF1*—clear cell sarcoma, angiomatoid fibrous histiocytoma
    - t(17;22)—*COL1A1, PDGFB1*—dermatofibrosarcoma protuberans
    - **t(2;13)**—*PAX3, FOXO1*—**alveolar rhabdomyosarcoma**
    - t(1;13)—*PAX7, FOXO1*—alveolar rhabdomyosarcoma
    - **t(12;16)**—*TLS, CHOP*—**myxoid liposarcoma**
    - **t(X;18)**—*SYT, SSX*—**synovial sarcoma**
    - t(X;17)—*ASPL, TFE3*—alveolar soft-parts sarcoma
  - Additional genetic abnormalities
    - Ring chromosome 12
      - Atypical lipomatous tumor/well-differentiated liposarcoma
      - Low-grade osteosarcoma
    - *GNAS*
      - Fibrous dysplasia
    - Colony-stimulating factor-1 (CSF-1)
      - Pigmented villonodular synovitis/giant cell tumor of tendon sheath
    - *EXT1, EXT2, EXT3* genes
      - Multiple hereditary exostoses

BENIGN BONE TUMORS

- Bone-forming tumors
  - Enostosis
    - Bone island
    - Small, asymptomatic
    - Typically cold on bone scan
    - No change over time
  - Osteopoikilosis
    - Heritable—autosomal dominant
    - Multiple enostoses
  - **Osteoid** osteoma (Figure 10.2)
    - **Small (<1.5 or <2 cm) nidus**
    - Osteoid seams with prominent osteoblastic rimming
    - Typically **cortically based**
    - Perilesional sclerosis and perilesional edema
    - Intensely painful

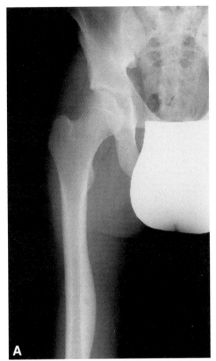

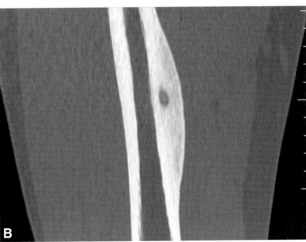

Figure 10.2 A, Osteoid osteoma may demonstrate a region of marked cortical thickening and benign periosteal new bone formation. B, Computed tomography is typically the best study to demonstrate the radiolucent cortically based nidus. C, A bone scan will typically demonstrate intense activity, similar to a stress reaction. D, Image-guided radiofrequency ablation has become the treatment of choice for most osteoid osteomas occurring in the appendicular skeleton. From Unni KK, Inwards CY. Osteoid osteoma. In: *Dahlin's Bone Tumors: General Aspects and Data on 10,165 Cases*. Philadelphia, PA: Lippincott Williams & Wilkins; 2010:102-111.

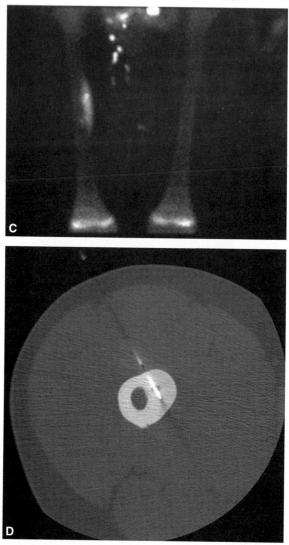

Figure 10.2 (*continued*)

- - **Relief with nonsteroidal anti-inflammatory drugs (NSAIDs)**
  - May worsen with ethyl alcohol
  - In spine, associated with **painful scoliosis**
- Best seen on CT
  - One of the few indications when axial CT will be used for diagnosis of a bone mass
- Treatment
  - NSAIDs (typically resolve after 2-3 years)
  - **Radiofrequency ablation** (standard of care, if location allows)
  - Surgical curettage or excision—need to remove entire nidus

- **Osteoblastoma**
  - Typically **larger than 2 cm**
  - Histology similar to osteoid osteoma
  - Typically more medullary
  - Less prominent cortical reaction on imaging than osteoid osteoma
  - Pain more variable
  - Frequently seen in posterior spine elements
- **Spine lesions**
  - **Posterior elements—typically benign**
    - Osteoid osteoma—painful scoliosis
    - Osteoblastoma (Figure 10.3A)

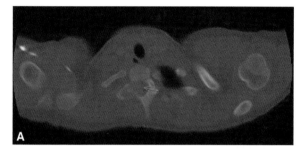

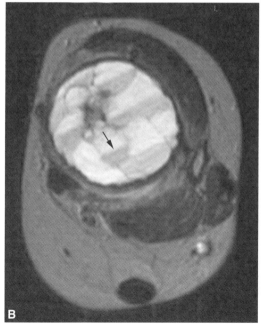

Figure 10.3 A, Osteoblastoma of the posterior elements of a 12-year-old girl, causing cord compression. B, Aneurysmal bone cysts (ABCs) demonstrate aneurysmal dilatation of the bone, as demonstrated in the cross-section. The arrow demonstrates a fluid-fluid level. There are typically numerous fluid-fluid levels within an ABC, as demonstrated. B: From Chew FS. Benign lesions. In: *Skeletal Radiology: The Bare Bones*. 3rd ed. Philadelphia, PA: Lippincott Williams & Wilkins; 2010:158-180.

- Aneurysmal bone cyst (ABC, Figure 10.3B)
- Osteochondroma
- **Anterior elements—often malignant**
  - Metastatic carcinoma
  - Plasmacytoma/multiple myeloma
  - Chordoma—classically clivus or sacrum but can be anywhere along the spine
  - Hemangioma—most common
  - LCH—vertebra plana in a child (Figure 10.4)
- Cartilage-forming tumors
  - **Enchondroma**
    - Benign, intramedullary cartilage lesion
    - Often metaphyseal
    - **"Ring and arc"** or popcorn-like calcifications
      - Hand/foot imaging may look more aggressive but remain benign.
      - Radiographic differential diagnosis includes:
        - Osteonecrosis—"smoke up a chimney" calcification
        - Chondrosarcoma
    - MRI
      - Dark T1
      - Bright T2
      - Variable gadolinium enhancement in a lobular pattern
    - Most common in the short tubular bones of the hands/feet (50%-60%)
      - Other common sites
        - Proximal humerus
        - Distal femur
        - Proximal tibia
      - Commonly asymptomatic and found incidentally while imaging for other nearby joint pathology

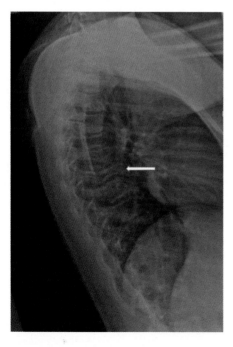

Figure 10.4 Langerhans cell histiocytosis may present with vertebra plana (arrow) in a young patient.

- Treatment
  - Observation
  - Avoidance with adjacent joint surgery
  - Curettage and local adjuvant treatment if necessary
- Malignant degeneration
  - Reports suggest approximately 1% lifetime risk for a solitary enchondroma
  - Increased concern for malignancy if:
    - >90% medullary fill by the tumor
    - Size > 5 cm
    - Pain related to the tumor rather than adjacent joint
    - Endosteal scalloping, cortical breach
    - Endosteal buttressing
    - Periosteal reaction
    - Measurable growth over time
    - Decreased mineralization over time—an indication of dedifferentiated chondrosarcoma
- **Ollier disease**
  - Multiple enchondromas
  - Often involves one limb or half of body
  - **Risk of malignancy (chondrosarcoma) approximately 30%**
- **Maffucci syndrome**
  - Multiple enchondromas with associated **angiomas**
  - **Risk of malignancy (chondrosarcoma, angiosarcoma)—almost 100%**
- **Osteochondroma**
  - Metaphyseal location
  - **Points away from physis**
  - Thought to represent physeal growth in an altered direction
  - May be sessile or pedunculated
  - Imaging with medullary and cortical continuity of bone with a cartilage cap
  - Cartilage cap mimics physeal cartilage in children
    - **Cartilage cap more than 1.5 to 2 cm concerning for malignancy** in adults
    - Cartilage cap growth after skeletal maturity concerning for malignancy
    - No limit to cartilage cap thickness in children
    - Reports suggest up to 1% lifetime risk of malignancy (chondrosarcoma) in solitary osteochondroma
    - Treatment
      - Observation
      - Excision at the base of the osteochondroma if symptomatic
      - Removal of entire cartilage cap and perichondrium necessary to prevent recurrence
- **Multiple hereditary exostoses/multiple hereditary osteochondromas** (Figure 10.5)
  - Heritable, autosomal dominant
    - *EXT1, EXT2, EXT3* **genes**
  - Multiple osteochondromas with variable severity
    - Often includes most long bones
  - May present with substantial deformity of the extremity and decreased range of motion
  - Up to 10% lifetime risk of malignancy (chondrosarcoma)
- Trevor disease (dysplasia epiphysealis hemimelica)
  - Similar to osteochondroma but found in the epiphysis
  - Typically noted in growing children
- **Chondroblastoma**
  - Typically in the **epiphysis** of **skeletally immature** adolescents
  - Often painful with **large inflammatory response** on imaging

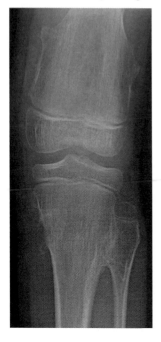

Figure 10.5 Multiple hereditary exostoses is associated with EXT mutations. This is characterized by osteochondromas in numerous bones, with characteristic deformities of the metaphyses.

- MRI
    - Appears lobular with similar characteristics to cartilage
    - Large surrounding edema pattern
    - May have a secondary ABC
    - On a short differential diagnosis list for "end-of-bone" or epiphyseal osseous lesions—same list as for apophyses
    - Chondroblastoma—often skeletally immature, chondroid
    - Clear cell chondrosarcoma—typically skeletally mature, chondroid
    - Giant cell tumor of bone
- Histopathology
    - Round chondroblasts with central nuclei—"**fried egg**" cells
    - Occasionally have some honeycombed mineralization—"**chicken wire**" calcifications
- Treatment
    - Curettage and local adjuvant
- Despite benign etiology, is capable of "**benign metastasis**" to the lung (like giant cell tumor of bone)
- **Chondromyxoid fibroma**
    - Most commonly in tibia of young adults
    - Lobulated, "**soap bubble**" appearance on imaging
    - Histopathology
        - Areas of low and high cellularity on low power
        - Higher power imaging with abundant myxoid background and stellate cells that look like helicopter propellers or "Mercedes-Benz" symbols
- Cystic lesions
    - **Unicameral bone cyst** (simple bone cyst)
        - Common pediatric condition (typically school-age at diagnosis)
        - Typically in the **proximal humerus**

- Largely self-limiting
- May present with pain or pathologic fracture
- **Pathologic fracture does not necessitate treatment** if alignment can be maintained
- Radiographs
  - Radiolucent lesion with thinned cortex
    - May have some mild expansion of the bone
    - Narrow zone of transition on imaging
  - Active—adjacent to the physis
  - Inactive—away from the physis
  - Can often have septations or with "fallen leaf" sign, representing a shelf of bone that has fallen within the cyst
- Histopathology
  - Thin cyst wall lined by a fibrocellular membrane
- Treatment
  - Observation
  - Aspiration and injection of corticosteroids
  - Aspiration and injection of marrow with demineralized bone matrix
  - Curettage and bone graft
- **ABC**
  - Typically seen in children and adolescents
  - May be **expansile** and may act aggressively locally
  - Often presents with pain
  - Typically in the long bones, although may be seen in the pelvis or posterior elements of the spine
  - Radiographs
    - Radiolucent, expansile lesion
    - Often lobulated
    - Typically wider than the physis
  - MRI
    - Typically with multiple septations
    - Multiple fluid-fluid levels on axial and sagittal imaging, representing blood products
  - Pathology
    - Multiloculated cyst wall with red blood cell within the cyst cavities
    - Multinucleated giant cells within the solid components
      - Note: Multiple etiologies demonstrate multinucleated giant cells, not just giant cell tumors.
  - **Radiologic differential diagnosis includes telangiectatic osteosarcoma.**
  - Treatment
    - Curettage and local adjuvant treatment
    - Wide excision if expendable bone
    - High local recurrence rate
- Intraosseous ganglion (geode)
  - Often related to nearby joint degeneration
  - Well-defined lytic lesion on imaging
  - Typically subchondral location
  - Clear, synovial or serous fluid
- Fibrous tumors
  - **Nonossifying fibroma (NOF, Figure 10.6)**
    - The most common benign bone tumor
    - Also known as xanthoma of bone; fibrous cortical defect
    - Typically noted in children, although may not be recognized until adulthood
    - **Often asymptomatic**, found incidentally for adjacent trauma
    - Radiographs

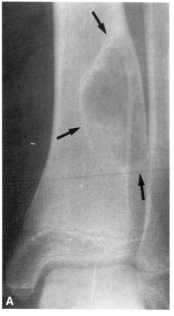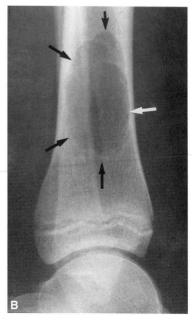

Figure 10.6 A nonossifying fibroma will typically be localized eccentrically in the metaphysis and demonstrates a thin cortical rim, as demonstrated by the arrows. AP (A) and lateral (B) radiographs of a distal tibial nonossifying fibroma in a skeletally immature patient. From Monu JU, Pope TL Jr. Diaphysis. In: Pope TL Jr, Harris JH Jr, eds. *Harris & Harris': The Radiology of Emergency Medicine.* 5th ed. Philadelphia, PA: Lippincott Williams & Wilkins; 2013:973-988.

- Cortical or eccentric
- Well-defined borders with a narrow cortical rim
- No periosteal elevation or reaction
- Histopathology
  - Bland, spindle cell proliferation in a fibrous stroma
  - Multinucleated giant cells and foamy histiocytes more common in adults
- Typically self-limiting, although may persist into adulthood
  - Often partially calcified over time
- Treatment
  - **Observation**
  - Curettage and bone graft if concern for risk of pathologic fracture
- Avulsive cortical irregularity
  - Similar to NOF
  - Thought to represent repetitive avulsive microtrauma at the medial gastrocnemius insertion
- Jaffe-Campanacci syndrome
  - Multiple NOFs
  - **Café-au-lait spots (Figure 10.7)**
    - Café-au-lait spots can be seen in multiple conditions
      · Jaffe-Campanacci syndrome
      · Neurofibromatosis type 1 (NF1)—"coast of California"
      · McCune-Albright syndrome
      · Tuberous sclerosis
      · Fanconi anemia

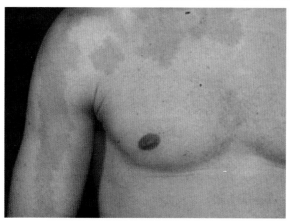

Figure 10.7 Café-au-lait spots may be seen in a number of conditions. This patient's spots have a rugged border, similar to the coast of Maine, in the setting of McCune-Albright syndrome. From Aronsson DD, Lisle JW. The pediatric orthopaedic examination. In: Weinstein SL, Flynn JM, eds. *Lovell and Winter's Pediatric Orthopaedics*. Vol 1. 7th ed. Philadelphia, PA: Lippincott Williams & Wilkins; 2014:87-128.

- Often with cognitive impairment
- Often with cryptorchidism
- May be associated with cardiac or ophthalmologic anomalies
- **Fibrous dysplasia**
  - Typically noted in school-age children and adolescents
  - May be solitary or multiple
  - Associated with *GNAS* **mutation**
    - Subunit of G protein
  - Can involve nearly any bone
  - Radiographs
    - Well-defined lytic lesion with a "**ground-glass**" hazy appearance
    - May be somewhat expansile
    - "Large lesion in a large bone"
  - Histopathology
    - Bland appearance of woven bone in a fibrous background without prominent osteoblastic rimming
    - Can be confused with low-grade osteosarcoma
  - May be associated with deformity of the bone or fracture
  - Often self-limiting with partial resolution into adulthood
    - May become cystic in adulthood
    - In the intertrochanteric region, some believe that **liposclerosing myxofibrous tumor** is a variant of fibrous dysplasia that has undergone fatty and cystic degeneration.
  - Treatment
    - Observation
    - Painful lesions or those with deformation may be treated with curettage and bone graft
      - Bone graft typically turns back into fibrous dysplasia with remodeling and creeping substitution
      - Often use cortical strut or coralline hydroxyapatite because of the slow turnover rate

- **McCune-Albright syndrome**
  - Polyostotic fibrous dysplasia
  - Café-au-lait spots
    - "Coast of Maine"—jagged edges
  - Endocrinopathies
    - Classically, precocious puberty
- **Mazabraud syndrome**
  - **Polyostotic fibrous dysplasia**
  - Soft tissue **myxomas**
- **Osteofibrous dysplasia (OFD)**
  - Typically, young, school-age children
  - Classically in the **anterior aspect of the tibia,** although may also involve adjacent fibula
  - Radiographs
    - **Anterior bowing of the tibia**
      - On the differential diagnosis for pediatric tibial bowing
    - Eccentric, anterior cortically based lytic lesion
    - Often with thin sclerotic border
    - May appear as multiple soap bubbles
    - No soft tissue involvement, although may erode the cortex
  - Histopathology
    - Similar to fibrous dysplasia with fragments of woven bone in a background of bland fibrous stroma
    - Prominent osteoblastic rimming—differentiates from fibrous dysplasia
  - Typically becomes less active into adulthood
  - Treatment
    - Observation
    - Biopsy if concern for malignancy
    - Curettage and bone graft, with or without open reduction and internal fixation, if fracture or progressive deformity
  - **Radiographic differential diagnosis includes adamantinoma**
- **Giant cell tumor of bone (Figure 10.8)**
  - Benign, often aggressive tumor

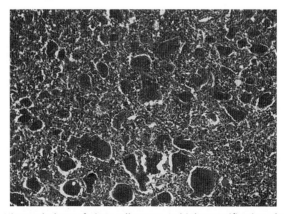

Figure 10.8 Histopathology of giant cell tumor. At high magnification, densely arranged tumor tissue consists of mononuclear cells intermixed with numerous uniformly distributed large giant cells (much larger than observed in other tumors) containing up to 50 or more nuclei (H&E, original magnification ×100). From Greenspan A, Borys D. Miscellaneous lesions. In: *Radiology and Pathology Correlation of Bone Tumors: A Quick Reference and Review*. Philadelphia, PA: Wolters Kluwer; 2016:298-352.

- Typically in young adults, although can be seen in adolescents or middle-aged patients
- Typically **epiphyseal**, often crossing the physeal scar
  - In rare pediatric cases, will start in metaphysis
  - On the differential diagnosis for end-of-bone or epiphyseal lesions
  - May be apophyseal (ie, greater trochanter)
- Radiographs
  - Well-demarcated lytic lesion with sharp zone of transition
  - Often without sclerotic rim
  - Common sites
    - Distal femur
    - Proximal tibia
    - Distal radius—commonly in young women on examinations
  - Campanacci staging (similar to Enneking benign tumor classification)
    - Latent—well-marginated border of a thin rim of mature bone; cortex intact or slightly thinned but not deformed
    - Active—well-defined margins but no sclerotic rim; cortical thinning or mild expansion but still present
    - Aggressive—cortical breach with soft tissue extension; permeative pattern
- MRI
  - May have secondary ABC component with fluid-fluid levels
- Histopathology
  - Dense collection of mononuclear cells with large, multinucleated giant cells
  - **Giant cells** have **nuclei that appear similar to nuclei of mononuclear cells** on histology
  - **Neoplastic cells are mononuclear cells** (not giant cells), which are of **osteoblastic** origin
- Treatment
  - **Curettage, local adjuvant**, packing
  - **Denosumab** may be used in difficult-to-treat masses, although neoplastic cells are not osteoclastic; denosumab induces a reactive shell but may not eliminate tumor
  - Wide excision in expendable bones
- Despite benign etiology, is capable of **benign metastasis to the lung** (like chondroblastoma)
- Rare cases of malignant giant cell tumor of bone
  - May be spontaneous, although most reported cases are after radiation
- Reactive lesions and other tumors
  - Osteomyelitis
    - On the differential diagnosis for most tumors, particularly in children
    - May have a wide presentation on imaging and clinical features
      - Increase suspicion with surrounding edema/inflammation
      - May have elevated inflammatory markers
        - Erythrocyte sedimentation rate
        - C-reactive protein
        - White blood cell count—and high neutrophil count or bands on differential
      - One of the "great mimickers"
  - **LCH**
    - Broad spectrum or presentations
      - Eosinophilic granuloma—most common, typically monostotic
      - Another of the **great mimickers** because of widely variable presentation
    - On the clinical and radiographic differential diagnosis for nearly any childhood lesion
    - Spine involvement
      - Typically in vertebral body—**vertebra plana** in a child

- **Calvarial involvement**
  - Lytic skull lesion
    - High index of suspicion on examination if showing a lateral skull radiograph in a child
    - In adults, lateral skull radiograph will often be either multiple myeloma ("punched-out" lytic lesion) or Paget disease (thickened cortex)
- Histopathology
  - Proliferation of Langerhans cell histiocytes
  - Eosinophilia may be less evident on frozen section, although are typically prominent on fixated hematoxylin and eosin staining
  - Under electron microscopy—**Birbeck granules** (look like tennis rackets)
    - LCH is one of the few diagnoses for which an electron micrograph may be shown on the board examination.
  - *CD1A*-positive staining
- Treatment
  - Typically will be biopsy to rule out other diagnosis because of variable presentation and imaging
  - Observation versus curettage and grafting
- Hand-Schüller-Christian disease
  - More severe, systemic disease
  - Bone lesions, diabetes insipidus, exophthalmos (triad seen in about one in three patients)
  - Typically treated with systemic chemotherapy
- Letterer-Siwe disease
  - Most severe, systemic disease
  - Typically fatal in young childhood
- **Hemangioma (Figure 10.9)**

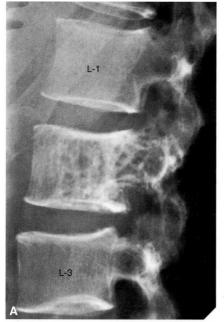

Figure 10.9 A, Lateral radiograph of the lumbar spine demonstrates a honeycomb pattern of hemangioma of L2 vertebra. B, Anteroposterior tomogram in another patient demonstrates vertical striations of hemangioma of L1 vertebra (arrows), referred to as a corduroy cloth pattern. From Greenspan A, Beltran J. Benign tumors and tumor-like lesions IV: miscellaneous lesions. In: *Orthopedic Imaging: A Practical Approach.* 6th ed. Philadelphia, PA: Wolters Kluwer Health; 2015:789-834.

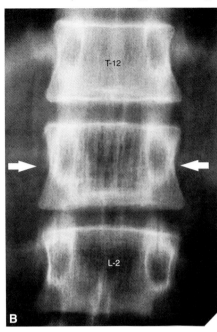

T-12

L-2

B

Figure 10.9 (*continued*)

- Most commonly seen in the spine—most common spine bone lesion
- Typically asymptomatic
- Radiographs/CT
  - Typically with a "jail-cell" trabecular pattern on lateral/sagittal imaging
    - One of the few indications for a coned in sagittal CT image on examination
  - May have **phleboliths** (small, round calcifications)
- MRI
  - High vascular flow, typically enhancing on postgadolinium images
- Treatment
  - Often can be managed with observation
  - If symptomatic or concerning—biopsy with possible curettage
  - Could consider embolization for difficult-to-treat locations

MALIGNANT BONE TUMORS

- **Osteosarcoma (Figure 10.10)**
  - **Most common primary bone sarcoma**
    - Most common primary bone malignancy is multiple myeloma.
  - Age
    - **Two peaks**—adolescent and late adulthood
      - Late adult peak often associated with Paget disease or after radiation
  - Associations
    - Paget disease
    - Previous radiation to the same field (postradiation sarcoma)
    - Bone infarcts
    - P53 mutations (**Li-Fraumeni** syndrome)
    - Retinoblastoma **(Rb)** tumor suppressor
      - 100-fold increase
    - Rothmund-Thomson syndrome
    - Werner syndrome

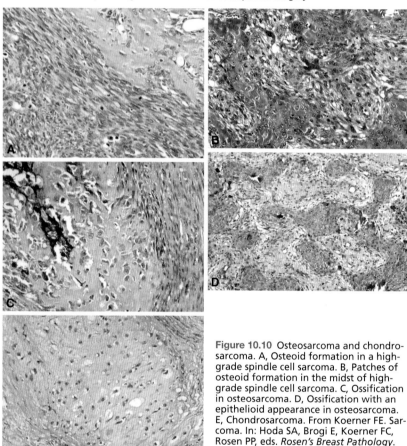

Figure 10.10 Osteosarcoma and chondrosarcoma. A, Osteoid formation in a high-grade spindle cell sarcoma. B, Patches of osteoid formation in the midst of high-grade spindle cell sarcoma. C, Ossification in osteosarcoma. D, Ossification with an epithelioid appearance in osteosarcoma. E, Chondrosarcoma. From Koerner FE. Sarcoma. In: Hoda SA, Brogi E, Koerner FC, Rosen PP, eds. *Rosen's Breast Pathology.* 4th ed. Philadelphia, PA: Lippincott Williams & Wilkins; 2014:1095-1165.

- Location
  - Typically metaphyseal (Figure 10.11)
  - More than 50% near the knee
  - Distal femur > proximal tibia > proximal humerus (Figure 10.12)
- Classification
  - Can be categorized by histologic subtype
    - Chondroblastic—chondroid features
    - Fibroblastic
    - Osteoblastic—heavy osteoid features
    - Telangiectatic—may be confused for ABC
    - Small cell—a small-round-blue-cell tumor (SRBCT)
  - Can be categorized by anatomic location
    - Conventional (high-grade intramedullary)
    - Low-grade central
    - Juxtacortical/surface

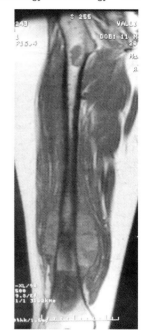

Figure 10.11 Whole-bone T1-weighted image of a patient with a distal femur osteosarcoma demonstrates soft tissue extension as well as extensive involvement of the diaphysis. There is evidence of a skip metastasis in the proximal femur. From Choong PF. Megaprosthesis after tumor resection. In: Sim FH, Choong PF, Weber KL, eds. *Master Techniques in Orthopaedic Surgery: Orthopaedic Oncology and Complex Reconstruction*. Philadelphia, PA: Lippincott Williams & Wilkins; 2011:125-136.

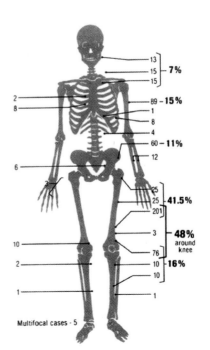

Figure 10.12 The skeletal distribution of primary osteosarcomas in patients treated on the Neoadjuvant Cooperative Osteosarcoma Study Group protocols of the Cooperative German-Austrian-Swiss Osteosarcoma Study Group. The majority of osteosarcomas are localized around the knee. From Meyers PA, Gorlick R. Osteosarcoma. *Pediatr Clin North Am.* 1997;44:973-989.

- · **Parosteal**
  - – On examination this will typically be presumed to be **low-grade**,
  - – **osteoblastic**, unless otherwise noted.
- · **Periosteal**
  - – On examination this will typically be presumed to be **intermediate-grade, chondroblastic**, unless otherwise noted.
- · High-grade surface
- • Treatment
  - · Most commonly treated with **neoadjuvant chemotherapy**, followed by wide surgical resection, followed by adjuvant chemotherapy
    - ▪ No data to support improved survival by altering order of treatment
    - ▪ High-dose methotrexate, doxorubicin, cisplatin
  - · **Low-grade osteosarcoma** treated with wide surgical resection alone, **no chemotherapy**
- • Histology—by definition, any sarcoma that makes osteoid is an osteosarcoma.
- • Prognostic factors
  - · Metastasis—lung most common, followed by bone (poor prognosis)
  - · **Histologic response to chemotherapy**—Huvos scale
    - ▪ Grade 1 response: ≤50% necrosis after neoadjuvant chemotherapy
    - ▪ Grade 2 response: 51% to 89% necrosis
    - ▪ Grade 3 response: 90% to 99% necrosis (good prognosis)
    - ▪ Grade 4 response: 100% necrosis (good prognosis)
  - · Factors associated with poor prognosis
    - ▪ Age ≤14 years
    - ▪ Tumor size >8 cm
    - ▪ Tumor growth on chemotherapy
    - ▪ Elevated alkaline phosphatase
    - ▪ Elevated lactate dehydrogenase
- ● **Chondrosarcoma (see Figure 10.10E)**
  - • Second most common primary bone sarcoma
  - • Most closely resembles cartilage
  - • Classified by grade
    - · Enchondroma—benign chondroid lesion (not chondrosarcoma)
    - · Low-grade chondrosarcoma/atypical chondroid lesion
    - · Intermediate-grade chondrosarcoma
    - · High-grade chondrosarcoma
    - · **Dedifferentiated chondrosarcoma (Figure 10.13)**
      - ▪ Very poor prognosis
      - ▪ **Juxtaposition of low-grade cartilage with high-grade sarcoma**
  - • Secondary chondrosarcoma
    - · Can be seen in the setting of osteochondromas and enchondromas
  - • **Clear cell chondrosarcoma**
    - · Rare variant of chondrosarcoma
    - · On the short differential diagnoses for **epiphyseal/apophyseal** lesions
  - • Clinical findings
    - · Size >5 cm
    - · Intramedullary fill >90%
    - · Interval growth
    - · Pain related to the tumor (rather than other intra-articular pathology)
    - · Periosteal reaction
    - · Cortical scalloping or invasion
    - · Decreased mineralization over time (indicative of aggressiveness and possible dedifferentiation)
  - • Radiologic appearance
    - · Popcorn calcification or ring and arc calcifications

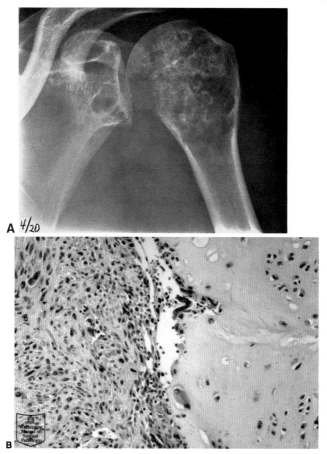

Figure 10.13 A, Radiographic features of a dedifferentiated chondrosarcoma, with a lytic destructive high-grade component eroding the cortical bone. B, Photomicrograph of the histopathology evaluation. Note the juxtaposition of high grade sarcoma to a low-grade chondroid lesion in the proximal humerus. A: From Vigorita VJ. Cartilage tumors, Fig 10-41A. In: *Orthopaedic Pathology*. 3rd ed. Philadelphia, PA: Wolters Kluwer; 2016:427-488. B: From Hameed O, Klein MJ. Bone neoplasms and other non-metabolic disorders. In: Humphrey PA, Dehner LP, Pfeifer JD, eds. *The Washington Manual of Surgical Pathology*. Philadelphia, PA: Lippincott Williams & Wilkins; 2008:630-652.

- Histologic appearance
  - Increased cellularity of chondroid tissue
  - May have increased myxoid appearance
  - Aggressive appearance or mitotic figures suggests higher grade
    - **In the short bones of the hand or foot, these may have a more aggressive appearance** and still be considered benign
  - Typically stains for S-100 proteins (as do many other tumors)
- Treatment
  - Wide resection alone (chemotherapy and radiation are largely ineffective in chondrosarcoma)
  - Low-grade tumors can be treated successfully with intralesional curettage and an adjuvant (eg, liquid nitrogen)

- **Ewing sarcoma (Figure 10.14)**
  - Ewing family of tumors encompasses Ewing sarcoma, primitive neuroectodermal tumor (PNET), and Askin tumor.
  - Age
    - Typically adolescents and young adults
  - Classically is **diaphyseal** location in long bones or **flat bones** (pelvis, scapula)
  - Histology
    - High-grade **SRBCTs** in bone
  - Radiographic appearance
    - Tends to have a permeative appearance
    - Onion-skin-like periosteal reaction
    - Often with an osseous and soft tissue mass
    - May have a "**hair-on-end**" radiographic appearance
  - Treatment
    - Most commonly treated with **neoadjuvant chemotherapy, followed by wide surgical resection and/or radiation therapy, followed by adjuvant chemotherapy**
    - Radiation and surgery are acceptable local control methods.
      - Local recurrence is slightly higher with radiation only.
- Other primary bone malignancies
  - **Adamantinoma**
    - Rare malignant neoplasm
    - Most commonly in adulthood
    - Typically in the **tibia**
    - Can be confused with OFD, by location
      - OFD typically seen in children

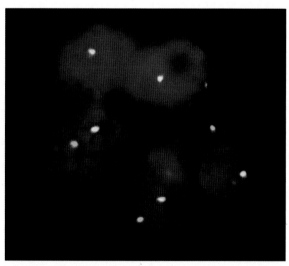

Figure 10.14 Interphase florescence in-situ hybridization with the *EWSR1* (22q12) break-apart probe in Ewing sarcoma demonstrating split red and green signals in addition to a fused red/green (yellow) signal of the intact 22q12 region, indicating the presence of an *EWSR1* gene rearrangement. *EWSR1* gene rearrangements are not specific for Ewing sarcoma, as they are also found in other tumors. From Bovée JVMG, de Andrea CE. Bone tumors. In: Mills SE, ed. *Sternberg's Diagnostic Surgical Pathology*. Vol 1. 6th ed. Philadelphia, PA: Wolters Kluwer Health; 2015:273-316.

- Histology
  - **Biphasic**—epithelial and mesenchymal features
- Treatment includes wide resection
- **Undifferentiated pleomorphic sarcoma of bone**
  - Previously called malignant fibrous histiocytoma
  - Typically in adulthood
  - May be secondary to radiation or **infarcts**, although can be spontaneous
  - Often treated like adult osteosarcoma
- **Chordoma**
  - Derived from **notochordal** tissues
  - Most commonly are low-grade malignancies
  - Classically in **clivus or sacrum**, although can occur anywhere between along the spinal column
  - Parachordoma—chordoma that occurs outside the vertebral axis
  - Stains with **T-brachyury, S-100 proteins**
  - Treatment
    - Wide excision, with or without radiation
- Myeloma and lymphoma
  - **Myeloma**
    - Systemic disease of multiple plasmacytomas
      - Malignancy of **plasma cells**—terminally differentiated B-lymphocytes that make antibodies
    - Pathology with sheets of plasma cells
      - Round cells with clock-faced, eccentric nuclei
      - Perinuclear halo
    - Most common primary bone malignancy
    - Multiple **punched-out lytic lesions** of bone—may be diagnosed in setting of unknown primary lesion of bone
    - Serum protein electrophoresis **(SPEP)** and urine protein electrophoresis **(UPEP)** with **immunofixation** for monoclonal spike of proteins from antibody light chains
    - May cause end-organ damage
      - Bone
      - Renal
    - Increased risk of **hypercalcemia of malignancy**
      - Treat with hydration and antiresorptive therapy (eg, bisphosphonate)
    - Systemic chemotherapy, with or without bone marrow transplantation
    - Prophylactic stabilization for impending/completed fractures
      - **30% false-negative bone scans**
        - Skeletal survey (radiographs) more sensitive for osseous disease
        - PET/CT or whole-body MRI are most sensitive
    - Highly radiation sensitive
  - **Lymphoma**
    - Malignancy of **lymphocytes**
    - Pathology: SRBCT with sheets of lymphocytes
    - Often with enlarged lymph nodes or "**B-symptoms**"
    - Cells are fragile, making **biopsy sometimes difficult**
      - Highly sensitive to corticosteroids, which may impair biopsy
      - **Flow cytometry** may be helpful with biopsy for characterization
    - Radiographs often with a poorly defined margin and **permeative appearance**
      - May have soft tissue mass around bone with relative preservation of the cortex—commonly seen in SRBCTs
    - **Highly radiation sensitive** and often respond well to systemic chemotherapy
    - Primary lymphoma of bone
      - Solitary lesion or few lesions originating in bone
      - Often treated with wide excision with curative intent

- Treatment principles for malignant bone tumors
  - **Margins of resection**
    - **Intralesional**—cutting into the tumor and removing piecemeal (ie, curettage)
      - Useful for benign tumors or removing metastatic lesions
    - **Marginal**—en bloc resection through the reactive zone
    - **Wide**—en bloc resection through normal tissue around
      - The mainstay of resections of primary malignancies
    - **Radical**—en bloc resection of the entire involved compartment
      - Historically performed for all sarcomas without an effective adjuvant treatment, although not frequently performed anymore
  - **Chemotherapy**
    - Used in most intermediate or high-grade bone sarcomas
      - **Exception is chondrosarcoma**, which is typically unresponsive to chemotherapy (or radiation).
    - For primary bone sarcomas, often will give chemotherapy before (neoadjuvant) and after (adjuvant) surgery
      - For osteosarcoma, neoadjuvant chemotherapy has not shown a survival benefit over early surgery with all chemotherapy given postoperatively but does give prognostic information regarding response to chemotherapy
        - Grade 1 response (poor, or standard); <50% necrosis
        - Grade 2 response (poor or standard); 50% to 89% necrosis
        - Grade 3 response (good); 90% to 99% necrosis
        - Grade 4 response (good); >99% necrosis
      - This is true for Ewing sarcoma as well.
    - Common chemotherapy medications
      - Methotrexate—interferes with folate metabolism
      - Doxorubicin (Adriamycin)—anthracycline
      - Cisplatin—DNA crosslinking agent
      - Ifosfamide—nitrogen mustard alkylating agent
      - Etoposide—topoisomerase inhibitor
      - Cyclophosphamide—nitrogen mustard alkylating agent
      - Vincristine—vinca alkaloid

BENIGN SOFT TISSUE TUMORS

- Adipocytic tumors
  - **Lipomas and atypical lipomatous tumors** are soft, compressible
    - May transilluminate like fat if superficial
    - On MRI, **looks like normal subcutaneous fat on all sequences** (Figure 10.15)
      - **Uniformly suppress on fat-suppression** sequences
      - No enhancement on MRI
      - Atypical lipomatous tumors may become large with some fibrous stranding
        - Higher local recurrence rate
    - May be observed if no clinical symptoms; if classic imaging, then no need for biopsy
    - Marginal excision if necessary
  - Angiolipomas
    - Sometimes cause local discomfort
    - Often superficial
    - Increased blood flow to the area—may be multifocal
  - **Hibernomas**
    - Rests of benign **brown fat**
    - Typically without other symptoms
    - Increased blood flow, may enhance slightly
    - Looks different from normal subcutaneous fat on imaging
    - May need biopsy to discern from malignancy on occasion

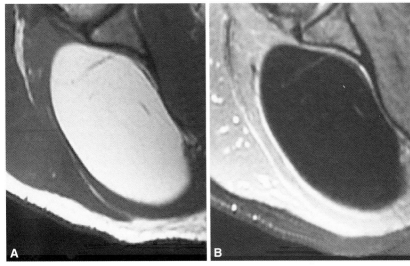

Figure 10.15 An intramuscular lipoma will demonstrate a uniform fat signal on all sequences, and will uniformly suppress on fat-suppressed sequences. T1 (A) and fat-saturated T2 (B) axial MRI demonstrating a uniform fat signal on both, with uniform suppression on fat-suppressed sequences. From Kransdorf MJ, Murphey MD. Lipomatous tumors. In: *Imaging of Soft Tissue Tumors*. 3rd ed. Philadelphia, PA: Lippincott Williams & Wilkins; 2014:95-177.

- Fibrous tumors
  - Nodular fasciitis
    - Typically adolescents and young adults, although can be any age
    - Can be infiltrative, firm, fixated along the fascia
      - Often poorly defined margins
    - Often tender with appreciable growth over short time
    - Pathology—plump myofibroblasts, may be cellular but without atypical mitoses
    - Treatment—observation versus marginal excision
  - **Extra-abdominal desmoid**
    - Infiltrative proliferation of dense fibrous tissue
    - May be related to previous trauma
    - Often in young adults, although can be any age
    - Imaging—isointense to muscle on T1, hyperintense on T2, may enhance
    - Clinical—may be painful, may spontaneously stop growing for long periods
    - Pathology—dense connective tissue with bland fibroblasts (looks like scar)
    - Associated with **Gardner syndrome (familial adenomatous polyposis)**
    - May be hormone responsive (ie, estrogen), NSAID-responsive
    - High local recurrence rate after surgery
  - Solitary fibrous tumor/hemangiopericytoma
    - Typically benign, although some follow a malignant course
    - Imaging features similar to sarcoma—isointense to muscle on T1, hyperintense on T2, heterogeneous enhancement
    - Pathology—may be hypercellular areas admixed with collagen bundles, may have prominent immature vessels (hemangiopericytoma)
    - Treatment—wide excision
  - **Elastofibroma**
    - Frequently asked on examinations
    - Typically in adults
    - Classically localized deep to the **inferior border of the scapula**

- May be bilateral
- Imaging
  - Poorly defined soft tissue mass with fibrous appearance and some internal fatty signal and indistinct borders along the posterolateral thoracic border, deep to the distal scapula
  - May be symptomatic (snapping, pain), although most are incidentally noted
- Histology
  - Bland fibroblasts in dense fibrous tissue, stains for elastin
- Treatment
  - May observe, marginal excision if symptomatic
- **Ganglion cyst**
  - May be related to adjacent joint pathology (paralabral, meniscal, popliteal)
  - Cystic extravasation of adjacent joint capsule, filled with clear, viscous fluid (apple-jelly appearance)
  - If superficial, will **transilluminate**
  - Imaging
    - Isointense to muscle on T1, uniformly hyperintense on T2 or short-tau inversion recovery (STIR), **peripheral enhancement only**
  - Treatment
    - Attempted trephination or aspiration, with or without corticosteroid injection
    - Surgery for refractory ganglia—marginal excision of cyst wall, sometimes with debridement of the underlying joint pathology or tying off the stalk
- Vascular tumors
  - **Hemangiomas and vascular malformations**
    - Common, seen at any age
    - May be tender or painful, may swell at times—intermittent symptoms
    - May have discoloration if close to the skin
    - Rarely may cause platelet dysfunction or high-output heart failure
    - Imaging
      - Radiographs may show **phleboliths**
      - MRI with heterogeneous appearance and indistinct borders
      - Some internal fat appearance
      - Often with avid enhancement because of high flow
      - Doppler ultrasound will often demonstrate the flow of multiple vessels
      - One of the few masses that can often be diagnosed on imaging
    - Treatment
      - Symptomatic management
      - Embolization
      - Surgical excision—high local recurrence rate
  - **Glomus tumors**
    - Typically in young adults
    - Classically **subungual**, but can be anywhere
    - Often extremely **painful**
    - Typically purplish-blue nodules
    - Imaging—small nodules, avidly enhance
    - Treatment—complete excision
- Neural tumors
  - **Schwannoma**
    - Round, firm, mobile in transverse more than longitudinal directions
    - If in sensory nerve, typically tender with **Tinel sign**
    - Benign peripheral nerve sheath tumor, which can be separated from the rest of the nerve fibers
    - Imaging
      - Isointense to muscle on T1, bright on T2 or STIR, enhancement

- **Tail sign**—tails proximal and distal in the plane of the nerve
  - **Target sign**—hypointense central signal on T2 imaging in some patients
- Histology
  - Biphasic
  - **Antoni A**—compact spindle cells in dense collagen background; Verocay bodies
  - **Antoni B**—loose myxoid stroma with less cellularity
- Typically strongly **S100 positive**
- Can be multiple
- Treatment
  - Marginal excision
- **Neurofibroma**
  - May be localized or multiple
  - Often associated with **NF1**
    - Café-au-lait spots
    - Lisch nodules
  - Often painful, may be deforming (eg, pediatric tibia)
  - Imaging—may appear similar to schwannoma, although often without clear tail
  - Histology—mixture of Schwann cells and fibroblasts; strongly **S100 positive**
  - Increased malignant potential, particularly in NF1
- Other benign soft tissue tumors
  - Leiomyoma
    - In uterus, called a fibroid
    - Firm soft tissue mass
    - Benign mass of smooth muscle
    - Smooth muscle actin (SMA) positive
  - **Pigmented villonodular synovitis/giant cell tumor of tendon sheath**
    - **Nodular**—isolated mass in the synovial lining
    - **Diffuse**—disseminated involvement of the entire joint or tendon sheath
    - Often with intermittent pain and swelling, with hemarthrosis
    - Imaging—"**blooming artifact**"; may be dark on T1 and T2 if hemosiderin deposits, enhancement
    - Appears to be driven by *CSF1* mutation
    - Treatment
      - Arthroscopic versus open synovectomy
      - Medications targeting *CSF1* are being tested
  - **Myxoma**
    - Firm, round, mobile soft tissue mass
    - Often nontender
    - May be associated with **Mazabraud** syndrome
    - Imaging—isointense to slightly hyperintense to muscle on T1, uniformly bright on T2 or STIR
    - Treatment
      - Observation or marginal excision

SOFT TISSUE SARCOMAS

- Staging and workup
  - History and physical examination
    - Firm, large, deep tumors more concerning for sarcoma
    - Interval growth concerning
    - Beware of spontaneous hematoma without reason and without prompt resolution
    - Often without pain—unless nerve or bone involvement
  - MRI of the limb segment
    - Most are isointense to muscle on T1 and hyperintense on T2 or STIR
    - Most will have heterogeneous enhancement (particularly on examination)

- Staging workup
  - Most common metastatic site is lung—CT chest as part of standard staging
  - Use of PET/CT less universal for most soft tissue sarcomas
  - Some subtypes more likely for **nodal spread**
    - Possible role for PET/CT versus sentinel node biopsy in these
    - Classically taught as "**SCARE**"
      - Synovial sarcoma (some literature questions this)
      - Clear cell sarcoma
      - Angiosarcoma
      - Rhabdomyosarcoma
      - Epithelioid sarcoma
- Staging systems
  - **Surgical staging system** (Enneking, MSTS)—most predictive of surgical or treatment plan
  - **AJCC**—most prognostic
- Histologic subtypes
  - Nearly 50 subtypes are recognized by the World Health Organization
  - **Liposarcoma**
    - May not look like fat on MRI
    - **Dedifferentiated liposarcoma**
      - Liposarcoma **arising within a lipoma or atypical lipomatous tumor**
      - Imaging and pathology will likely show area of aggressive tumor adjacent to normal fat
    - **Myxoid/round cell liposarcoma**
      - Continuum of aggressiveness
      - **t(12;16)** *TLS, CHOP*
      - Myxoid—low number of round cells per high-power field (<5%), lower grade
      - **Round cell (>5% round cells)—higher grade**
      - May have a myxoid appearance (similar to schwannoma or myxoma, with bright signal on T2 or STIR)
    - Pleomorphic liposarcoma
      - Aggressive-appearing soft tissue sarcoma with some admixed adipocytes on pathology
  - Fibroblastic/myofibroblastic
    - Infantile fibrosarcoma
      - May be congenital or occur in infancy
    - Myxoinflammatory fibroblastic sarcoma
      - Unlikely to be asked on examinations
      - Rare tumor, typically in fingers and toes
    - Fibrosarcoma
      - Classically with pathology demonstrating herringbone pattern of malignant spindle cells
    - **Myxofibrosarcoma**
      - Unlike most other sarcomas, this tends to be more **superficial**
      - **Spreads along fascial planes**
      - **High local recurrence rate**
      - May have a myxoid appearance (high T2 or STIR signal) with surrounding edema
  - Undifferentiated pleomorphic sarcoma
    - Used to be called malignant fibrous histiocytoma
    - Typically with a highly pleomorphic appearance on pathology
  - **Leiomyosarcoma**
    - Malignancy of smooth muscle lineage
      - Most commonly of uterus, although can be of any other smooth muscle (vein)
    - **SMA** positive on pathology

- **Rhabdomyosarcoma**
  - Malignancy of skeletal muscle lineage
  - Most common soft tissue sarcoma in children
    - **Embryonal**—more common
      - Paratesticular is frequent primary site.
      - Pathology—rhabdomyoblasts in a fibrous or myxoid stroma
        - More immature cells appear to have small tails (tadpole cells)
    - **Alveolar**—more likely to be asked on examinations
      - **t(2;13)** *PAX3*, **FOXO1**
      - t(1;13) less common
      - Small, round blue cells often after an alveolar pattern
  - **Desmin**, actin, myoD stains positive
- Vascular malignancies
  - **Epithelioid hemangioendothelioma**
    - Unlike most sarcomas, these are often painful
    - **t(1;3)** *WWTR1*, *CAMTA1*
  - **Angiosarcoma**
    - Malignant mass of spindle or endothelial cells arranged in immature vascular channels
    - May be associated with other conditions
      - **Postradiation** (breast carcinoma)
      - Klippel-Trenaunay syndrome
      - **Chronic lymphedema** (Stewart-Treves syndrome)
      - Maffucci disease
- Extraskeletal osteosarcoma
  - Rare variant of osteosarcoma, found in soft tissues
  - Need to differentiate
    - **Myositis ossificans—zonal pattern of calcification** is key finding
      - Commonly asked examination question
    - Juxtacortical osteosarcoma—attachment to bone is key finding
    - Other masses with calcifications
      - Synovial sarcoma—may have calcifications
      - Tumoral calcinosis
      - Hemangioma
  - Soft tissue sarcoma that makes bone or osteoid
- **Synovial sarcoma**
  - Commonly in young adults
  - High-grade malignancy
  - Most common sarcoma of the **foot**
  - **t(X;18)** *SYT*, *SSX*
  - Classically taught as having increased risk of nodal metastasis
  - May be **monophasic** (typically spindle cells) or **biphasic** (spindle and epithelial cells) (Figure 10.16)
  - Biphasic may stain for **epithelial membrane antigen (EMA)**
- **Epithelioid sarcoma**
  - High risk of **nodal metastasis**
  - Most common sarcoma of the **hand**
  - Often in young adults
  - Stains for **EMA and cytokeratin**
- **Malignant peripheral nerve sheath tumors**
  - About half are associated with **NF1**
  - May be painful
  - Stains for **S100 proteins**

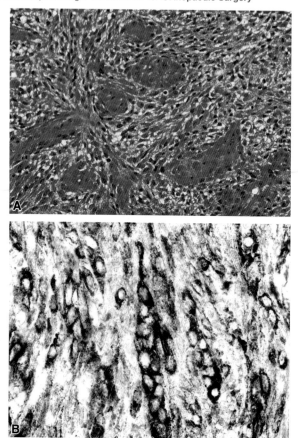

Figure 10.16 A, High-power magnification may demonstrate a biphasic growth pattern in synovial sarcoma, with areas of spindle cells and areas of epithelioid cells. B, Epithelial membrane antigen (EMA)-positive neoplastic cells in biphasic synovial sarcoma. Note that adamantinoma may also be biphasic and may also demonstrate EMA positivity. Other EMA-positive malignancies include carcinomas and epithelioid sarcomas. A: From Maleszewski JJ, Burke AP. Sarcomas of the heart and great vessels. In: Burke AP, Aubry M-C, Maleszewski JJ, et al, eds. *Practical Thoracic Pathology: Diseases of the Lung, Heart, and Thymus*. Philadelphia, PA: Wolters Kluwer; 2017:851-857. B: From Requena L, Kutzner H. Synovial sarcoma. In: *Cutaneous Soft Tissue Tumors*. Philadelphia, PA: Wolters Kluwer; 2015:206-214.

- **Clear cell sarcoma**
  - Increased risk of **nodal metastasis**
  - **t(12;22)** *EWS, ATF1*
- **Extraskeletal myxoid chondrosarcoma**
  - Behaves like a soft tissue sarcoma, not like a chondrosarcoma
  - **t(9;22)** *EWS, CHN*
- Molecular genetics
  - t(9;22) *EWS, CHN*—extraskeletal myxoid chondrosarcoma
  - t(11;22) *EWS, FLI1*—Ewing family of tumors

- t(12;22) *EWS, ATF1*—clear cell sarcoma; angiomatoid fibrous histiocytoma
- t(17;22) *COL1A1, PDGFB1*—dermatofibrosarcoma protuberans
- t(2;13) *PAX3, FOXO1*—alveolar rhabdomyosarcoma
- t(1;13) *PAX7, FOXO1*—alveolar rhabdomyosarcoma (less common)
- t(12;16) *TLS, CHOP*—myxoid liposarcoma
- t(X;18) *SYT, SSX*—synovial sarcoma
- t(X;17) *ASP, TFE3*—alveolar soft-part sarcoma
- *MDM2*—**well-differentiated liposarcoma/atypical lipomatous tumor**; well-differentiated osteosarcoma
  - Associated with ring chromosome 12
- Treatment principles for soft tissue sarcomas
  - Wide surgical excision
  - High-grade, large, deep—typically with radiation to decrease local recurrence
    - **Preoperative radiation**, compared with postoperative radiation
      - **Smaller dose** (approximately 50 Gy vs. 56-66 Gy)
      - **Smaller field size**
      - **Decreased stiffness** near joints
      - **Increased wound complications** (35% vs. 17%)
  - Low grade—typically without radiation (weigh risks and benefits)
  - Chemotherapy
    - Small improvement in overall survival in high-grade sarcomas
    - Some soft tissue sarcoma subtypes more frequently treated with chemotherapy
      - Ewing family of tumors
      - Angiosarcoma
      - Extraskeletal osteosarcoma
      - Synovial sarcoma
    - Used in metastatic disease and in healthier patients with aggressive tumors

OSSEOUS METASTASIS

- Presentation and workup
  - Should be high on the differential for a destructive bone lesion in an adult over age 40
  - Most patients with osseous metastases have a known history of carcinoma.
  - If **unknown, primary** neoplasm
    - **CT chest, abdomen, pelvis**
    - **MRI** of the limb segment
    - **Labs**
      - Complete blood count
      - Comprehensive metabolic panel
      - SPEP, UPEP (with immunofixation)
    - **Bone scan**
    - **Biopsy** should be the **final confirmatory diagnostic procedure**
  - Lung carcinoma is the most common primary malignancy to present as an unknown primary.
  - If no confirmed metastatic disease, a biopsy is necessary before intervention.
  - Pathology
    - Different tumors have different histopathologic characteristics.
    - For examinations, typically will show an adenocarcinoma, with nests or glands of epithelial cells
      - May show thyroglobulin inside a glandular architecture for thyroid carcinoma
    - Often will show carcinoma inside trabecular bone, highlighting osseous destruction
  - Imaging
    - May have a varied appearance
    - Typically, poorly defined lytic lesion

- Myeloma—punched-out appearance
- Lymphoma—permeative appearance with haziness to the cortex
- Prostate carcinoma—usually blastic, sclerotic lesions
- Pathophysiology
  - **Most common carcinomas to metastasize to bone**
    - Breast
    - Lung
    - Prostate
    - Renal cell
    - Thyroid
    - Melanoma
  - Local bone destruction via osteoclastic resorption
    - "**Vicious cycle**" of osteolysis
      - Transforming growth factor-beta **(TGF-β)** acts on carcinoma cells to produce interleukin-11 and parathyroid hormone-related protein **(PTHrP).**
      - PTHrP acts on osteoblasts to increase receptor activator of nuclear factor κ-B ligand **(RANKL)** and decrease osteoprotegerin
      - RANKL promotes osteoclastic differentiation
      - Osteoclasts degrade bone, releasing TGF-β—cycling back to 1
- Treatment principles
  - **Antiresorptive therapy**
    - **Bisphosphonates** (zoledronic acid) or **denosumab** (anti-RANKL) to block osteoclastic bone resorption
    - Very useful for hypercalcemia of malignancy
    - Decreases skeletal-related events—for example, fracture, need for radiation
  - Radiation
    - Good for slowing tumor progression locally
    - Good for pain control
  - Surgery
    - To prevent fracture, to restore/maintain function
    - One bone, one operation—typically will attempt to stabilize the limb segment with one operation
    - Immediate stability—expectation that the patient will be full weight bearing postoperatively
    - Construct should be durable to last the patient's lifetime

APPENDIX Test-Taking Strategies

Bashir A. Zikria and Francis Hwang

BOARD EXAMINATIONS

- Written, cognitive examination covering entire field of orthopaedics
- Multiple-choice questions
- The total time is 8 hours of testing time.
- **Practice timing for examination**

Part I Examination

- Information from entire 5 years of residency
- Approximately 33%—basic knowledge stays consistent.
- Approximately 67%—clinical knowledge
- 30% to 35% of questions have been used previously.
- Review self-assessment exams (SAE) and orthopaedic in training exam (OITE) questions.

Part I Examination Statistics

- Criterion-referenced examination
  - Defines the performance of each test taker without regard to the performance of others
  - **Implies that all candidates with requisite knowledge can pass**

Part I Boards Pass Rate: (All test takers)			
	Test takers	Passed	Failed
2018	835	91%	9%
2017	850	92%	8%
2016	837	86%	14%

General Statistics

- Approximately 97% of first-time test takers passed last 3 years
- **First time test takers 2017 and 2018: 97% passed**
- **First time test takers 2016: 96% passed**
- Approximately 79% second time
- Approximately 50% third time

Why Do People Not Pass?

- **Poor preparation**
- Remember to **review subjects**.
- Very difficult to learn new subjects or concepts at this time
- Since should have learned subject from 5 years of residency
- Takes valuable time from actually reviewing subject
- Set a schedule of studying.
- **Poor test-taking skills**
- **High anxiety-stress**

STANDARDIZED TESTS: ORTHOPAEDIC RESIDENTS

- One of the most competitive specialties
- Previous standardized testing includes the SAT, MCAT, USMLE Steps I, II, and III.
- **Thus, it can be inferred that orthopaedic residents generally performed well on those examinations.**

United states medical licensing exam (USLME) versus Part I Boards

- Studies are conflicting regarding the USLME Step-I and Step-II scores as being a predictor of Part I examination performance.
- **Evidence suggests that scoring in the lowest third of the OITE in PGY-3 and PGY-4 stand a greater chance of failing the ABOS Part I examination.**

OITE versus Part I Boards

- Differences in psychometrics between the examinations may limit the ability to find a correlation for performance.
- OITE questions are submitted based on subspecialties.
- **General knowledge**
- **Help guide your studying**
- **Practice test—timing**
- Part I questions have been previously administered to board-certified orthopaedic surgeons, analyzed statistically, and selected for inclusion on the basis of their psychometrics.
- Reliability and validity
- Analysis
  - Difficulty
  - Discriminate between those students who really knew the material from those that did not.
    - Rank test scores from highest to lowest, so the highest is at the top of the list.
    - Define high group (top 20%).
    - Define low group (bottom 20%).

Types of Questions: Cognitive Level

- Taxonomy I—recall
  - Anatomy
  - Basic science
- Taxonomy II—interpretation or comprehension
  - Written description
  - Image
- Taxonomy III—problem-solving
  - Knowledge application
  - Complications

Construction of a Question

- Stem
  - Question
- Responses
  - One preferred response
  - Four distractors
- Figures—may or may not be included

TEST-TAKING FOR MULTIPLE-CHOICE FORMATS

- **Research has indicated that adequate preparation in test-taking skills can improve test performance.**
- Familiarity with **characteristics and content of tests**
- Test **preparation**
- Test-**wiseness**
- Management of **test anxiety**

Familiarity with Characteristics Contents of Tests

- Purpose of test
- **Qualified** (responsible) orthopaedic surgeons
  - Anatomy and basic science
  - Diagnosis
    - Imaging—exact
    - Arthroscopic anatomy
  - Treatment
    - Non operative
    - Surgical
    - Indications
  - Complications
- Areas to be covered
  - **33%—basic knowledge—stays consistent throughout the years**
  - **Memorization questions**
  - 17%—pediatrics
  - 25% to 30%—trauma
  - 15% to 20%—adult reconstruction
  - **5% to 10%—sports medicine**

TEST PREPARATION

- There is debate over whether or not enrolling in a test preparation course will improve performance (at the very least it cannot hurt).
  - **Helps with organizing and at least reviews all topics once**
- **Time-management skills—answer all questions**
- Study strategies—quality more important than quantity
  - It's not the amount of time studying but the actual time reviewing the material in depth!
- Study location—Select a specific place and do not use it for nonstudy activities.
- Preferred learning styles—visual, auditory, tactile
- Study groups—versus independently (study with someone who is serious about doing well and can contribute; may not be a friend)—can really help you or hurt
- **Use old examinations to identify frequently used "signal" words and practicing correctly.**
- Memory strategies
  - Use information as quickly as it is learned.
  - Associate new information with learned information.
  - Visual imagery (ie, Italy is shaped like a boot)
  - Overlearn—and keep track of repetitions required to do this
  - Mnemonics
- Study of student's test-taking
  - Reading and highlighting (final test mark 77%)
  - Reading and taking notes (final test mark 79.50%)
  - **Reading and generating questions (final test mark 89.10%)**
  - **If a student goes back to a question and asks why the correct answer is correct, the student is much more likely to uncover a flaw in his original thinking.**

TEST-WISENESS

- **Refers to the ability to use characteristics and format of a test to improve performance**
- Standardized, multiple-choice examinations test recognition of information, not recall, over a short period of time to evaluate knowledge, comprehension, and application (requires both speed and accuracy)

- Strategies for multiple-choice tests
  - Read carefully but answer quickly—**answer all questions.**
  - Look for clue words in the stem—establish diagnosis or treatment.
    - **Atraumatic versus traumatic**
    - **Chronic versus acute**
  - Complete the easiest questions first.
  - Eliminate the incorrect options first—**must be absolutely sure.**
  - Eliminate responses that are the same.
  - Eliminate absurd or humorous options.
  - Eliminate absolute options (always and never).
  - Pure guess versus educated guess
  - SPLASHDOWN technique—write down information difficult to recall when examination is received (ie, brachial plexus)
  - Underline relevant options in a complex stem.
  - "All of the above are true" is a good guess if two correct options can be identified.
  - "None of the above" cannot be correct if one correct option can be identified.
- Do not read too much into questions or try to find hidden meanings (even best test takers can fall into this trap).
  - Do not second-guess the motivation of test developers.
  - Do not assume anything (ie, no way there can be three "B" in a row).
  - Suspend judgment until all options have been read (all may be true but only one will be the best or most important).
- "**SCORER**" technique
  - **S**—Schedule your time.
    - Practice test—Time yourself.
  - **C**—Use clue words.
    - JERK test, KIM test = Posterior instability
  - **O**—Omit difficult questions with the first pass—**at least pure guess—have to answer all questions.**
  - **R**—Read carefully.
  - **E**—Estimate answers by writing "E" beside estimated answers.
  - **R**—Review test and make sure *all questions have been answered.*
- When you have no clue . . . do not punt.
- *Answer all questions!*
  - Pure guess
  - Select the nonparallel option.
  - Select the longest option.
  - Try to narrow it down to two best choices and select the one you first thought was correct.
  - If you cannot do that, then go with the letter of the day.

MANAGEMENT OF TEST ANXIETY

- DTA (Debilitating Test Anxiety)
  - **Failure to pass professional licensing examinations despite sufficient energy and time spent in preparation**
  - No evidence of health problems, learning disabilities, clinical depression, drug/alcohol dependency, and so on
  - Except for performance on multiple-choice tests, there is realistic sense of being competent in professional setting.
  - Other demanding academic, extracurricular, and clinical activities are not impaired by anxiety.
- Behavioral modifications
  - Behavioral rehearsal
    - **Cannot think failure**
    - Reduce potential distractions caused by anxiety on test day.

- Imagine feelings that would be present on test day.
- Practice run through all steps.
  - Progressive muscle relaxation, systematic desensitization, the behavioral rehearsal, and a psychoeducational component—93% passed examination
- Psychoeducational techniques
  - Error analysis—Identify areas of relative strength and weakness.
  - Maximize probability of correct answer.
    - Cover answers while reading question.
    - Choose first of two answers if all but two possible choices can be eliminated.
    - When no idea which of 3+ answers is correct, use "letter of the day" strategy (eg, answer all questions with B).
- Relaxation approaches
  - Self-control triad
    - Thought stopping
    - Deep relaxing breaths
    - Visualizing a pleasant scene
- Count backward from 5 to 1.
- Maintain a healthy lifestyle—fitness, nutrition, rest, limited caffeine.
- Prayer and meditation
- Seek professional help
- Other interventions
  - **Regular moderate exercise:** lower anxiety, improved mood, enhanced self-concept, quicker reaction time, better attention, stronger reasoning skills
  - **Cognitive techniques: reduce negativism, self-criticism, helplessness**
- Mentor—preceptor
- Regular review of outlined study plan
- Individualized coaching
- Problem-based study groups
- Evaluation of study skills
- Weekly reading assignments/test
- **Get organized and have a plan of attack.**

EXAMINATION PREPARATION CHECKLIST

- Components
  - Knowledge
  - Preparation
  - Test-taking skill
- Knowledge: study materials
  - Old examinations
  - OKU (two most recent)
  - American Academy of Orthopaedic Surgeons (AAOS) self-assessment examinations
  - Review course(s)
  - Review books
  - Residency curriculum
    - Handouts
    - Journal club material
    - Personal notes
- Preparation
  - Strategic study plan leading up to examination
  - **Spend final week reviewing basic knowledge, areas of weakness as determined by OITE.**
  - BASIC SCIENCE—mostly memorization
  - Structured study habits
  - **Review tutorial on ABOS website.**

The Day before Checklist

- Review test instructions and know where to be for the test:
  - Brief review
  - Gather materials
  - Limit medications
  - Eat a light dinner
  - Reduce caffeine
  - **Good night's sleep**

Examination Day

- Eat a breakfast high in complex carbohydrates.
- Arrive early but not too early
- The total time allotted for the examination is 9 hours.
  - 8 hours of testing time
  - 40 minutes of break time
  - 20 minutes for lunch
- Answer all questions
- Be confident and maintain stamina
- Postexamination
  - Relax

INDEX

Note: Page numbers followed by *f* and *t* indicate material in figures and tables respectively.